D1446918

LIBRARY
THE UNIVERSITY OF TEXAS
AT BROWNSVILLE
Brownsville, TX 78520-4991

OXFORD MEDICAL PUBLICATIONS

Obstetric Ultrasound 1

Editorial Board

Frank A. Chervenak (New York); Michael Connor (Glasgow); Margaret Furness (Adelaide); Reynir Geirsson (Reykjavik); Michael Harrison (San Francisco); Henry Irving (Leeds); Philippe Jeanty (Nashville); Jean Keeling (Edinburgh); Norman McDicken (Edinburgh); Stephen Munjanja (Harare); John Newnham (Perth); Stuart Nicholson (Calgary); Roberto Romero (New Haven); Martin Whittle (Birmingham); Juri Wladimiroff (Rotterdam).

LIBRARY
H. DAVIS. S OF TEXAS
A. EL ANALLE
Brownsvi . TX PECSeon

Obstetric Ultrasound 1

Edited by

JAMES P. NEILSON

Professor of Obstetrics and Gynaecology
University of Liverpool;
Consultant Obstetrician and Gynaecologist
Royal Liverpool University Hospital and Liverpool Maternity Hospital,
Liverpool, UK

and

S. E. CHAMBERS

Consultant Radiologist
Simpson Memorial Maternity Pavilion and
Royal Infirmary of Edinburgh,
Edinburgh, UK

LIBRARY
ıHE UNIVERSITY OF TEXAS
AT BROWNSVILLE
Brownsville, TX 78520-4991

OXFORD   NEW YORK   TOKYO
OXFORD UNIVERSITY PRESS
1993

Oxford University Press, Walton Street, Oxford OX2 6DP

Oxford New York Toronto
Delhi Bombay Calcutta Madras Karachi
Kuala Lumpur Singapore Hong Kong Tokyo
Nairobi Dar es Salaam Cape Town
Melbourne Auckland Madrid
and associated companies in
Berlin Ibadan

Oxford is a trade mark of Oxford University Press

Published in the United States
by Oxford University Press Inc., New York

© *James P. Neilson and S. E. Chambers, 1993*

All rights reserved. No part of this publication may be reproduced, stored in a retrieval system, or transmitted, in any form or by any means, without the prior permission in writing of Oxford University Press. Within the UK, exceptions are allowed in respect of any fair dealing for the purpose of research or private study, or criticism or review, as permitted under the Copyright, Designs and Patents Act, 1988, or in the case of reprographic reproduction in accordance with the terms of licences issued by the Copyright Licensing Agency. Enquiries concerning reproduction outside those terms and in other countries should be sent to the Rights Department, Oxford University Press, at the address above.

A catalogue record for this book is available from the British Library

Library of Congress Cataloging in Publication Data
(Data applied for)
ISBN 0 19 262224 2

Typeset by
EXPO HOLDINGS, Malaysia
Printed in Hong Kong

Preface

Obstetric ultrasound is a multidisciplinary subject. That is its strength and its weakness. The contributions of radiologists and radiographers, obstetricians and midwives, physicists, pathologists, paediatricians, and geneticists have, by expressing their various professional skills, made obstetric ultrasound a rich and exciting subject. Too often in the past, however, the potential for collaborative endeavours and the sharing of knowledge went unexploited because of petty interdisciplinary suspicions. We are committed to obstetric ultrasound as an effective multidisciplinary subject, as seen from our own professional backgrounds of obstetrics and radiology. This is shared by the members of the editorial board, whose backgrounds are varied, professionally and geographically.

Because obstetric ultrasound is a multidisciplinary subject, there are especial difficulties in keeping abreast of new developments as important publications appear in such a wide variety of journals. There has seemed to us a clear need for a regular series of books both to review progress at the cutting edges of the subject and to include authoritative critiques of important topics — hence, this series. Those involved in obstetric ultrasound nowadays need to understand much more than the mere mechanics of producing the ultrasound image, and we shall feel no inhibition about including contributions which are directly relevant to, if not specifically about, obstetric ultrasound.

The speed of development of ultrasound has been testament to its value. The first published report (by Professor Stuart Campbell) of the prenatal diagnosis by ultrasound of a major fetal malformation (anencephaly) resulting in pregnancy termination appeared a mere 20 years ago (in 1972). Imaging capabilities of equipment then were extremely crude by modern standards, but they were in turn much better than the original machines of the 1950s and 1960s. The vision and commitment of the pioneers of diagnostic ultrasound who saw promise in these appallingly unclear images, can only be an inspiration to us all. James Willocks was a pioneer and we are most grateful to him for contributing a chapter giving his personal recollections of the greatest pioneer of them all, the late Professor Ian Donald.

As imaging has improved, new challenges have emerged — new structures are seen; smaller defects are identified in the fetus; earlier diagnoses become possible. Dr John Hobbins was, and still is, an important pioneer of obstetric ultrasound and, with Dr Mark Cullen, has contributed to this book a valuable account of the promise and pitfalls of first trimester prenatal diagnosis using the transvaginal probe. It is important to detect the sometimes subtle dysmorphic features associated with chromosomal abnormalities if we wish to make a major impact on this source of perinatal death and damage, and of long-term handicap;

Dr Nicolaides, Professor Gosden, and Dr Snijders have made a significant contribution to this volume, by updating their analyses of the unique data on clinical problems, ultrasound findings, and tissues sampled at King's College Hospital, London. Other difficult prenatal diagnostic problems are also addressed by authorities of international distinction, from the United States and from Australia. The contributions are scholarly, but also aim to provide practical guidance for the obstetric ultrasonographer; none more so than Professor Connor's unique database of prenatal diagnoses. Here is real help with the difficult problems that confront us all.

In all countries, we are being asked more and more by our patients, and by those who control the medical purse strings, to justify our actions and procedures. Critical thought, and audit of results, are both vital if obstetric ultrasound is to remain a robust subject. Dr Walkinshaw and Dr Munjanja have written thoughtful reviews, the former on the biophysical profile, and the latter on the use of ultrasound in developing countries where resource limits, human and economic, are especially acute. Dr Munjanja provides a thought-provoking model for the critical appraisal of all ultrasound services, including those in more affluent countries. Also included are very new ultrasound applications — the colour flow Doppler ultrasound study of the human fetal circulation, in fetal sheep (the source of most of our concepts of fetal physiology), and in the veins of the mother.

In 1978, one of us had just begun to learn the art of ultrasound in the Queen Mother's Hospital, Glasgow. One afternoon was made memorable by the dramatic appearance of the then retired Regius Professor of Midwifery, Ian Donald. He had fallen on his yacht and now had a red, swollen, and painful leg. Was this, he demanded of the bemused ultrasound novice, a deep venous thrombus or a haematoma? As Professor Greer and Dr Allan show in this volume, ultrasound investigation has become much more sophisticated, but the idea has been around for a while!

Liverpool and Edinburgh   J. P. N.
January 1993   S. E. C.

Contents

Contributors

Paul L. Allan, Department of Medical Radiology, University of Edinburgh, Royal Infirmary of Edinburgh, Edinburgh, UK

H. M. Chambers, Department of Pathology, Women's and Children's Hospital, Adelaide, South Australia 5067

S. E. Chambers, Simpson Memorial Maternity Pavilion and Royal Infirmary of Edinburgh, Edinburgh, UK

J. M. Connor, Department of Medical Genetics, University of Glasgow, Duncan Guthrie Institute of Medical Genetics, Glasgow, UK

Mark T. Cullen, Division of Maternal–Fetal Medicine, Jacksonville College of Medicine, University of Florida, Jacksonville, Florida, USA

M. E. Furness, Department of Radiology, Women's and Children's Hospital, Adelaide, South Australia 5067

D. L. Gordon, Department of Microbiology and Infectious Diseases, Flinders Medical Centre, Bedford Park, South Australia 5042

Christine M. Gosden, MRC Human Genetics Unit, Western General Hospital, Edinburgh, UK

Ian A. Greer, Department of Obstetrics and Gynaecology, University of Glasgow, Glasgow Royal Infirmary, Glasgow, UK

John C. Hobbins, Department of Obstetrics and Gynecology, Yale University School of Medicine, New Haven, Connecticut, USA

Philippe Jeanty, Department of Radiology, Vanderbilt University, Nashville, Tennessee, USA

Robert W. Kelly, Sheep and Wool Division, Department of Agriculture, South Perth, Western Australia 6151

S. P. Munjanja, Department of Obstetrics and Gynaecology, University of Zimbabwe, Harare, Zimbabwe

James P. Neilson, Department of Obstetrics and Gynaecology, University of Liverpool, Royal Liverpool University Hospital, Liverpool, UK

John P. Newnham, Department of Obstetrics and Gynaecology, King Edward Memorial Hospital for Women, Subiaco, Western Australia 6008

K. H. Nicolaides, Harris-Birthright Research Centre for Fetal Medicine, King's College Hospital, London, UK

David A. Nyberg, Ultrasound Associates, 1229 Madison — Suite 1150, Seattle, Washington, USA

R. J. M. Snijders, Harris-Birthright Research Centre for Fetal Medicine, King's College Hospital London, UK

S. Vyas, Department of Obstetrics and Gynaecology, King's College Hospital, Denmark Hill, London, UK

S. Walkinshaw, Department of Feto-Maternal Medicine, Liverpool Maternity Hospital, Liverpool, UK

S. Wesselingh, Department of Microbiology and Infectious Diseases, Flinders Medical Centre, Bedford Park, South Australia 5042

T. Wheeler, Department of Obstetrics and Gynaecology, Vanderbilt University, Nashville, Tennessee, USA

James Willocks, 16 Sutherland Avenue, Pollokshields, Glasgow, UK

Plates

1

Ian Donald and the birth of obstetric ultrasound

James Willocks

The success of obstetric ultrasound, its transformation in 30 years from a rather crazy experimental idea to a routine and welcome part of antenatal care, is truly astonishing. There are a number of reasons for its popularity:

1. It is patient-centred — not a remote laboratory test.
2. It is atraumatic and non-invasive, so women accept it gladly.
3. It is safe. After more than 30 years there is no substantial evidence of damage to mother or baby.
4. It is reliable — although it *can* be wrong and has to be interpreted in a clinical context.
5. Results are immediately available and can be directly communicated to the woman *with care and sensitivity*. The pregnant woman with her hopes and fears (often unspoken) is constantly alert. 'Is my baby all right?' is the question to be answered.

All these features appealed to Ian Donald, without whose work this book might never have been written (Fig. 1.1).

The whole history of ultrasound is quite short. The first practical application of ultrasound was the effort made by the French physicist, Paul Langevin, to detect submarines during the First World War. Results were not achieved in time for use in the war but his work formed the basis of sonar (sound navigation and ranging) detection which was developed during the Second World War. In the 1940s Karl Dussik, in Austria, began to try to measure the transmission of ultrasound through the brain and produced images which he believed were the ventricles, and in 1952 Tanaka and Wagai, from Japan, using an A-scan technique, reported detection of intracerebral haematomas and brain tumours. Dr J. J. Wild and his physicist colleague, J. M. Reid, of Minneapolis, constructed a prototype B-mode contact scanner in 1951. In the same year Dr D. Howry of Denver, Colorado, introduced a compound scanning method which produced impressive pictures, but he ran into difficulties because of the need to immerse the naked body of his subject in a large tank of water and this for obvious reasons was unsuitable in clinical practice.

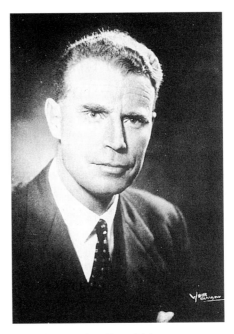

Fig. 1.1. Ian Donald in 1955.

The real breakthrough of ultrasound into clinical practice came in gynaecology and obstetrics. In gynaecology, tumour masses, such as ovarian cysts and
fibroids, are often revealed by laparotomy within a few days of ultrasound
examination and a diagnosis can therefore be quickly confirmed or revised. In
pregnancy, the outcome of the case is likely to be known within a matter of
weeks, and again there is a ready feedback of information. In this way it was
possible to rapidly develop extensive experience over the space of a few years.
Mistakes were as instructive as successes.

The founding father of ultrasound in gynaecology and obstetrics, and consequently in much of clinical medicine and surgery, was undoubtedly Ian
Donald, whose vision, persistence, and eloquent advocacy was responsible for
the important place that diagnostic ultrasound occupies today. I had the privilege
of knowing him as a friend for more than 30 years and of working closely with
him for nearly 20. What follows is a personal account of the man and his work.
Pasteur wrote that success in research came to the prepared mind, and others
have written of serendipity, the happy chance which brings success. Both played
a part in Ian Donald's career.

Ian Donald was born in Cornwall in December 1910, the son and grandson of
Scottish doctors. His early schooling was in Edinburgh at Fettes College. The

family moved to South Africa and Ian's father died when he was only 16. He finished his school education at the Diocesan College, Rondebosch and afterwards graduated BA in the University of Capetown. During these years he acquired his deep knowledge of literature. The Bible and Shakespeare were second nature to him and quotations constantly illustrated his conversation and his writing. This breadth of education is in striking contrast to what is on offer to medical students nowadays. He returned to England in 1931 and studied Medicine at St Thomas' Hospital Medical School. He graduated in 1937 and in the same year married the love of his life, Alix. She was also from South Africa and was born in Bloemfontein during the great influenza pandemic at the end of the First World War.

At one stage Ian thought he might become a psychiatrist but his career was interrupted by the outbreak of war. In 1939 he joined the RAF where his service was distinguished. He was decorated for gallantry for entering a burning bomber, with the bombs still in it, to rescue injured airmen. On a less dramatic level, service in the RAF stimulated his interest in gadgetry of all kinds and he became familiar with radar.

On returning to London at the end of the war he took up Obstetrics and Gynaecology and held appointments in St Thomas' Hospital, The Chelsea Hospital for Women, and Hammersmith Hospital. His talents developed rapidly under the stimulating influence of great masters of the profession, such as A. J. Wrigley, Victor Bonney, and Sir Charles Reid, all strong characters with marked eccentricities. Ian Donald's first publications gave no idea of the originality that was to come. They were on subjects such as 'The aetiology and investigation of vaginal discharge'. However, in 1952 he became fascinated by the problems that babies face passing through what he called the 'valley of the shadow of birth' and directed enthusiastic research efforts towards the problem of respiration in the newborn. He measured experimentally the very first breath of life and devised apparatus to help babies breathe when respiration did not get off to a flying start. His work was a forerunner of modern methods used in neonatal paediatrics, and in 1954 he gave the Blair–Bell Lecture at the Royal College of Obstetricians and Gynaecologists on the subject of '*Atelectasis neonatorum*' (Donald 1954). He developed a patient cycled respirator which went by the name of the Pneumotron. He brought this instrument with him when he came to Glasgow and I remember many evil hours spent in trying to get it to work.

Because of his interest in machines Ian was known as 'mad Donald' by some of his London colleagues, who caricatured him as a crazy inventor, but his talent was eventually spotted by Sir Hector Hetherington, Principal and Vice-Chancellor of the University of Glasgow. Principal Hetherington was a great university statesman who was committed to the concept of a modern Glasgow Medical School where full time professors would have adequate teaching and research facilities. He was also committed to the idea of cooperation between the University and the new National Health Service. He was prepared to go to great lengths to secure his objective and realized that a new teaching Maternity Hospital was essential. Ian Donald was appointed to the Regius Chair of Midwifery at the University of Glasgow in 1954, and the new Maternity Hospital became a reality 10 years later.

At the time of his appointment Ian was working on his great book, *Practical obstetric problems*, which was first published in 1955 (see Donald 1979). Young, enthusiastic, dynamic, restless, and irreverent, he was eager to challenge the established practice of his predecessors. 'The art of teaching is the art of sharing enthusiasm' was his motto. Clinical excellence was his aim. When the book came out we who were young read it from cover to cover like a novel. We could not put it down. Had diagnostic ultrasound never been developed, Ian Donald would be remembered as a great clinical teacher. *Practical obstetric problems* had an enormous impact internationally, and through it the name of Donald became as famous on the banks of the Nile and the Ganges as on those of the Clyde.

Professor Donald's clinical appointments were as Obstetrician to the Glasgow Royal Maternity Hospital and Gynaecologist to the Western Infirmary. These were proud Victorian Hospitals with great traditions but in the 1950s both were intensely conservative. The Royal Maternity Hospital at Rottenrow was famous for the work on Caesarean section performed by Murdoch Cameron and Munro Kerr and for the pathological studies of Harold Sheehan. Obstetric abnormalities of all kinds were rife. The Western Infirmary, built in 1874 at the other end of the city as the teaching hospital attached to the new University building at Gilmorehill, was famous for the pioneering work in thoracic and brain surgery performed by Sir William Macewen at the turn of the century.

Into this traditional atmosphere Ian Donald exploded like a display of fireworks. His lectures provided a feast of dramatic entertainment to which students responded by enthralled silence alternating with side-splitting laughter. In his book he referred to the value of overstatement. In his lectures he elevated this into an art form where all characters were larger than life. In the wards, Professor Donald clung to the traditional 'grand round' but revitalized it beyond belief. It became a forum for new ideas and debate. He was never pompous and would engage in serious or humourous discussion with the most junior members of the staff. He was always keen to acquire new knowledge and try things out. The effect on patients was variable. Sometimes tears had to be dried after the Chief's visit, but some Glasgow women are tough and the observation that the fetal head could not be felt could be greeted by the comment, 'My Goad! A heidless wean! I'll be the talk of the steamie!' Ian Donald was interested in every aspect of the subject and demanded logical reasons for every procedure. The answer that 'we have always done it that way', would be greeted by a torrent of abuse, largely unprintable. He maintained that an academic unit had to be clinically better than its colleagues but that clinical excellence in itself was not enough for:

...the pen is mightier than the knife and the gutters of Europe are littered with those who can perform hysterectomies and Caesarean sections.

On his appointment to the Chair, research was mainly centred on neonatal respiration, but soon his interest turned to the idea that sonar could be used for medical diagnosis. In the early 1950s there was no apparatus available for the medical use of ultrasound. At the Royal Cancer Hospital in London a modified industrial flaw detector was being used in efforts to detect brain tumours without much success. The start of diagnostic ultrasound in Glasgow began on 21 July 1955 (Donald 1974*a*, *b*) when Ian Donald visited the Research Department of the boiler makers, Babcock and Wilcox at Renfrew on the invitation of one of the directors, the husband of a grateful patient. He took with him two cars, the boots of which were loaded with recently excised fibroids, large, small, and calcified, and a very large ovarian cyst. He carried out some experiments with an industrial ultrasonic flaw detector on these tumours and on a large lump of steak which the company had kindly provided as control material. He was encouraged by the results, although no-one apparently had the appetite for the steak afterwards. Later he managed to borrow the old Kelvin and Hughes Mk II supersonic flaw detector which had been in use in London. Professor Donald became greatly involved with the Kelvin and Hughes Scientific Instrument Company and a word about its origins is worthwhile. The Scottish part of the company was founded by William Thomson, Lord Kelvin, Professor of Natural Philosophy at the University of Glasgow, five times President of the Royal Society and a giant of Victorian science. Innovation was very much part of the heritage of the company. In 1951 the firm engaged an 18-year-old technical apprentice called Tom Brown. In the following five years he gained some experience in developing an ultrasound metal flaw detector for use on boilers, railway lines, aircraft parts, and other metal components. Quite by accident he heard the strange tale of a professor who was attempting to use a metal flaw detector on patients from some of his colleagues who had been fitting a new theatre lamp in the Gynaecological Department at the Western Infirmary. Tom Brown was fascinated by the apparently bizarre idea of detecting flaws in women and, with great daring, telephoned Professor Donald at home that evening (Brown 1988). Professor Donald was very courteous and invited Brown to come and see what he was doing. He found the Professor using a very old and rather battered A-scope instrument which had been modified along the way and was not really working very well. Soon afterwards Professor Donald wrote to the firm of Kelvin and Hughes as follows:

I ought to let you know that a young chap in your firm in Glasgow, to wit Mr Thomas Graham Brown, has of his own initiative taken an interest in our ultrasonic experiments with different tissues and has managed to scrounge from his firm first of all a Mk V which we had for a few days on loan and now a Mk IV detector with camera attachment which appears rather more suitable.

The Mk IV instrument was a contact scanner. This meant that the ultrasound probe could be applied directly to the skin of the patient's abdomen which had been previously smeared with olive oil. Echo patterns could be clearly seen on a cathode ray screen which Tom Brown had rigged alongside the bed. This contact scanning method, which everyone takes for granted today, was a great advance. Previous methods necessitated passing the ultrasound beam through water in flexible buckets and other bizarre containers balanced precariously on the patient's abdomen with consequent profanity as water inevitably emptied itself on the bed, the Professor, and the patient.

Professor Donald with his Registrar, Dr John MacVicar (until recently Professor of Obstetrics and Gynaecology in the University of Leicester), plunged into an intensive investigation of the value of ultrasound in differentiating between cysts, fibroids, and any other intra-abdominal tumours that came their way. They were able to do this work because of the great wealth of clinical material. Plenty of patients were available because of Ian Donald's powerful position as a Scottish clinical professor. 'In America', he used to say, 'they call a guy who plays the piano in a brothel a Professor but in Scotland a divinity hedges a Professor as it does a King'. At the Western Infirmary the procedure used by Donald, MacVicar, and Brown was as follows. The patient was examined by ultrasound and a finding was recorded. The patient and the Professor would then go to theatre and a few minutes later John MacVicar would have the grisly proceeds in a basin to examine in his water tank. Early results were disappointing and the enterprise was greeted with a mixture of scepticism and ridicule. John MacVicar recorded,

...hours of continuous work often late at night became usual. Examination of countless patients and experiments with mechanical developments and picture display took up much of our time. Feelings of fatigue and frustration, despair and delusion, excitement and elation became well known to us. Recognition of the birth of a new science was slow (MacVicar 1988, personal communication).

But Ian Donald's vision of ultrasound as a new diagnostic science never faded. Undeterred by remarks from eminent colleagues who announced to hilarious students that ultrasound might be of value to a deaf, dumb, and blind gynaecologist who had lost the use of his hands and that in Glasgow they had an expensive machine to make a diagnosis that could be made with a twopenny glove, he pressed towards the mark and the vision became a reality.

A stroke of luck came early in 1957. Professor Donald was invited by Sir Edward Wayne, Professor of Medicine, to examine a patient on his wards who was believed to be dying with massive ascites due to secondaries from carcinoma of the stomach. Haematemesis and weight loss were dominant features. Her abdomen was so distended that it was difficult to examine her. Ian Donald passed the probe over the abdomen, expecting to see echoes from the bowel but all that was seen was a large clear space where the cancer should have

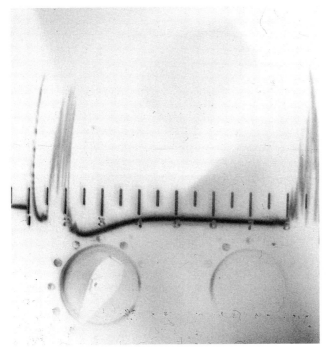

Fig. 1.2. A-scan image of a massive ovarian cyst, 1957.

been and a strong echo at the edge (Fig. 1.2). Donald's conclusion was that the apparatus was faulty, but at that moment John MacVicar, passing the bed looking for his Chief, saw the picture and said in a voice of certainty, 'seems like a big cyst'. The Professor was convinced, had the courage of his convictions, persuaded his medical colleagues that their diagnosis might just be wrong and, with their agreement, transferred the patient upstairs to the gynaecological department. A massive benign ovarian cyst was removed and the patient made an uninterrupted recovery. Undoubtedly ultrasound saved her life. 'From this point', Ian Donald wrote, 'there could be no turning back'.

It became clear to Tom Brown that although a lot of information was coming back from inside the abdomen the A-scope display was not really suitable. He was familiar with radar technology and the use of sector scanning. A contact sector-scanning system was used for the first time around the spring of 1957. The first scan made with the machine was on a patient suffering from ovarian carcinoma. It was a transverse scan just below the umbilicus. It is an unimpressive picture by modern standards but it was the first (Fig. 1.3). The investigators were quite willing to use themselves for experiments and some hilarity was caused by estimating the amount of fat on some people's abdomens. When I became involved it was gleefully reported that my head contained no solid material.

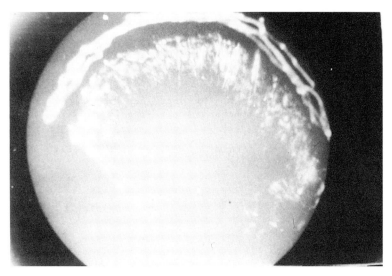

Fig. 1.3. The first compound sector scan of a patient with ovarian carcinoma, 1957.

Results eventually appeared in print in the *Lancet* of 7 June 1958 under the rather dry title, 'Investigation of abdominal masses by pulsed ultrasound' (Donald *et al.* 1958). The tone of the paper was modest. It stated:

...our experience of 78 cases in which diagnosis was quickly verified by laparotomy and subsequent histology indicates that ultrasonic diagnosis is still very crude, and that the pre-operative diagnosis of histological structure is still far off, although such a possibility in the future is an exciting prospect. The fact that recordable echoes can be obtained at all has both surprised and encouraged us, but our findings are still of more academic interest than practical importance and we do not feel that our clinical judgement should be influenced by our ultrasonic findings. The illustrations shown herewith are among the very best that we have so far been able to produce out of about 450. The possible harmful effects of diagnostic ultrasound are discussed; they appear to be negligible... Further refinements in technique may provide a useful diagnostic weapon in cases in which radiological diagnosis with ionising radiations is either impracticable or undesirable.

This was probably the most important paper on medical diagnostic ultrasound ever published.

Ten years later all doubt had been cast away and Ian Donald was able to review the early history of ultrasound in a more characteristically forthright fashion (Donald, 1969).

It is possible that the dazzling start of the first half century of radiology may yet be overtaken by the more steady and highly controlled growth of ultrasonic diagnosis... We should not forget the original pioneer work in the United States by Wild, Howry, Reid and Bliss in the early 1950s. We ourselves were relative late comers, only entering the field in 1955. Wild for example sought to measure the thickness of bowel wall and hence signs of carcinomatous ulceration of the stomach using a quartz transducer within the lumen of the gut. His experiments were carried out on dead dogs' intestines and post-mortem room material. Having never had to waste time myself on animals and corpses, both of which I detest in experimental work, I was able to cut a lot of the corners which they had first to round. Howry and Bliss produced, I believe, the first 2-dimensional sonograms in 1950s. Again their work unfortunately was confined largely to post-mortem room material, although they noted that better pictures could be obtained from fresh specimens of living subjects than formalin-fixed specimens. We soon found this out ourselves and threw our tanks onto the top of the most inaccessible cupboards. As soon as we got rid of the back room attitude and brought our apparatus fully into the department with an inexhaustible supply of living patients with fascinating clinical problems we were able to get ahead really fast...

Any new knowledge or technique becomes more attractive if its clinical usefulness can be demonstrated without harm, indignity or discomfort to the patient, better still if it requires not the eye of faith to comprehend it. Comprehension is well within the range of any average clinician...

In medicine today there are two main types of research, the animate and the inanimate. Inanimate research usually involves the measurement of some property, be it trace element, enzyme or structural feature, on a portable specimen removed far from the scene of the patient's illness. Such specimens may include blood, serum, urine, faeces and a variety of expendable tissues. While not denying its importance there are many of us for whom such activities hold very little attraction and we prefer a more animated type of research, on the patient, with the patient, as far as possible by the patient and always for the patient...

Anyone who is satisfied with his diagnostic ability and with his surgical results is unlikely to contribute much to the launching of a new medical science. He should first be consumed with a divine discontent with things as they are. It greatly helps, of course, to have the right idea at the right time and quite good ideas may come, Archimedes fashion, in one's bath.

Ian Donald often used to say, 'The easiest part of any experiment is the idea. Its application is more difficult and most difficult of all is its financial support.' The enterprise of diagnostic ultrasound was backed by the Deputy Chairman of Kelvin and Hughes, Mr William T. Slater, who gave it an initial budget of £500. As Tom Brown stated, 'It turned out to be a remarkably elastic sum of money'. Slater kept the budget going, sometimes in near defiance of the rest of the Board and of the Chairman himself. But by late 1959 he had to announce that the end had come. In this crisis Professor Donald approached the Principal of the University, Sir Hector Hetherington.

This wonderful and wise old man always knew perfectly well that I could smell there was money under the counter and after letting me expostulate for a while he suddenly produced £750 and advised me to hurry over and see the Scottish Hospital Endowments Research Trust which provided continuing support.

Tom Brown went on to build a completely automated, motorized contact scanning machine which was the size of a grand piano. This went into service in 1959 and was used by Professor Donald and his team until 1965. This particular machine was also constructed to be able to perform three-dimensional scanning, although the necessary three-dimensional display system was never completed.

In 1959 there was another leap forward with conversion to polaroid photography yielding instant results while the patient was still on the examination couch.

About this time too came Dr Bertil Sunden from the University of Lund, Sweden. Ian Donald taught him all he knew and Sunden later approached Kelvin and Hughes with a purchase order for a hand-operated machine which was to become the prototype for the later diasonograph family of instruments. Sunden's machine was delivered in 1961 — the first commercial delivery anywhere of an ultrasonic contact scanner. Dr Sunden had a particular interest in twins and produced some beautiful pictures with this machine (Sunden 1964).

In 1959 Ian Donald noted that clear echoes could be obtained from the fetal head *in utero* and began to apply this information (Donald and Brown 1961). I became involved in this work shortly afterwards and indeed was given the project to play with on my own for the reason that the work had to be done where the pregnant patients were, namely in the Royal Maternity Hospital at the other end of the City from the Western Infirmary where the Professor had made

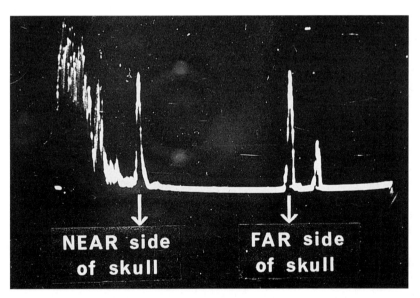

Fig. 1.4. Measurement of the fetal biparietal diameter by A-mode ultrasound, 1962.

his headquarters and which housed the compound sector scanner. At Rottenrow, there was no separate room to examine the patients in and not even a cupboard in which to keep the apparatus, so we pushed it about on a trolley and approached patients in the wards for permission to examine them at the bedside. Glasgow women are wonderful and they accepted all this without demur. A lady approached me many years later and told me that her family whose births I had supervised were doing well and added, 'I mind ye fine coming roon Rottenrow wi' yer wee barra.' There was no time off for research in those days and it had to be done amidst an enormous workload of emergencies in Obstetrics and Gynaecology, huge clinics, and the teaching of undergraduates. Results were written up through the night. In this I was greatly assisted by the selfless devotion of my wife, Elma. At the hospital the physicist, Mr Tom Duggan, was responsible for all the technical developments and attended the examination of the patients in the wards often at great inconvenience to himself. Work was often interrupted by clinical crises and I remember one particular dramatic day when we were trying out a new method of measurement and the whole thing had to be abandoned because the woman in the next bed started pouring blood from placenta praevia and I had to take her to theatre.

However, we were able to complete experiments comparing the time taken by ultrasound to traverse the biparietal diameter in the neonate with the actual measurement of that diameter and to estimate the proportion of the various components, scalp, skull, and brain in the fetal head. This latter experiment involved post-mortem work. Later we applied this information to echo-encephalography in the newborn. We then went on to apply the method clinically with three objectives:

(1) to confirm the presentation

(2) to assess the size of the fetus

(3) to follow fetal growth.

This last idea was completely original and owed much to Tom Duggan's development of the ultrasonic caliper principle which made more accurate measurement possible (Willocks *et al.* 1964)

Our results were presented at a memorable meeting of the Royal Society of Medicine in London on Friday 12 January 1962 (Donald *et al.* 1962). Professor Donald was just recovering from his first cardiac operation and was technically still an in-patient in the Western Infirmary, Glasgow. John MacVicar and I were in attendance and were somewhat apprehensive about making presentations to this august body and even more apprehensive about the state of health of our Chief. It was a cold foggy night, not the best atmosphere for a cardiac invalid. Our film had broken into bits on rehearsal and we had to make some emergency repairs. The Professor collapsed with acute dyspnoea half-way through the presentation and John MacVicar had to continue with his paper, 'Illustrative examples of ultrasonic echograms', showing pictures of ovarian cysts, fibroids, hydatidiform mole, and early pregnancy. I then gave my paper, 'Ultrasonic cephalometry as a measure of fetal growth in normal and abnormal pregnancy'. We were all relieved when the meeting ended successfully.

When the Queen Mother's Hospital opened in 1964 it became possible to do cephalometry both by A-scan and B-scan techniques because of the availability of apparatus (Willocks *et al.* 1967) (Fig. 1.5). My registrar, Dr Stuart Campbell (now Professor at King's College Hospital, London) expressed an interest in fetal cephalometry and greatly refined the method (Campbell 1968). It was widely applied and became the standard biophysical method for the study of fetal growth for many years.

Further developments were proceeding apace. A chance observation made by Professor Donald in 1963 had opened the way to studies of early pregnancy (MacVicar and Donald 1963). A patient who had been kept waiting had a very full bladder. This had the effect of displacing the intestine out of the way and providing a clear sounding tank through which the pelvic viscera including the uterus could be examined. This was the first application of the full bladder technique which later proved such a diagnostic success, although rather a nuisance to patients (Fig. 1.6). The first triumph with this technique was with a patient who had a sequence of four spontaneous abortions and who did not even know she was pregnant. When she was examined through the full bladder, a

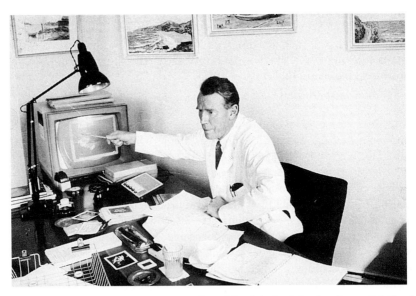

Fig. 1.5. The 'actor–manager' — Ian Donald at his desk in the Queen Mother's Hospital.

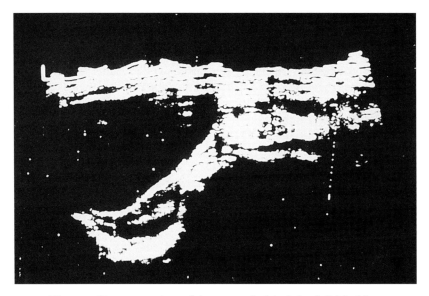

Fig. 1.6. Demonstration of the uterus behind the full bladder.

curious white ring was seen within the uterus which at first perplexed Ian Donald until he realized that he was looking at a very early gestation sac. This caused great excitement because pregnancy could now be studied from beginning to end. Ultrasound could define the rate of growth from the fifth week onwards, the site of implantation, the phenomenon of blighting of the ovum, and even the process of abortion. The very early recognition of twins became possible, and when Stuart Campbell moved to Professor Dewhurst's Department at Queen Charlotte's Hospital he made the dramatic demonstration of quintuplets at the ninth week of pregnancy (Campbell and Dewhurst 1970). From 1966 ultrasound became the method of choice for placentography and this work, following the lead of the Denver group (Gottesfeld *et al.* 1966) was published by Professor Donald and Dr Usama Abdulla (Donald and Abdulla 1967, 1968). All cases of antepartum haemorrhage and unstable lie in the hospital were examined for placenta praevia, and ultrasound placentography was soon a prerequisite for amniocentesis at any stage of pregnancy.

Dr Hugh Robinson, than a junior member of the Department, was looking for a research project and I suggested to him that he could use ultrasound in the assessment of cases of threatened and incomplete abortion who took up a lot of space in the Gynaecology Department in the Western Infirmary. This went on to a wide ranging study of problems in early pregnancy and eventually to the display of fetal heart activity from the seventh week of amenorrhoea (Robinson 1972 *a* and *b*, 1973).

Ultrasound barely avoided a severe crash in 1966 when the Kelvin Hughes Glasgow factory now part of Smith's Industrial Division was closed. Professor Donald wrote, 'Desperately I could see our apparatus suffering the fate of so much electronic apparatus in medicine — namely the dust sheet phenomenon.' Again he approached the University Principal, now Sir Charles Wilson, who to his astonishment and delight instructed him to set up his own Ultrasound Department and to engage John Fleming and Angus Hall, members of the original team, as research engineers. Angus Hall later went on to pursue a distinguised career in Leeds. John Fleming has continued at the Queen Mother's Hospital where he has remained as the technical genius behind all ultrasonic developments, continuously providing ideas, ingenuity, and endless patience. Practically all the ultrasound apparatus in current use is now Japanese in origin but the contribution of Scottish engineering in the development of diagnostic ultrasound should never be forgotten.

Professor Donald had many friends in the United States where he was a frequent visitor. He was particularly associated with the research groups in Denver, Colorado, under Professor Joseph Holmes and those in New York under Professor Louis Hellman. Work in Denver dated back to the time of D. Howry with whom Professor Holmes had worked. In 1962 Ian Donald was told that Professor Holmes had been doing some pioneer work in the upper abdomen and planned to follow Glasgow workers into the field of obstetrics and gynaecology. A very happy association, with friendly rivalry, grew up between Glasgow and Denver. Ian Donald's only regret was that Denver is at such an appalling altitude at the base of Rockies. When he visited there he had to have cylinders of oxygen always available. During the first of his American lecture tours in 1961 he collapsed with cardiac failure and over subsequent years had three major heart operations, one valvotomy, and two mitral valve replacements. Professor Louis Hellman from New York came to Glasgow as a guest professor in 1965. He was an extrovert character who was a good match for Ian Donald and learned with great gusto all that Ian could teach him. He had strong opinions on everything and was great fun to work with. His last achievement was to diagnose a large hydatidiform mole, although he missed the associated fetus found on later scanning. He left to return to the USA muttering, 'I may be wrong but I am not in doubt.' This was soon adopted by Ian Donald as one of his own favourite phrases. On returning to New York Hellman established an ultrasound department of his own and later collaborated with the Departments in Glasgow and in Lund in a study on the safety of ultrasound in obstetrics (Hellman *et al.* 1970). The results showed a slightly lower incidence of fetal abnormality than might have been expected from a cross-section of the population; moreover the period of gestation at which the first examination was carried out did not seem to be a significant factor. This was one of a number of investigations into the safety of ultrasound in which Ian Donald was involved. He was never blasé about the subject. On the last page of the last edition of his *Practical obstetric problems* he wrote:

...Present day ultrasonic diagnostic machines use such small levels of energy that they would appear to be safe, but the possibility must never be lost sight of that there may be safety threshold levels possibly different for different tissues, and that with the development of more powerful and sophisticated apparatus these may yet be transgressed (Donald 1979).

The long promised new maternity hospital opened in 1964. Situated near the University and Western Infirmary and on the same campus as the Royal Hospital for Sick Children, the Queen Mother's Hospital was ideally sited for research endeavour. Ian Donald, who believed that the ideal committee was a committee of one, had been intimately involved in the design from the earliest stages and took the opportunity of breaking with tradition in many respects. The hospital served as a model for many others elsewhere. The new hospital gave full scope for Ian Donald's enthusiasms and histrionic skill. He ran it like an actor–manager of the old school, directing the productions, and playing all the leading parts himself.

From the opening of the Queen Mother's Hospital until long after his retirement Ian Donald was a famous international figure. His unfailing sense of occasion was well suited to his role as a guest Professor and Lecturer and the list of his appointments of this kind occupies two closely typed foolscap pages.

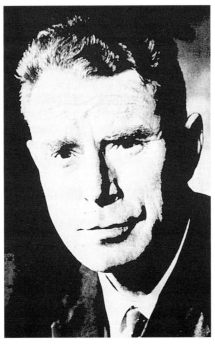

Fig. 1.7. Professor Ian Donald in his later years.

Among the distinctions that he particularly prized were his appointment as Joseph Price Orator to the American Association of Obstetricians and Gynaecologists, the award of the Eardley Holland Gold Medal of the Royal College of Obstetricians and Gynaecologists in 1968, the Blair–Bell Gold Medal of the Royal Society of Medicine in 1970, the Victor Bonney Prize of the Royal College of Surgeons of England in 1973, and the McKenzie Davidson Medal of the British Institution of Radiology in 1975. In 1980–81 he was the guest of the Brazilian, Egyptian, Yugoslavian, Japanese, and Australian Societies of Ultrasound in Medicine. He was made an Honorary DSc of the Universities of Glasgow and London in 1981. He had been awarded the CBE by the Queen in 1973 and in 1982 he was awarded the Order of the Yugoslav Banner with Gold Star. He loved the pomp and circumstance of academic occasions and was delighted when he met princes either of the Realm or the Church. On the subject of his meeting with the Pope he said proudly, 'His Holiness talked to me for nearly an hour', on which his friend Wallace Barr commented, 'I have never known anyone get away from Ian Donald in under an hour.' He was a great talker and exulted in his intellectual strength and dexterity. He could wield the conversational rapier or the polemical bludgeon with equally devastating effect on colleagues and opponents alike. Telling phrases would be carefully polished on ward rounds and in theatre and later delivered with dramatic effect in public to his favourite and often unsuspecting prey, visiting professors and examiners. He was masterly at the game of one-upmanship and had a great talent for assimilating technical jargon which he could deliver authoritatively to wide-eyed visitors. All this was done with great good humour. He was always fun to be with and there were lots of laughs.

His recreations were sailing, music, and landscape painting. Of his ability as a sailor I cannot speak but he was certainly intrepid. He was a competent and spirited, if slightly inaccurate, pianist with a particular liking for the works of Beethoven and Chopin. His paintings reflected his love of the sea and shore. These works were generally in watercolour, gouache, or wax crayon. Oil paint was too slow a medium for him.

He faced failing health with astonishing courage. If he did not wear his heart upon his sleeve he certainly exposed it to view in a series of publications, the most comprehensive of which was in the *Scottish Medical Journal* in 1976 and is entitled, 'At the receiving end. A doctor's personal recollections of second time cardiac valve replacement' (Donald 1976). This account concludes, 'For most of my life I have thought it fun to be alive and now I am more sure of it than ever.'

In all his troubles Ian was sustained by his Christian faith which was never rigid or puritanical. His outspoken opposition to the increasing practice of abortion from the mid 1960s onwards provoked an intense reaction from those who were committed to its liberalization. His opinions were often caricatured by his opponents. In fact he had no absolute views on the matter of abortion. He saw no problem where the mother's health or life were at severe hazard nor

when the child was proved to be severely defective mentally or physically, but he wrote:

…The destruction of perfectly healthy unborn life in healthy women because of the great nuisance value foreseen, rightly or more usually wrongly is something which one could never regard as God's work (Donald 1978).

Ian's personal kindness to his patients and friends knew no bounds and he would always respond when people were in trouble. Alix and he were married for nearly 50 years and she was with him when he died at home on 19 June 1987. This gracious, gentle, and truly heroic lady made Ian's success possible. Ian Donald was a man of faith, a man of courage, and a man of vision. In my opinion he never received the public honour due to him. A title would have given him much innocent pleasure, and fitting international recognition would have been the Nobel Prize in Medicine. But honours and titles are buried with the man. If you seek Ian Donald's memorial look around you and in every maternity hospital you will see ultrasound in use.

References

Brown, T. G. (1988). *Ultrasound in Glasgow*. Paper read at History of Ultrasound Symposium, Washington DC.

Campbell, S. (1968). An improved method of fetal cephalometry by ultrasound. *Journal of Obstetrics and Gynaecology of the British Commonwealth*, **75**, 568–76.

Campbell, S. and Dewhurst, C. J. (1970). Quintuplet pregnancy diagnosed and assessed by ultrasonic compound scanning *Lancet*, **i**, 101–3

Donald, I. (1954). Atelectasis neonatorum. *Journal of Obstetrics and Gynaecology of the British Empire*, **61**, (6), 725–37.

Donald, I. (1969). On launching a new diagnostic science. *American Journal of Obstetrics and Gynecology*, **103**, 609–28.

Donald, I. (1974a). Apologia: how and why medical sonar developed. *Annals of the Royal College of Surgeons of England*, **54**, 132–40.

Donald, I. (1974b). Sonar — the story of an experiment. *Ultrasound in Medicine and Biology*, **1**, 109–17.

Donald, I. (1976). At the receiving end. A doctor's personal recollections of second time cardiac valve replacement. *Scottish Medical Journal*, **21**, 49–57.

Donald, I. (1978). *Does Christianity help?* Unity Press, London.

Donald, I. (1979). *Practical obstetric problems* (5th edn). Lloyd–Luke (Medical Books) Ltd, London.

Donald, I. and Abdulla, U. (1967). Ultrasonics in obstetrics and gynaecology. *British Journal of Radiology*, **40**, 604–11.

Donald, I. and Abdulla, U. (1968). Placentography by sonar. *Journal of Obstetrics and Gynaecology of the British Commonwealth*, **75**, 993–1006.

Donald, I. and Brown, T. G. (1961). Demonstration of tissue interfaces within the body by ultrasonic echo-sounding. *British Journal of Radiology*, **34**, 539–46.

Donald, I., MacVicar, J., and Brown, T. G. (1958). Investigation of abdominal masses by pulsed ultrasound. *Lancet*, **i**, 1188–95.

LIBRARY
THE UNIVERSITY OF TEXAS
AT BROWNSVILLE
Brownsville, TX 78520-4991

Donald, I., MacVicar, J., and Willocks, J. (1962). Sonar: a new diagnostic echo-sounding technique. Illustrative example of ultrasonic echograms. The use of ultrasonic cephalometry. *Proceedings of the Royal Society of Medicine*, **55**, 637–40.

Gottesfeld, K. R., Thompson, H. E., Holmes, J. H., and Taylor, E. S. (1966). Ultrasonic placentography — a new method for placental localisation. *American Journal of Obstetrics and Gynecology*, **96**, 538–47.

Hellman, L. M., Duffus, G. M., Donald, I., and Sunden, B. (1970). Safety of diagnostic ultrasound in obstetrics. *Lancet*, **i**, 1133–4.

MacVicar, J. and Donald, I. (1963). Sonar in the diagnosis of early pregnancy and its complications. *Journal of Obstetrics and Gynaecology of the British Commonwealth*, **70**, 387–95.

Robinson, H. P. (1972*a*). Sonar in the management of abortion. *Journal of Obstetrics and Gynaecology of the British Commonwealth*, **79**, 90–4.

Robinson, H. P. (1972*b*). Detection of fetal heart movement in first trimester of pregnancy using pulsed ultrasound. *British Medical Journal*, **4**, 466–8.

Robinson, H. P. (1973). Sonar measurement of fetal crown–rump length as a means of assessing maturity in first trimester of pregnancy. *British Medical Journal*, **4**, 28–31.

Sunden, B. (1964). On the diagnostic value of ultrasound in obstetrics and gynaecology. *Acta Obsetrica et Gynaecologica Scandinavica*, **43**, Suppl 6, 190.

Willocks, J., Donald, I., Duggan, T. C., and Day, N. (1964). Foetal cephalometry by ultrasound. *Journal of Obstetrics and Gynaecology of the British Commonwealth*, **71**, 11–20.

Willocks, J., Donald, I., Campbell, S., and Dunsmore, I. R. (1967). Intrauterine growth assessed by ultrasonic foetal cephalometry. *Journal of Obstetrics and Gynaecology of the British Commonwealth*, **74**, 639–47.

2
Transvaginal ultrasound in early prenatal diagnosis
Mark T. Cullen and John C. Hobbins

Introduction

Prenatal diagnostic ultrasound is employed to identify specific structural abnormalities, or subtle morphological changes associated with genetic syndromes in the fetus. The traditional period in which to perform a targeted ultrasound examination of the fetus is from 16 to 20 menstrual weeks; a time when the fetus is large enough that anatomical structures may easily be evaluated, and data are available on the sensitivity of the examination.

Patient expectations and technical advances in ultrasound equipment have facilitated the trend for earlier antenatal diagnosis. 'Earlier' diagnostic methods practised include chorionic villus sampling, amniocentesis and recently, diagnostic ultrasound. All have been successfully performed employing transvaginal sonography.

First trimester diagnosis alleviates the anxiety of waiting for second trimester evaluation and allows the option for safer, and more humane pregnancy termination. While ultrasound evaluation of the early conceptus has been accomplished with transabdominal transducers; its use to diagnose congenital abnormalities in the first trimester has only recently been explored.

It is the purpose of this discussion to explore the role of transvaginal ultrasound in early prenatal diagnosis, from the early identification of viable pregnancy to the diagnosis of complex structural anomalies in the fetus.

Advantages and disadvantages

Transvaginal transducers have added a significant new dimension to the ultrasound examination, permitting a detailed image of the first and early second trimester fetus, that is unparalleled. The technique offers several advantages over traditional abdominal imaging. Resolution is often improved because the fetus is closer to the transducer allowing higher frequencies to be used. Fewer tissue interfaces are traversed with less beam scatter. The bladder does not need to be filled which improves patient comfort. The examination is well tolerated by the patient. The transvaginal approach is especially valuable in the evaluation of the very early conceptus, in cases where a retroverted uterus is encountered, when maternal obesity is a factor, or when the structure to be evaluated is deep in the pelvis (Cullen *et al.* 1989).

Equipment

Transvaginal transducers are now available from most ultrasound manufacturers. Sizes and shapes vary, as does the field of view (60–180 degrees), and transducer angle. Colour Doppler is available on some models. Five MHz to 7.5 MHz mechanical sector and curvilinear transvaginal probes are commonly used for detailed imaging. The highest frequency probe should be employed when possible.

The disadvantages of the examination are minimal. In some instances it may be difficult to obtain specific anatomical views due to limited manoeuvrability of the probe. In addition, since the focal zone of most transducers approximates 8–10 cm, if the fetus is out of the focal zone, as with a pelvis mass, resolution can be impaired. The inexperienced operator may experience difficulty with the unique orientation of the anatomy. Coordination of the examining room, patient, and sonographer is important for maximum efficiency.

The examination

The transvaginal examination is best performed in a private room equipped with a gynaecological examining table with stirrups. The patient is asked to empty her bladder prior to being placed in the lithotomy position and draped. The transducer is coated with coupling gel and then covered with a condom or the finger of a glove. Sterile lubricant is then placed on to the tip of the probe which is introduced into the vagina. The examination, while object directed, should be complete and systematic. The entire pelvis should be evaluated as well as the conceptus in an obstetric scan. Some vaginal transducers yield a small effective field of view, and pelvic pathology could potentially be missed. The optimal focal point is achieved by advancing the probe toward the object being studied. Additional views are obtained by rotation of the transducer, or by limited lateral and vertical movement. Uterine and fetal position can be changed with gentle pressure of a hand on the maternal abdomen. Universal precautions should be practised, cleaning the probe between patients with a sterilizing solution recommended by the manufacturer of the equipment.

While there is a significant body of literature objectively comparing vaginal and abdominal sonography in gynaecolology, for follicle induction evaluation (Meldrum *et al.* 1984; Vermesh *et al.* 1987; Yee *et al.* 1987; Gonzalez *et al.*

1988) and the diagnosis of ectopic pregnancy (Nyberg *et al.* 1987; Rempen 1988; Shapiro *et al.* 1988; Cacciatore *et al.* 1989), limited prospective comparisons exist for evaluating the fetus. In a prospective study of 120 fetuses evaluated between 5–13 weeks, vaginal scanning was judged as good or superior to the abdominal approach both subjectively and objectively for:

(1) visualizing the fetus (75 per cent)

(2) obtaining biometric parameters (90 per cent)

(3) visualizing detailed anatomy (70 per cent).

These differences were not as pronounced as gestational age increased (Cullen *et al.* 1989). D'Amelio *et al.* (1990), in a study evaluating transvaginal scanning for early fetal echocardiography in fetuses between 11 and 18 weeks, was able to obtain specific cardiac views more often than transabdominally. A recent comparison of 800 patients, scanned both abdominally and vaginally between 9–13 menstrual weeks, to diagnose congenital anomalies suggested that vaginal scanning was more sensitive and specific (Achiron and Tabmor 1991).

Developmental embryology

Applying vaginal scanning to the second and third trimester fetus requires familiarization with a new orientation to anatomy. Antenatal diagnosis in the first trimester on the other hand, requires a thorough understanding of developmental embryology. Green and Hobbins (1988), using an abdominal approach, and Timor-Tritsch *et al.* (1989), using transvaginal sonography, have chronicled the normal embryonic and fetal developmental anatomy (Table 2.1). This background of normal sonographic anatomy is necessary prior to undertaking early diagnosis.

A 2 mm gestational sac is the first direct sonographic evidence of early pregnancy. It can be visualized as early as 2 days after a missed period and always by the end of the fourth menstrual week when it appears as a symmetrical double echogenic ring or 'doughnut'. The diagnosis of pregnancy can be made with transvaginal scanning earlier, and therefore correlates with a lower level of human chorionic gonadotropin than originally described with transabdominal techniques (Bernascheck *et al.* 1988; Crespigny *et al.* 1988; Fossum *et al.* 1988). The gestational sac will grow throughout gestation in a near-linear fashion (Goldstein *et al.* 1991). Small for gestational age sacs have been suggested as predicting poor pregnancy outcome (Bromely *et al.* 1991). A fetal pole with cardiac activity can be seen reliably with a sac diameter of 1–1.2 cm (Crespigny 1987). Correlation of HCG values and sac diameter has been suggested as a predictor of normal early pregnancy outcome (Nyberg *et al.* 1986). The amniotic sac remains distinct within the chorionic cavity until 12–13

Table 2.1 Gestational age in menstrual weeks when anatomical structures are reliably seen sonographically

Anatomical landmark	Gestational age (weeks)
Gestational sac	4–5
Secondary yolk sac	5
Embryonic pole	5
Heart beat	5–6
Tail remnant	7
Limb buds	8
Fetal movements	8–9
Physiological bowel herniation	8–10
Kidneys	10
Mineralization long bones	10
Calvarium calcified	10–11
Face	10–11
Stomach	10–11
Digits	11
4 Chamber view of heart	11–12
Bladder	11–12
Diaphragm	12
Genitalia	12–13

weeks, when it becomes juxtaposed to the chorion. The amniotic fluid volume increases nearly linearly from 8 weeks to 12 weeks, occupying a larger percentage of the total uterine cavity. This information can be useful in deciding the amount of amniotic volume to be removed during early amniocentesis.

The secondary yolk sac, a remnant of the primary yolk sac, remains an extra-embryonic structure. It is visible at five menstrual weeks as a 4 mm spherical ring, sometimes seen attached to the vitelline vessels coursing to the embryo. When the gestational sac is as small as 7 mm it is possible to visualize the yolk sac. This is in contrast to previous observations by abdominal scanning suggesting that the yolk sac is seen when the gestational sac diameter reaches 1 cm in diameter (Jain *et al.* 1988). The yolk sac can often be seen throughout the first trimester in the extra-coelomic space until the space is obliterated by growth of the amniotic cavity (Fig. 2.1). Growth of the secondary yolk sac follows a curvilinear pattern described by a simple quadratic regression (Reece *et al.* 1989). Small sclerotic yolk sacs, those that are less than 2 mm in diameter, and macrosomic yolk sacs greater than 8 mm have been found with early pregnancy failures and aneuploidy (Green and Hobbins 1988; Ferrazzi *et al.* 1988; Cullen *et al.* submitted; Brambati 1991).

The embryo is visible as early as 5–6 menstrual weeks as a 2 mm flat disc. Heart pulsations are seen as early as 25 days from ovulation and almost always

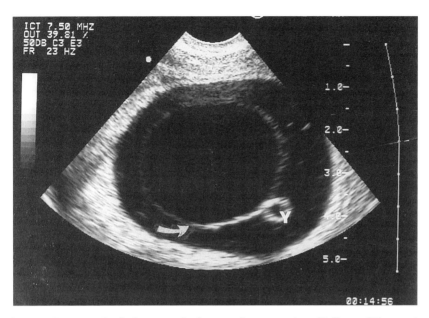

Fig. 2.1. Transvaginal ultrasound of 10 week conception. Yolk sac (Y) seen in the extracoelomic cavity. Amnion (arrow).

by 30 days (Fossum *et al.* 1988; Levi *et al.* 1990; Schats *et al.* 1990), approximately one week prior to transabdominal detection. Embryonic and technical factors, including the smoothing effects of the ultrasound equipment, might account for this discrepancy. The crown–rump length at this time is between 1.5–5 mm (Fig. 2.2). The embryo grows rapidly and is seen completely inside the amniotic sac at 7 weeks. The transvaginal approach allows for earlier and perhaps, a more accurate reference chart for crown–rump length (Schats *et al.* 1991) than the nomograms generated (Robinson 1973) using a compound B-scanner, although this difference is minimal. Studies correlating crown–rump length and gestational age have varied depending upon the ultrasound techniques used and historical factors. For example, dating methods have included last menstrual period, LH surge, and embryo transfer date from *in vitro* fertilization programmes. It has been suggested that initial studies using menstrual dating might have underestimated true gestational age by 3.2 (± 3.9) days (Evans 1991).

Embryonic heart rate, while initially detected at 100–120 beats per minute (b.p.m.) at 5–6 menstrual weeks, increases to a rate of 170–180 by 12 weeks. Bradycardia, with fetal heart rates more than two standard deviations below the mean may predict poor pregnancy outcome (Hertzberg *et al.* 1988; Laboda *et al.* 1989; Achiron *et al.* 1991).

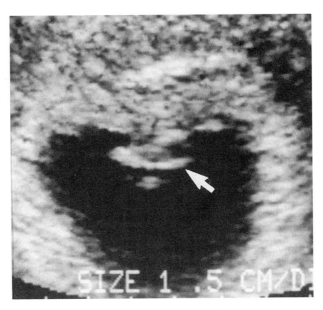

Fig. 2.2. Image of 5 weeks and 6 days embryo.

At eight menstrual weeks anatomical detail of specific organ systems can be delineated. Diagnostic criteria for the prenatal diagnosis in the first trimester of pregnancy and developmental limitations are discussed below by anatomic location.

Head and neck

At 8 weeks, the cranium contains a single ventricle and a large hypoechoic rhombencephalon posteriorly. The echogenic falx cerebri divides the midline, and two prominent choroid plexus are seen bilaterally at 9 weeks. Calcification of the calvarium and visualization of the cerebellum become apparent in the tenth week (Green and Hobbins 1988). The ventricles and prominent choroid plexus fill much of the calvarium throughout the first trimester, although a thin mantle of cerebral cortex is often seen as early as 10 weeks and certainly by the end of the twelfth week. The corpus callosum does not fully develop until the second trimester.

From the above observations of normal neuroanatomical development, acrania (Fig. 2.3) cannot be diagnosed until the completion of the tenth or eleventh week when the calvarium is calcified. Anencephaly (Fig. 2.4), which is diagnosed by the absence of a calvarium and cerebral cortex, is thought to be a progression from exencephaly through tissue degeneration and might appear at a later gestation. Exencephaly (Fig. 2.5) is pathologically defined as disorganized neural and vascular tissue. The diagnosis of an encephalocele should be

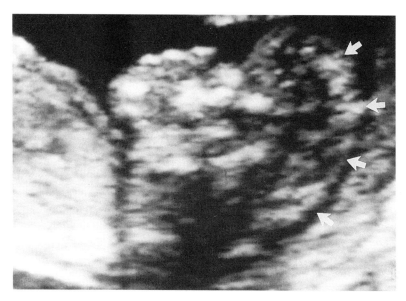

Fig. 2.3. Sagittal scan in an 11 week pregnancy with exencephaly. Disorganized neural tissue (arrows) and the absence of the calvarium is noted.

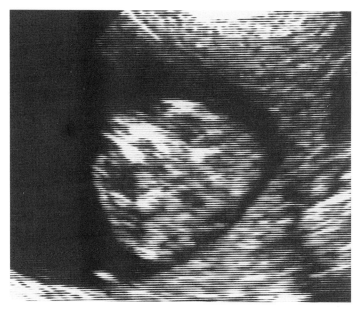

Fig. 2.4. Transverse scan of the head at the level of the orbits in a 12 week embryo with anencephaly.

considered when a calcified cranium is seen with protruding neural tissue. In fetuses with acrania, normal cerebral cortex is seen without a bony calvarium. Choroid plexus cysts occur infrequently in the first trimester and appear as well-defined sonolucencies in the choroid plexus. The significance of their presence is unclear. Hydrocephaly without craniomegaly has been diagnosed in the first trimester, but is difficult to ascertain due to the relatively large proportions of the lateral ventricles to the calvarium. Compression and or deviation of the choroid plexus might be the only indication.

Anencephaly, exencephaly, encephaloceles, acrania, hydrocephaly, Dandy-Walker syndrome, and holoprosencephaly (Vergani *et al.* 1987; Benacerraf 1988; Cullen *et al.* 1990*b*; Rottem and Bronshtein 1990; Achiron and Tabmur 1991, Bronshtein and Weiner 1991; Bronshtein and Zimmer 1991; Timor-Tritsh *et al.* 1991) have all been reported in the literature in the first trimester and early second trimester.

Face

The mandible and maxilla are visualized sonographically at 10 weeks, fusion of the midline structures occurs after the seventh week. Facial clefting may also be evident at this time. The prominent cephalic curve and small size limits examination prior to this period. The external ears are visualized as early as 8

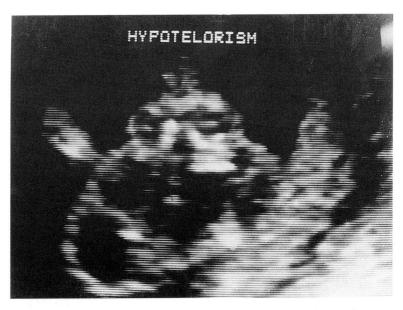

Fig. 2.5. Transverse scan at the level of the orbits showing hypotelorism in a 12 week embryo with exencephaly.

weeks; initially they are found at the level below the mandible, but assume their final more cephalad position in the second trimester. Low set ears can be diagnosed using a measurement from the lower auricular insertion to the apex of the head at midcalvarium and comparing it to a nomogram (Green 1988). The orbits are initially seen at 11 weeks followed by the lens by at 12 weeks. Hypotelorism (Fig. 2.5) has been described in the first trimester (Cullen *et al.* 1990*b*). Bronshtein *et al.* (1991*a*) in a report of eight ocular defects diagnosed by transvaginal sonography in the first and second trimester observed strabismus, cataracts, and microphthalmia. Anopthalmia was not appreciated on an initial scan. In our first trimester screening programme, a diabetic mother whose embryo was scanned at 10.5 weeks prior to long bone mineralization, appeared normal, but at 18 weeks the fetus was found to have micrognathia and mesomelic limb dysplasia.

Cleft lip, cyclopia, and abnormalities of the nose, including proboscis, have not been reported at this time but are potentially detectable in early pregnancy.

Spine

The dorsal wall can be imaged at seven menstrual weeks. Closure of the neural pore with calcification of the lamina of the spine does not occur until six and ten weeks, respectively, at which time the potential exists to diagnosis open spina bifida. Kyphoscoliosis has been diagnosed by demonstrating misalignment of the lamina and spinal body (Cullen 1990*b*) and spinal bifida by laminar splaying (Rottem *et al.* 1989).

Ventral wall

The ventral wall of the developing embryo is apparent at 6–7 menstrual weeks. Physiological herniation of the bowel into the proximal portion of the umbilical cord can be demonstrated between 8 and 11 weeks as a thickening of the cord insertion (Fig. 2.6) (Green and Hobbins 1988; Timor-Tritsch *et al.* 1989). Midgut herniation noted after 12 weeks should suggest an omphalocele. Gastroschisis (Fig. 2.7), a lateral herniation of the bowel through an anterior abdominal wall defect, is easily differentiated in the first trimester. Omphaloceles, gastroschisis, and anterior folding defects have been reported in the first trimester (Curtis and Watson 1988; Gray *et al.* 1989; Cullen 1990*b*; Achiron and Tabmor 1991).

Cystic hygromas

Nuchal cystic hygromas are being reported with increasing frequency in the first trimester (Gustavii and Edvall 1984; Exalto *et al.* 1985; Reuss *et al.* 1987; Bronshtein *et al.* 1989; Cullen 1990*a,b*).

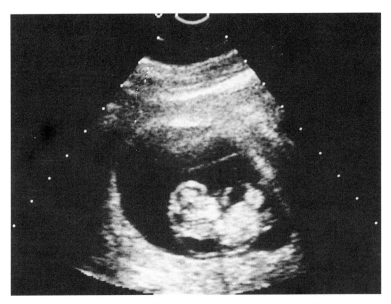

Fig. 2.6. 10 week fetus with physiologic gut herniation and posterior cystic hygroma.

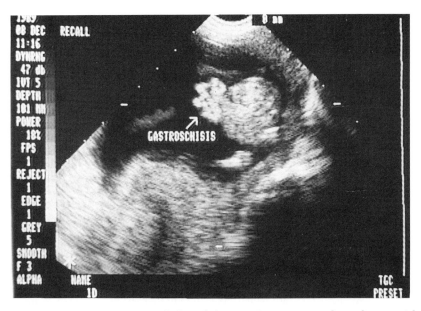

Fig. 2.7. Transverse scan of the abdomen in a 11 week embryo with gastroschisis. Umbilical cord can be seen in midline.

Cystic hygromas are fluid-filled sacculations of the lateral neck and nuchal region, resulting from lymphatic dysplasia (Chervenak *et al.* 1983). Our experience, and most series in the literature have shown that these are the most common structural anomalies diagnosed in the first trimester. In a recent series (Cullen *et al.* 1990*a*), 30 cases of nuchal cystic hygromas were reported and described by anatomical location as lateral nuchal, posterior nuchal (Fig. 2.8), or either location associated with hydrops (Figs 2.9, 10). The incidence of aneuploidy in this series and in a follow-up series was about 60 per cent, and was not influenced by location or the presence of septation or hydrops. This data is in contrast to that of other authors who have suggested that septations were a poor prognostic finding associated with a higher risk of aneuploidy (Bronshtein *et al.* 1989). This difference may be due to the relative small numbers studied and differences in gestational ages. Karyotypic abnormalities observed with this condition are varied in the first trimester. Experience has shown that hygromas without aneuploidy can resolve, often by 18 weeks without neonatal phenotypic findings. Noonan syndrome must be considered when counselling patients with affected fetuses.

Cystic hygromas must be differentiated from defects of the fetal spine and calvarium. Positioning of the dorsal wall of the embryo in close proximity to the amnion or the yolk sac, as well as the 'nuchal bleb', a normal anatomical finding present in embryos up to 10 weeks, can give an appearance similar to a posterior hygroma and must be avoided.

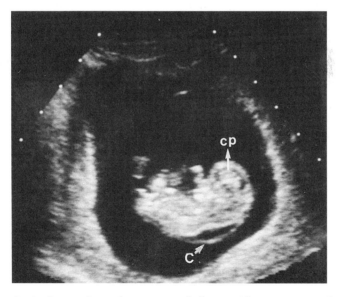

Fig. 2.8. Sagittal scan through a 10.5 week fetus with posterior nuchal cystic hygroma (C), choroid plexus (CP).

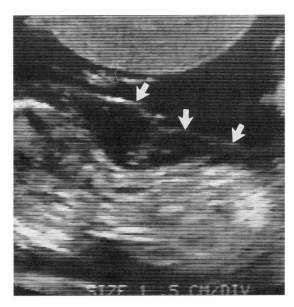

Fig. 2.9. Fetus with diffuse cystic hygroma and hydrops (arrows).

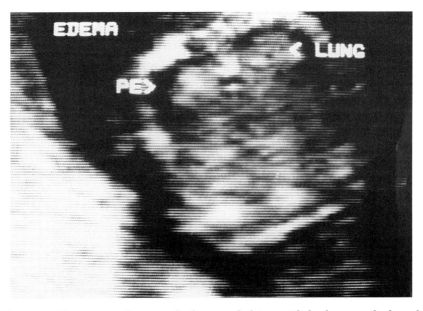

Fig. 2.10. Transverse ultrasound of 11 week fetus with hydrops and pleural effusions (PE).

When a cystic hygroma is found in the first trimester we advocate chromosomal testing, a complete anatomical screen, and follow-up examinations in the euploid fetus to determine if the lesions resolve.

Extremities and digits

Distinct limb paddles can be seen at 8 weeks, with the long bones appearing to calcify at 10 weeks. Early antenatal diagnosis of fetuses affected with a short limb dysplasia has been reported (Benacerraf *et al.* 1988; Gray *et al.* 1989) as well as club feet (Bronshtein and Zimmer 1989). We have had experience of a fetus with a mesomelic dysplasia in which the diagnosis was not apparent at 10.5 weeks. At that time the extremities appeared normal in size and morphology, but were not yet mineralized. Currently it is not known when specific limb dysplasias become manifest.

Digits are well delineated at 11 weeks. Polydactyly and syndactyly have been observed in the first trimester.

Heart

A four-chamber view of the heart and great vessels can be obtained as early as 11 weeks and consistently at 13 weeks (D'Amelio *et al.* 1990). Recently, Gembruch *et al.* (1990) reported the antenatal diagnosis of an atrioventricular canal defect with complete heart block at 11 weeks. In a recent report, Bronshtein *et al.* (1991*b*) describe their results in the evaluation of 3899 patients screened for congenital heart disease between 12 and 16 weeks. An adequate examination was accomplished in 80 per cent at the initial examination. Ten cardiac abnormalities were found; these included aortic override, hypoplastic left heart, single atrium, ventricular, and atrial septal defects. Despite these promising reports, alterations in chamber size may not be apparent until later in pregnancy, making the diagnosis of subtler defects difficult. We are aware of two cases where congenital heart defects were not seen in the first trimester but were discovered on a follow-up ultrasound examination. At this time, the sensitivity of transvaginal sonography for the diagnosis of early congenital heart disease is unknown.

Genitourinary system

The kidneys and bladder may be imaged as early as 10 weeks (Green and Hobbins 1988). Bronshtein *et al.* (1990*b*) have recently published normative data for kidney dimensions from 12 to 14 weeks. Obstructive uropathies diagnosed in the first trimester have included megacystis (Fig. 2.11) and hydronephrosis, these were diagnosed by observing dilatation of the urinary bladder and renal pelvis. While infantile polycystic and multicystic dysplastic

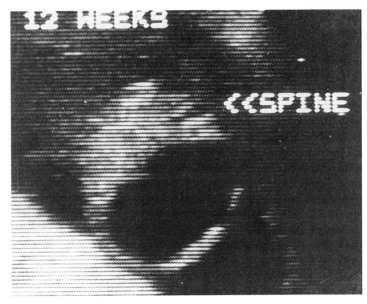

Fig 2.11. Transverse scan in a 12 week embryo with a bladder outlet obstruction.

kidney disease have also been reported, renal agenesis has not been observed. This diagnosis should be possible by 11 weeks. Care must be exercised in not confusing the adrenal gland with the kidneys. The adrenals are of similar size at this gestation but, unlike the kidneys, have a sonolucent cortex and dense medullary region.

Anatomical differentiation of the fetal genitalia is not complete until 11 weeks. Identification of the male phallus can be made at 12–13 weeks when fetal position permits. Bronshtein *et al.* (1990*a*) in a study evaluating identification of genitalia using vaginal sonography reported a 99.5 per cent specificity at 13–14 weeks during the latter part of their experience. No abnormalities of this system have been recorded to date in the first trimester.

Gastrointestinal

The stomach is seen as a hypoechoic structure inferior to the diaphragm on the left side of the abdomen, first seen at 10–11 weeks. Identification of duodenal atresia is rare in the first trimester despite the large number of trisomy 21 fetuses that undergo ultrasound at the time of chorion villus sampling. We have had experience with one case of duodenal atresia in an aneuploid fetus identified at the end of 13 weeks' gestation. Oesophageal and small bowel atresias have not been observed.

Prominent bowel patterns are often observed in the fetal abdomen at 10–11 weeks after the return of the bowel in the abdomen, and should not be mistaken as abnormal.

Placenta and umbilical cord

The chorion frondosum is demarcated at seven weeks. A partial mole has been reported in the first trimester (Romero *et al.* 1989), and the placenta was noted to have multiple small sonolucent areas associated with an elevated maternal HCG level.

The umbilical cord is seen at the seventh week. Transient umbilical cord cyst (Fig. 2.12) and a short abnormal umbilical cord associated with a ventral wall folding defect has been described (Cullen *et al.* 1990*b*).

Multiple gestations

Identification of twin gestational sacs is possible as early as 5 weeks. Zygosity can at times be determined by identification of sac number and position as well as membrane thickness. The reports of early scanning studies suggest a much

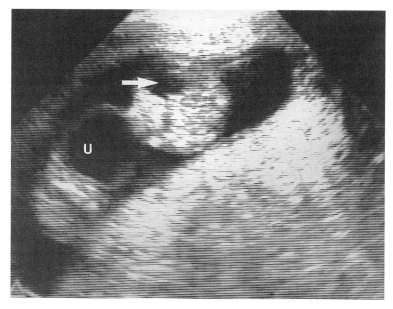

Fig. 2.12. Ultrasound of fetus with transient umbilical cyst (U). Arrow indicates ventral wall folding defect.

higher incidence of twinning than previously thought with a 21 per cent incidence of early loss, the so called 'vanishing twin syndrome' (Landy 1986). Structural abnormalities reported in multiple gestations have included exencephaly (Cullen *et al.* 1992), twin reverse arterial perfusion syndrome (Stiller *et al.* 1989), and conjoined twins (Maggio *et al.* 1985).

With enhanced visualization, care must be given not to misinterpret artefacts or normal variations in first trimester anatomy as first pointed out by Hill *et al.* (1988) and echoed in most studies investigating early prenatal diagnosis.

Antenatal diagnosis in the first trimester

Few antenatal series have been published using transvaginal ultrasound for diagnosis. These series are difficult to assess objectively for several reasons. Large experiences are often reported separately by specific anatomical locations. Pathological correlation has not always been available. Follow-up of fetuses thought to be morphologically normal is often not presented, and the gestational ages being reported as 'early' are varied.This makes estimates of the sensitivity and specificity of early transvaginal diagnosis impossible at this time. Cullen *et al.* (1990*a–d*) reported on 33 structural anomalies detected in a transvaginal screening programme of 622 patients in the first trimester; three additional anomalies were not detected in that series. Achiron and Tabmor (1991) reported 14 malformations detected in a prospective comparison of abdominal and vaginal sonography. Eight anomalies (57 per cent) were detected in the first trimester. Abdominal sonography identified four but was non-specific in diagnosis. Rottem *et al.* (1989) detected three abnormal fetuses in a population of 141 patients without a false-negative report. In a subsequent report, 40 fetuses between the ages of 9–16 weeks were found to have 61 malformations in a population of 1652 patients screened for a reported detection rate of 2.6 per cent.

Pathological correlation with ultrasound findings, especially during the early investigating period of first trimester detection, is imperative. Since routine suction curettage often makes pathological confirmation difficult, prostaglandin induction or embryoscopy (Cullen *et al.* 1990*c*) can be used as an alternative.

Early diagnosis and the prediction of aneuploidy

The association of structural abnormalities, growth retardation, and abnormal biometric ratios with chromosomally abnormal fetuses is well documented in the second and third trimesters of pregnancy. These findings form the basis for suggestions that ultrasound may be useful as a screening tool for identifying fetuses with aneuploidy. The first trimester is an intriguing time to look for aneuploid fetuses as the incidence of chromosomal aberrations is higher, being directly related to maternal age, and inversely related to gestational age. While the incidence of aneuploidy in live births is 0.6 per cent, it has been shown that the loss rate of first trimester aneuploid embryos is as high as 21–33 per cent (Hook *et al.* 1988).

There are few data on aneuploidy detection in the first trimester. In a series of 1760 patients referred for chorion villus sampling, 54 aneuploid fetuses were identified (3 per cent). Eight additional aneuploid fetuses were identified from a transvaginal ultrasound screening programme. Forty structural anomalies were identified in both groups, of which 35 had karyotypes available, and 16/35 (45 per cent) had aneuploidy. Of the 62 aneuploid fetuses identified, 15 (24 per cent) had an identifiable structural anomaly. Cystic hygromas were the most common anomalies identified and were associated with a risk of aneuploidy of 61 per cent.

Early growth retardation (Benacerraf 1988; Lynch and Berkowitz 1989) has previously been associated with trisomy 18 and triploidy. This has not been observed in our experience. These findings are consistent with recently reported work (Brambati 1991) in which early growth retardation was observed with impending fetal demise, but not with chromosomally abnormal fetuses. No association was observed in that study with yolk sac size and aneuploidy.

The recent identification of one case of low set ears associated with trisomy 18 and cystic hygroma is promising but requires more prospective evaluation.

It is our assumption that as more first trimester fetuses undergo early ultrasound examinations, more aneuploid fetuses will be scanned, and more anomalies will be detected.

Invasive early prenatal diagnosis using transvaginal ultrasound

For similar reasons that transvaginal ultrasound allows a more detailed evaluation of the pelvis and the early developing fetus, it also permits easy access to the fetal placental unit. Transvaginally guided amniocentesis, chorion villus sampling (Popp and Ghirardini 1990) as well as multifetal reductions have all been successfully performed by this route. Whether there is an advantage to this approach is unclear.

Colour Doppler and early diagnosis

Colour flow Doppler problems are currently being evaluated on a research basis to evaluate physiological flow patterns in the fetus, arcuate arteries, placental and uterine arteries. Alteration in flow pattern might predict poor pregnancy outcome and conditions of altered uteroplacental blood flow.

Later diagnosis

Transvaginal scanning is not only limited to the first trimester fetus but can be applied to later gestations (Hilpert and Kurtz 1990). The lower uterine segment and cervix are easily evaluated by this approach. The transducer is introduced under direct observation approximately 2–3 cm into the introitus yet away from the cervix. By using a sagittal plane the cervical length can be evaluated while cervical dilatation is seen on a transverse cut. The endocervical canal appears as an anechoic line. Funnelling of the internal os or ballooning of the lower uterine segment with bulging of the amniotic sac can be suggestive of premature labour or cervical incompetence (Brown *et al.* 1986). Placenta previa can be appreciated using the same approach without the influence of the bladder (Farine *et al.* 1988; Lim *et al.* 1989).

Fetal anatomy that is deep in the maternal pelvis lends itself to the vaginal approach (Benacerraf 1989). Neuroanatomical detail is often excellent when the beam is directed through a fontanel. Case reports of an anterior parietal encephalocele (Fig. 2.13) (Cullen *et al.* 1990d) and caudal regression syndrome (Baxi *et al.* 1990) diagnosed by the transvaginal route support its use. Oligohydramnios is a condition in which transvaginal sonography offers additional information (Benacerraf 1990).

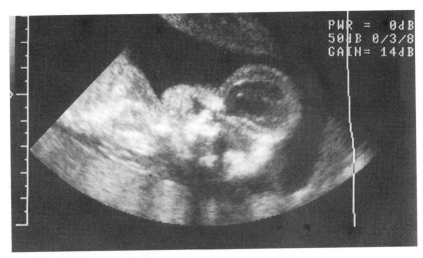

Fig. 2.13. Transvaginal scan of 17 week fetus deep in the maternal pelvis with an anterior parietal cephalocele.

Conclusion

Exploration of early prenatal diagnosis has been greatly enhanced by the development of the vaginal transducer. It is clear that many congenital abnormalities can now be diagnosed earlier in pregnancy using this approach. As vaginal scanning is more widely applied for early pregnancy detection and dating, the fetal anatomical survey will likely become incorporated into the evaluation. It should be cautioned that a first trimester vaginal evaluation should not represent a substitute for a carefully performed second trimester examination in a patient at risk for a fetal anomaly.

References

Achiron, R. and Tabmor, O. (1991). Screening for fetal anomalies during the first trimester of pregnancy: transvaginal versus transabdominal sonography. *Ultrasound Obstet. Gynecol.,* **1**, 186–91.

Achiron, R., Tabmor, O., and Mashiach, S. (1991). Heart rate as a predictor of first trimester spontaneous abortion after ultrasound proven viability. *Obstet. Gynecol.,* **78**, 330–3.

Baxi, L., Warren, W., Collins, M., and Timor-Tritsch, I. E. (1990). Early detection of caudal regression syndrome with transvaginal scanning. *Obstet. Gynecol.,* **75**, 486–9.

Benacerraf, B. (1988). Intrauterine growth retardation in the first trimester associated with triploidy. *J. Ultrasound Med.,* **7**, 153–4.

Benacerraf, B., Lister, J., and DuPonte, B. (1988). First trimester diagnosis of fetal anomalies: A report of three cases. *J. Rep. Med.,* **33**, 777–80.

Benacerraf, B. (1989). Transvaginal sonographic imaging of the low fetal head in the second trimester. *J. Ultrasound Med.,* **8**, 325–8.

Benacerraf, B. (1990). Examination of the second trimester fetus with severe oligohydramnios using transvaginal scanning. *Obstet. Gynecol.,* **75**, 491–3.

Bernascheck, G., Rubelstorfer, R., and Csaicsich, P. (1988). Vaginal sonography versus serum human chorionic gonadatropin in early detection of pregnancy. *Am. J. Obstet. Gynecol.* **158**, 608–12.

Brambati, B. (1991). Ultrasound measurements of GS volume, YS diameter and CRL for screening aneuploidies and predicting early failure. *Ultrasound Obstet. Gynecol.,* **1**, 75.

Bromely, B., Harlow, B., Laboda, L., and Bernacerraf, B. (1991). Small sac size in the first trimester: A predictor of poor fetal outcome. *Radiology,* **178**, 375–7.

Bronshtein, M. and Zimmer, E. (1989). Transvaginal ultrasound diagnosis of fetal clubfeet at 13 weeks, menstrual age. *J.C.U.* **17**, 518–20.

Bronshtein, M., Rottem, S., Yoffe, N., and Blumenfeld, Z. (1989). First-trimester and early second-trimester diagnosis of nuchal cystic hygroma by transvaginal sonography: diverse prognosis of the septated from the nonseptated lesion. *Am. J. Obstet. Gynecol.,* **161**, 78–82.

Bronshtein, M., Rottem, S., Yoffe, N., Blumenfeld, Z., and Brandes, J. M. (1990*a*). Early determination of fetal sex using transvaginal sonography: technique and pitfalls. *J.C.U.,* **18**, 302–6.

Bronshtein, M., Kushnir, O., Ben, R. Z., Shalev, E., Nebel, L., Mashiach, S. and Shalev, J. (1990b). Transvaginal sonographic measurement of fetal kidneys in the first trimester of pregnancy. *J.C.U.*, **18**, 299–301.

Bronshtein, M. and Weiner, Z. (1991). Early transvaginal sonographic diagnosis of alobar holoprosencephaly. *Prenat. Diagn.*, **10**, 459–62.

Bronshtein, M., and Zimmer, E. (1991). Transvaginal sonographic follow up on the formation of fetal cephalocele at 13–19 weeks gestation. *Obstet. Gynecol.*, **78**, 528–30.

Bronshtein, M., Zimmer, E., Gershoni, B., Yoffe, N., Meyer, H., and Blumenfeld, Z. (1991a). First and second trimester diagnosis of fetal ocular defects and associated anomalies: report of eight cases. *Obstet. Gynecol.*, **77**, 443–9.

Bronshtein, M., Zimmer, E., Milo, S., Ho, S., Lorber, A., and Gerlis, L. (1991b). Fetal cardiac abnormalities detected by transvaginal sonography at 12–16 weeks' gestation. *Obstet. Gynecol.*, **78**, 374–8.

Brown, J. E., Thieme, G. A., Shah, D. M., Fleisher, A. C., and Boehm, F. H. (1986). Transabdominal and transvaginal endosonography: Evaluation of the cervix and lower uterine segment in pregnancy. *Am. J. Obstet. Gynecol.*, **155**, 721–6.

Cacciatore, B., Hakan, U., and Ylostalo, P. (1989). Comparison of abdominal and vaginal sonography in suspected ectopic pregnancy. *Obstet. Gynecol.*, **73**, 770–4.

Chervenak, F., Isaacson, G., Blakemore, K., Breg, R., Hobbins, J., Berkowitz, R., Tortora, M., and Mahoney, J. (1983). Fetal cystic hygroma. Cause and natural history. *N. Engl. J. Med.*, **309**, 822–5.

Crespigny, L. C., (1987). Early diagnosis of pregnancy failure. *Am. J. Obstet. Gynecol.*, **159**, 408–9.

Crespigny, L. C., Cooper, D., and McKenna, M. (1988). Early detection of intrauterine pregnancy with ultrasound. *J. Ultrasound Med.*, **7**, 7–10.

Cullen, M. T., Green, J. J., Reece, E. A., and Hobbins, J. C. (1989). A comparison of transvaginal and abdominal ultrasound in visualizing the first trimester conceptus. *J. Ultrasound Med.*, **8**, 565–9.

Cullen, M. T., Gabrielli, S., Green, J. J., Rizzo, N., Mahoney, M., Salafia, C., *et al.* (1990a). Diagnosis and significance of cystic hygroma in the first trimester. *Prenat. Diagn.*, **10**, 643–51.

Cullen, M. T., Green, J., Whetham, J., Salafia, C., Gabrielli, G., and Hobbins, J. C. (1990b). Transvaginal ultrasonographic detection of congenital anomalies in the first trimester. *Am. J. Obstet. Gynecol.*, **163**, 466–76.

Cullen, M. T., Reece, E. A., Whetham, J., and Hobbins, J. C. (1990c) Embryoscopy: desciption and utility of a new technique. *Am. J. Obstet. Gynecol.*, **162**, 82–6

Cullen, M. T., Anthenosiotis, A., Green, J. J., and Hobbins, J. C. (1990d) Prenatal diagnosis of anterior parietal encephalocele with transvaginal sonography. *Obstet. Gynecol.*, **75**, 489.

Cullen, M. T., Green, J., Scioscia, A., Mahoney, M., Hobbins, J. C., and Sanchez-Ramos, L. (1992). Ultrasound evaluation of the first trimester aneuploid fetus. *Obstet. Gynecol.* (In press).

Curtis, J., and Watson, L. (1988). Sonographic diagnosis of omphalocele in the first trimester of fetal gestation. *J. Ultrasound Med.*, **7**, 97–100.

D'Amelio, R., Giorlandino, C., Marsal, L., Garofalo, M., Martinelli, M., Anelli, G. *et al.* (1990). Fetal echocardiography using transvaginal and transabdominal probes during the first period of pregnancy: A comparative study. *Prenat. Diagn.*, **11**, 69–75.

Evans, J. (1991). Fetal crown-rump length values in the first trimester based upon ovulation timing using the luteinizing hormone surge. *Br. J. Obstet. Gynaecol.*, **98**, 48–51.

Exalto, N., Zalen, R. V., and Brandenburg, W. V. (1985). Early prenatal diagnosis of cystic hygroma by real-time ultrasound. *J. Ultrasound Med.*, **5**, 165–8.

Farine, D., Fox, H., Jakobson, S., and Timor-Tritsh, I. E. (1988). Vaginal ultrasound for the diagnosis of placenta previa, *Am. J. Obstet. Gynecol.*, **159**, 566–9.

Ferrazzi, E., Brambati, B., Lanzani, A., Oldrini, A., Stripparo, L., Guerneri, S., *et al.* (1988). The yolk sac in early pregnancy failure. *Am. J. Obstet. Gynecol.*, **158**, 137–42.

Fossum G., Davajan, V., and Kletzky, O. (1988). Early detection of pregnancy with transvaginal ultrasound. *Fert. Steril.*, **49**, 788–91.

Gembruch, U., Knopfle, G., Chatterjee, M., Bald, R., and Hansmann, M. (1990). First trimester fetal congenital heart disease by transvaginal two-dimentional and doppler echocardiography. *Obstet. Gynecol.*, **75**, 496–8.

Goldstein, I., Zimmer, E., Tamir, A., Peretz, A., and Paldi, E. (1991). Evaluation of normal gestational sac growth: Appearance of embryonic heartbeat and embryo body movements using the transvaginal technique. *Obstet. Gynecol.*, **77**, 885–8.

Gonzalez, C., Curson, R., and Parsons, A. (1988). Transvaginal versus transabdominal ultrasound scanning of ovarian follicles: are they comparable? *Fert. Steril.*, **50**, 657–9.

Gray, D., Martin, C., and Crane, J. (1989). Differential diagnosis of first trimester ventral wall defects. *J. Ultrasound Med.*, **8**, 255–8.

Green, J. and Hobbins, J. C. (1988). Abdominal ultrasound examination of the first trimester fetus. *Am. J. Obstet. Gynecol.*, **159**, 165–75.

Gustavii, B. and Edvall, H. (1984). First trimester diagnosis of cystic nuchal hygroma. *Acta Obstet. Gynecol. Scan.*, **63**, 377–8.

Hertzberg, B. S., Mohony, B. S. and Bowie, J. D. (1988). First trimester fetal cardiac acivity: Sonographic documentation of a progressive early rise in heart rate. *J. Ultrasound Med.*, **7**, 573.

Hill, L., Thomas, M., Kislak, S., and Runco, C. (1988). Sonographic assessment of the first trimester fetus: A cautionary note. *Am. J. Perinatol.*, **5**, 13–15.

Hilpert, P. L., and Kurtz, A. B. (1990). The role of transvaginal ultrasound in the second and third trimesters. *Seminars in Ultrasound CT MRI.*, **1**, 59–70.

Hook, E., Cross, P., Jackson, L., Pergament, E., and Brambati, B. (1988). Maternal age specific rates of 47, +21 and other cytogenetic abnormalities diagnosed in the first trimester of pregnancy in chorionic villus biopsy specimens: Comparison with rates expected from observations at amniocentesis. *Am. J. Human Genet.*, **15**, 797–807.

Jain, K., Hamper, U., and Sanders, R. (1988). Comparison of transvaginal and transabdominal sonography in the detection of early pregnancy and its complications. *Am. J. Roentgenology*, **151**, 1139–43.

Laboda, L. A., Estroff, J. A., and Benacerraf, B. R. (1989). First trimester bradycardia. A sign of impending fetal loss. *J. Ultrasound Med.*, **8**, 561–3.

Landy, H., Weiner, S., Corson, S., Batzer, F., and Bolgnese, R. (1986). The 'vanishing twin': Ultrasonographic assessment of fetal disappearance in the first trimester. *Am. J. Obstet. Gynecol.*, **155**, 14–16.

Levi, C., Lyons, E., Zheng, X., Lindsay, D., and Holt, S. (1990). Endovaginal US: Demonstration of cardiac activity in embryos less than 5.0 mm in crown rump length. *Radiology*, **176**, 71–4.

Lim, B. H., Tan, C. E., Smith, A. P. M., and Smith, N. C. (1989). Transvaginal ultrasonography for diagnosis of placenta previa. *Lancet*, **i**, 444.

Lynch, L. and Berkowitz, R. (1989). First trimester growth delay in trisomy 18. *Am. J. Perinatol.*, 6, 237–9.

Maggio, M., Callahan, N., Hamond, K., and Saunders, R. (1985). The first trimester ultrasonographic diagnosis of conjoined twins. *Am. J. Obstet. Gynecol.*, **152**, 833–5.

Meldrum, D., Chetkowski, R., Steingold, K., and Randle, D. (1984). Transvaginal ultrasound scanning of ovarian follicles. *Fert. Steril.* **42**, 803–5.

Nyberg, D., Filly, R., Filho, L., Laing, H., and Mahoney, B. (1986). Abnormal pregnancy: Early diagnosis by US and serum chorionic gonadotropin levels. *Radiology*, **158**, 398–401.

Nyberg, D., Mack, L., Jefferey, R., and Laing, F. (1987). Endovaginal sonographic evaluation of ectopic pregnancy: A prospective study. *Radiology*, **149**, 1181–6.

Popp, L. W. and Ghirardini, G. (1990) The role of transvaginal sonography in chorion villus sampling. *J. Clin. Ultrasound*, **18**, 315–22.

Reece E. A., Scioscia A., Green J. C., and Hobbins, J. C. (1989). Prognostic significance of the human yolk sac assessed by ultrasound. *Am. J. Obstet. Gynecol.*, **159**, 1191–4.

Rempen, A. (1988). Vaginal sonography in ectopic pregnancy. *J. Ultrasound Med.*, **7**, 381–7.

Reuss, A., Pijpers, L., Swaaij, E. V., Jahoda, M. and Wladimiroff, J. (1987). First trimester diagnosis of cystic hygroma using a vaginal ultrasound transducer. *Eur. J. Obstet. Gynecol. Reprod. Biol.*, **27**, 271–3.

Robinson, H. P. (1973). Sonar measurements of fetal crown-rump length as means of assessing maturity in the first trimester. *Br. J. Obstet. Gynaecol.*, **82**, 707–10.

Romero, R., Ghidini, A., Siritori, M., Cullen, M. T., Fisher, N., and Hobbins, J. (1989). First trimester diagnosis of a partial mole with the combined use of ultrasound and chorion villus sampling. *Am. J. Perinatol.*, **6**, 314–15.

Rottem, S., Bronshtein, M., Thaler, I., and Brandes, J. (1989). First trimester transvaginal sonographic diagnosis of fetal anomalies. *Lancet*, **i**, 445–6.

Rottem, S. and Bronshtein, M. (1990). Transvaginal sonographic diagnosis of congenital anomalies between 9 weeks and 16 weeks, menstrual age. *J. Clin. Ultrasound*, **18**, 307–14.

Schats, R., Jansen, C., and Wladimiroff, J. (1990). Embryonic heart activity: appearance and development in early human pregnancy. *Br. J. Obstet. Gynaecol.*, **97**, 989–94.

Schats, R., Os, H. V., Jansen, C., and Wladimiroff, J. (1991). The crown-rump length in early human pregnancy: a reappraisal. *Br. J. Obstet. Gynaecol.*, **98**, 460–2.

Shapiro, B., Cullen, M. T., Taylor, K., and DeCherney, A. (1988). Transvaginal ultrasonography for the diagnosis of ectopic pregnancy. *Fertil. Steril.*, **50**, 425–9.

Stiller, R., Romero, R., Pace, S., and Hobbins, J. (1989). Prenatal identification of twin reverse arterial perfusion syndrome in the first trimester. *Am. J. Obstet. Gynecol.*, **160**, 1194–6.

Timor-Tritsch, I. E., Warren, W. B., Peisner, D. B., and Pirrone, E. (1989). First-trimester midgut herniation: a high-frequency transvaginal sonographic study. *Am. J. Obstet. Gynecol.*, **161**, 831–3.

Timor-Tritsch, I. E., Monteagudo, A., and Warren, W. B. (1991). Transvaginal ultrasonographic definition of the central nervous system in the first and early second trimesters. *Am. J. Obstet. Gynecol.*, **164**, 497–503.

Vergani, P., Ghindini, A., Sirtori, M., and Roncaglia, N. (1987). Antenatal diagnosis of fetal acrania. *J. Ultrasound Med.*, **6**, 715–17.

Vermesh, M., Kletzky, O., Davajan, V., and Isreal, R. (1987). Monitoring techniques to predict and detect ovulation. *Fert. Steril.*, 47, 259–64.

Yee, B. R., Barnes, R. B., Vagyas, J., and Marrs, R. (1987). Correlation of transabdominal and transvaginal ultrasound measurements of follicle size and number with laproscopic findings for *in vitro* fertilization. *Fert. Steril.*, **47**, 828–32.

3

Ultrasonographically detectable markers of fetal chromosomal defects

K. H. Nicolaides, C. M. Gosden,
and R. J. M. Snijders

Introduction

Chromosomal abnormalities are major causes of perinatal death and childhood handicap. It is, therefore, not surprising that the risk for cytogenetic disorders constitutes the most frequent indication for invasive prenatal diagnosis. However, despite the widespread introduction of amniocentesis and more recently chorion villus sampling for fetal karyotyping, during the last 20 years there has been only a minor reduction in the birth incidence of chromosomally abnormal infants (Fig. 3.1). The main reason for this relative failure is that less

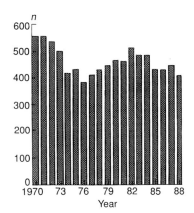 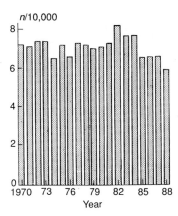

Fig. 3.1. Despite the widespread introduction of fetal karyotyping for advanced maternal age in England and Wales during the last 20 years there was no significant reduction in the number or incidence of live births with Down syndrome. (Data provided by the Office of Population Censuses and Surveys.)

than 3 per cent of chromosomally abnormal pregnancies have any preconceptu-
ally identifiable risk factor, such as parental translocation or the previous birth of
a chromosomally abnormal child. Furthermore, the well-recognized association
between advanced maternal age and fetal chromosomal defects, which constitutes the basis for current policies on screening, will at most identify 25–30 per
cent of the chromosomal defects. This policy is further complicated by the
relatively poor uptake of invasive fetal testing among the at-risk group, which
has been less than 50 per cent. Although there are many reasons for this poor
uptake, the fact that the procedure related risk for fetal loss from amniocentesis
or chorion villus sampling is at least 1 per cent, which is often substantially
greater than that of having an affected child, must not be underestimated.

The combination of maternal age and abnormal maternal serum biochemistry
could potentially identify more than 50 per cent of pregnancies with fetal
trisomy 21 (Wald *et al.* 1988). However, this test is currently available in very
few centres. Furthermore, it is unrealistic to expect that the vast majority of
parents would necessarily wish to undergo invasive fetal testing because their
risk of having a baby with trisomy 21 is < 0.3 per cent.

Most fetuses with major cytogenetic abnormalities have either external or
internal defects (Jones 1988), which can be recognized by detailed ultrasonographic examination. Since it is now well accepted that such a detailed
ultrasound examination should be offered routinely to all pregnant women
(RCOG 1990), it is very likely that ultrasonography will constitute the most
effective method of screening for chromosomal abnormalities.

This chapter reviews the association between fetal malformations and
chromosomal defects, and reports the findings of cytogenetic results in 2086
fetuses with a wide range of malformations that were detected at ultrasound
examination and were referred to our centre for further investigations during the
last eight years (Tables 3.1–5).

Brain abnormalities

Ventriculomegaly

Congenital hydrocephalus, with an incidence of 5–25 per 10 000 births, may
result from chromosomal and genetic abnormalities, intrauterine haemorrhage,
or congenital infection, although many cases have not as yet a clear-cut
aetiology. Prenatal diagnosis by ultrasonography is based on the demonstration
of dilated lateral cerebral ventricles.

Several reports on fetal hydrocephalus have established an association with
chromosomal defects (Table 3.6; Cochrane *et al.* 1984; Chervenak *et al.* 1985*a*;
Pretorius *et al.* 1985; Pilu *et al.* 1986; Serlo *et al.* 1986; Nyberg *et al.* 1987*a*;
Vintzileos *et al.* 1987; Hudgins *et al.* 1988; Drugan *et al.* 1989; Nicolaides *et al.*

Table 3.1 Ultrasonographically detectable brain and spinal abnormalities and incidence of chromosomal defects

Anomalies	Fetal anomalies Isolated (%)	Multiple (%)	Chromosomal defect				Triploidy	Sex chrom 45, X	XXX/Y	Deletions or translocations
			Trisomies 21	18	13	other				
Ventriculomegaly	1/35 (3)	39/151 (26)	7	12	3	1	12	3	—	2
Holoprosencephaly	—/7	15/51 (29)	—	3	11	—	—	—	—	1
Microcephaly	—/1	6/39 (15)	—	1	3	1	—	—	—	1
Choroid plexus cyst	1/48 (2)	33/73 (46)	2	30	1	—	—	—	—	1
Posterior fossa cyst	—/1	20/45 (44)	—	8	5	2	3	—	—	2
Porencephalic cyst	1/1 (100)	—/1	—	—	—	—	—	—	—	1
Absent corpus callosum	—/1	1/2 (50)	—	1	—	—	—	—	—	—
Iniencephaly	—/—	—/2	—	—	—	—	—	—	—	—
Anencephaly	—/3	—/5	—	—	—	—	—	—	—	—
Encephalocele	—/—	1/8 (13)	—	—	—	—	—	—	—	1
Spina bifida	—/1	6/20 (30)	—	3	—	—	3	—	—	—
Kyphoscoliosis	—	1/18 (6)	—	—	—	—	1	—	—	—
Sacrococcogeal teratoma	—/1	—/2	—	—	—	—	—	—	—	—

Table 3.2 Ultrasonographically detectable skull, facial, and nuchal abnormalities and incidence of chromosomal defects

Anomalies	Fetal anomalies Isolated (%)	Multiple (%)	Chromosomal defect Trisomies 21	18	13	other	Triploidy	Sex chrom 45,X	XXX/Y	Deletions or translocations
Brachycephaly	—	43/114 (38)	7	19	5	1	3	8	—	—
Strawberry shaped head	—	44/54 (81)	—	43	—	—	1	—	—	—
Clover leaf shaped head	—/1	2/4 (50)	1	—	—	—	—	—	—	1
Micrognathia	—	37/57 (65)	—	21	3	1	9	—	—	3
Facial cleft	—/8	31/56 (55)	1	10	15	2	1	—	—	2
Ocular defects	—	5/12 (42)	—	1	4	—	—	—	—	—
Nasal defects	—	6/20 (30)	—	—	5	—	—	—	—	1
Tumour	—/1	—/2	—	—	—	—	—	—	—	—
Macroglossia	—	10/13 (77)	9	—	—	1	—	—	—	—
Nuchal oedema	—/13	52/132 (39)	31	5	6	1	2	3	—	4
Cystic hygromata	—/3	35/49 (71)	1	1	—	—	—	33	—	—
Hydrops	7/105 (7)	19/109 (17)	14	1	2	—	2	2	2	3

Table 3.3 Ultrasonographically detectable fetal abnormalities of chest and abdomen and incidence of chromosomal defects

Anomalies	Fetal anomalies Isolated (%)	Multiple (%)	Chromosomal defect							
			Trisomies 21	18	13	other	Triploidy	Sex 45, X	chrom XXX/Y	Deletions or translocations
Diaphragmatic hernia	—/37	16/42 (38)	—	10	2	—	1	—	—	3
Cystic adenomatoid malf	—/8	1/12 (8)	—	1	—	—	—	—	—	—
Heart defect	—/3	100/153 (65)	21	37	13	2	4	16	1	6
Exomphalos	1/29 (3)	41/87 (47)	—	32	6	—	1	—	1	2
Gastroschisis	—/16	—/10 —	—	—	—	—	—	—	—	—
Duodenal atresia	1/6 (17)	9/17 (53)	10	—	—	—	—	—	—	—
Oesophageal atresia	—/1	18/23 (78)	1	17	—	—	—	—	—	—
Bowel obstruction	—/8	1/16 (6)	—	—	—	—	—	—	—	1
Abdominal cyst	—/18	1/9 (11)	1	—	—	—	—	—	—	—
Renal defects	9/473 (2)	86/368 (23)	23	25	19	5	5	8	2	8

Table 3.4 Ultrasonographically detectable fetal abnormalities of digits and extremities and incidence of chromosomal defects

Anomalies	Fetal anomalies Isolated (%)	Multiple (%)	Chromosomal defect Trisomies 21	18	13	other	Triploidy	Sex chrom 45, X	XXX/Y	Deletions or translocations
Syndactyly	—	31/39 (79)	1	—	—	—	30	—	—	—
Clinodactyly	—/1	16/30 (53)	15	1	—	—	—	—	—	—
Polydactyly	—	11/14 (79)	—	2	8	—	1	—	—	—
Oligodactyly	—	—/3 —	—	—	—	—	—	—	—	
Overlapping fingers	—	64/84 (76)	—	56	5	—	—	—	—	3
Flexed wrist	—/2	—/12 —	—	—	—	—	—	—	—	
Rocker bottom feet	—	18/26 (69)	—	14	3	—	—	—	—	1
Sandal gap	—/1	10/21 (48)	6	—	—	—	1	1	—	2
Talipes	—/12	38/94 (40)	3	25	5	—	3	—	—	2
Short femur	—/3	116/408 (28)	25	20	5	4	29	28	—	5
Phocomelia	—/1	—/4 —	—	—	—	—	—	—	—	
Radial aplasia	—/1	—/6 —	—	—	—	—	—	—	—	
Tibial aplasia	—	—/1 —	—	—	—	—	—	—	—	

Table 3.5 Chromosomal defects in 300 of the 2086 fetuses that underwent antenatal karyotyping because of malformations and/or severe growth retardation detected by ultrasound

Chromosomal abnormality	n	Chromosomal abnormality	n	Chromosomal abnormality	n
47,XY,+ 4q	1	45,X	38	46,XY,2q–	3
47,XX,+ 8	1	47,XXY	3	46,XY,3p–	1
47,XY,+ 9	2	47,XXY	2	46,XX,4p–, + der	1
47,XX,+ 11p	1	69,XXX	28	46,XY,4p–	4
47,XY,+ 12p	1	69,XXY	12	46,XX,5q–	1
47,XX,+ 13	15	92,XXYY	2	46,XY,5p–	1
47,XY,+ 13	15	46,XX,7q–	1	46,XY,6p–	1
47,XX,+ 18	29	46,XX,t (1; 1)	1	46,XX,7q–	1
47,XY,+ 18	53	46,XY,t (4;15)	1	46,XY,8p–	1
48,XXX,+ 18	1	46,XY,t (11;12)	1	46,XY,8q–	1
47,XX,+ 21	35	46,XY,t (13;14)	1	46,XY,9p–	1
47,XY,+ 21	32	46,XX,t (17;19)	1	46,XX,13q–	1
48,XYY,+ 21	1			46,XY,14q–	1
47,XX,+ 21q	1			46,XY,21q–	1
47,XX+ 22	1				
47,XX, ring(22)	1				
47,XY, + marker	1				

1990). However, in many of these studies there were no strict criteria for the diagnosis of ventriculomegaly and they included other brain abnormalities, such as holoprosencephaly or porencephalic cysts. Furthermore, data on the number of fetuses karyotyped, the presence of other defects, and the selection criteria used for undertaking the investigation were not clearly defined; the incidence of chromosomal defects varied from 2 per cent to 29 per cent.

In our study of 186 fetuses with ventriculomegaly (Table 3.1; Nicolaides *et al.* 1992*a*), the diagnosis was made if the ratios of the width of the anterior and/or posterior horn of the lateral cerebral ventricle to that of the cerebral hemisphere were above the 95th centile of the reference ranges for gestation (Van den Hof *et al.* 1990). Fetuses with ventriculomegaly secondary to spina bifida and without other defects were not karyotyped, because Gosden and Brock found no chromosomal abnormalities in 226 consecutive fetuses with isolated neural tube defects that were karyotyped at 16–18 weeks' gestation (personal communication).

Abnormal karyotypes were found in 1 of 35 (3 per cent) fetuses with isolated ventriculomegaly and in 39 of 151 (26 per cent) of those with additional malformations (Table 3.1). The commonest abnormal karyotypes were triploidy,

Table 3.6　Summary of reports on antenatally diagnosed hydrocephalus providing data on the presence of other defects (Holop, holoprosencephaly; NTD, neural tube defects). Under abnormal karyotype, data is provided, where possible, only for cases without holoprosencephaly.

Author		n	Other defects			Abnormal karyotype (%)	Alive (%)
			Total (%)	Holop (%)	NTD (%)		
Chervenak *et al.*	1985*b*	53	44 (83)		15 (28)	4/ ?	28
Cochrane *et al.*	1984	41	32 (78)	3 (7)	15 (37)	1/?	34
Pretorius *et al.*	1985	40	28 (70)	1 (3)	13 (33)	2/7　(29)	15
Pilu *et al.*	1986	30	9 (30)			3/30　(10)	?
Serlo *et al.*	1986	38	32 (84)	1 (3)		4/?	26
Nyberg *et al.*	1987*b*	61	51 (84)	13 (21)	23 (38)	2/21　(10)	16
Vintzileos *et al.*	1987	20	16 (80)	1 (5)	6 (30)	2/19　(11)	45
Hudgins and Edwards	1988	47	35 (74)	15 (32)		1/47　(2)	40
Drugan *et al.*	1989	43	31 (72)	3 (7)	18 (42)	5/19　(26)	44
Nicolaides *et al.*	1990	267	209 (78)		184 (68)	12/64 (19)	9

*　Trisomy 13, n=2; Trisomy 18, n=7; Ring 18, n=1; Trisomy 21, n=4; 46XY/48XY +7+8, n=1; Duplication 4p, n=1; Deletion 7q, n=1; Triploidy, n=1; Turner, n=1.

**　Trisomy 13, n=1; Trisomy 18, n=1; Trisomy 21, n=1; 48XYY+21, n=1; Duplication 9p, n=1; Deletion 6p, n=1; Triploidy, n=6.

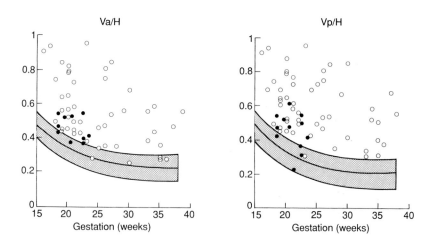

Fig. 3.2. Anterior (*Va/H*) and posterior (*Vp/H*) lateral cerebral ventricle to hemisphere ratio in 186 fetuses with ventriculomegaly that were karyotyped antenatally, plotted on the appropriate reference range (mean, 5th, and 95th centiles) for gestation. The chromosomally abnormal fetuses (o) tended to have mild ventriculomegaly.

trisomy 18, and trisomy 21. In the chromosomally abnormal fetuses, there was a tendency for the degree of ventriculomegaly to be mild (Fig. 3.2).

Holoprocencephaly

Holoprosencephaly, with an incidence of 0.6–1.9 per 10 000 births, encompasses a heterogeneous group of cerebral malformations resulting from either failure or incomplete cleavage of the forebrain. Although in many cases the cause is a chromosomal abnormality or a genetic disorder with an autosomal dominant or recessive mode of transmission in many cases the aetiology is unknown.

Prenatal diagnosis by ultrasonography is based on the demonstration of a single dilated midline ventricle replacing the two lateral ventricles. Although some authors have suggested that confident diagnosis requires the additional demonstration of facial abnormalities, such as hypotelorism, these abnormalities are not always present.

Fetal holoprosencephaly is associated with a high incidence of other morphological and chromosomal defects (Table 3.7; Filly *et al.* 1984; Chervenak *et al.* 1985*b*; Nyberg *et al.* 1987*b*; Berry *et al.* 1990). Furthermore, the incidence of chromosomal abnormalities is strongly related to the presence of multisystem malformations (Table 3.8). Thus, in our series of 58 cases none of the seven fetuses with isolated holoprosencephaly, as opposed to 15 of the 51 (29 per cent)

Table 3.7   Summary of major series on antenatally diagnosed holoprosencephaly providing data on the presence of associated malformations and chromosomal defects

Author	1	2	3	4
Number of cases	5	7	14	38
Facial cleft	0	0	3	14
Extrafacial defects	0	1	4	21
Abnormal karyotype*	1/?	4/7	6/11	11/38
Outcome: TOP	1	0	5	29
IUD	3	3	2	3
PND	1	4	5	4
ALIVE	0	0	2	2

1. Filly *et al.* 1984
2. Chervenak *et al.* 1985*b*
3. Nyberg *et al.* 1987*b*
4. Nicolaides *et al.* 1990

*   Trisomy 13, *n*=7; Triploidy, *n*=1; Deletion 13q, *n*=2; Duplication 5p, *n*=1.
**   Trisomy 13, *n*=8; Trisomy 18, *n*=1; 46XX − 18+i(18q), *n*=1, Deletion 21q, *n*=1.

Table 3.8 Gestation at diagnosis (GA), ultrasound findings, karyotype and outcome (O/C; TOP = termination of pregnancy, NND = neonatal death) of fetuses with holoprosencephaly. Facial defects included facial cleft (FC), absent nose (A), single nostril (1N) or proboscis (P) and hypotelorism (H) or cyclops (cycl). Extrafacial abnormalities included mild (H1) and severe hydronephrosis (H3), renal agenesis (RA), congenital diaphragmatic hernia (CDH), congenital heart disease (CHD), exomphalos containing bowel (Exom-B), and umbilical cord with 2 vessels (2V). The additional defects detected at post-mortem examination are given in brackets.

Case No	GA	Facial abnormalities			Extrafacial abnormalities				Karyotype	Outcome
		FC	Nose	Eyes	Skeletal	Renal	CHD	Other		
1	31								46XX	IUD
2	32								46XX	TOP
3	32								46XX	ALIVE
4	36								46XX	IUD
5	36								46XX	TOP
6	18								46XY	TOP
7	20								46XY	TOP
8	20								46XY	TOP
9	22								46XY	TOP
10	26								46XY	TOP
11	26								46XY	TOP
12	27								46XY	ALIVE
13	17	Y	A(1N)	H					46XY	TOP
14	18	Y	A						46XX	TOP
15	19		P	H					46XX	TOP
16	32	Y	A						46XX	NND
17	32	Y	A						46XX	NND

18	22			H	Talipes	H1–H1		Scalp oedema	46XX	TOP
19	23				Rocker-bottom feet		(CHD)	CDH	46XX	TOP
20	35	Y			Talipes	H1–H1 (RA)	CHD	46XX	NND	
21	19			H		H1–H1			46XY	TOP
22	22	Y				H1–H1		46XY		TOP
23	23					H1–H1		46XY		TOP
24	23	Y	A		Sandal gap	H1–H1		46XY		TOP
25	24		A		Talipes				46XY	TOP
26	24		1N						46XY	TOP
27	27			H	(Polydactyly)				46XY	NND
28	16	Y	A	Cycl	Polydactyly	H3		Exom-B	47XX + 13	TOP
29	19	Y	A	H	Polydactyly	H3	CHD		47XX + 13	TOP
30	20	Y			Polydactyly				47XX + 13	TOP
31	21		A(1N)		Polydactyly				47XX + 13	TOP
32	21					RA–RA	CHD	47XX + 13	TOP	
33	21	Y	A		Polydactyly		CHD	47XY + 13	47XX + 13	TOP
34	18	Y			Talipes	H1–H1		Exom-B	47XX + 13	TOP
35	20	Y			Overlap fingers		CHD	Exom-B	47XY + 13	TOP
36	27	Y			Rocker-bottom feet	RA	CHD	CDH Cord 2V	47XY + 18	TOP
37	19								46XX − 18 + i(18q)	TOP
38	20	Y					CHD	(Cord 2V)	46XY,21q −	TOP

with additional malformations, had chromosomal defects (Table 3.1; Nicolaides *et al.* 1992*a*). This is not surprising, because the most commonly found chromosomal defects are trisomy 13 and trisomy 18, which are usually associated with multisystem malformations that are easily recognizable by diligent ultrasonographic examination.

Microcephaly

Microcephaly has a birth incidence of 1–2 per 20 000. Prenatal diagnosis is based on the identification of a disproportionally reduced head circumference ratio and the associated abnormal intracranial pathology. However, the intracranial anatomy may be normal, in which case the condition is defined by a biparietal diameter of > 3 SD below the mean. In milder cases, diagnosis requires the demonstration of a progressive decrease in the head circumference until it falls below the 5th percentile, in the presence of a normal growth in the abdominal circumference. This difference may not become apparent before 26 weeks' gestation.

In our series of 2086 fetuses that were karyotyped because of fetal malformations or growth retardation, the diagnosis was made if the ratio of head circumference to femur length was below the 2.5th centile. Microcephaly was diagnosed in 40 cases and six (15 per cent) were chromosomally abnormal (Table 3.1; Nicolaides *et al.* 1992*b*).

Choroid plexus cysts

Choroid plexus cysts are found in 2–20 per 1000 fetuses at 16–18 weeks' gestation, but in more than 90 per cent of cases they resolve by 25 weeks and are of no pathological significance (Chudleigh *et al.* 1984). However, if the cysts are associated with other malformations, they may indicate the presence of an underlying chromosomal abnormality (Nicolaides *et al.* 1986*a*; Bundy *et al.* 1986; Chitkara *et al.* 1988; Khouzam and Hooker 1989; Gabrielli *et al.* 1989; Thorpe-Beeston *et al.* 1990).

In our series of 73 fetuses with choroid plexus cysts and additional malformations, 33 (46 per cent) had chromosomal defects. In contrast only 1 of the 48 cases with isolated choroid plexus cysts had an abnormal karyotype (Table 3.1; Nicolaides *et al.* 1992*a*). The commonest chromosomal defect was trisomy 18. There are three additional reported cases in which choroid plexus cysts were the only antenatal finding where the fetuses had either trisomy 18 or trisomy 21 (Ricketts *et al.* 1987; Furness 1987; Ostlere *et al.* 1989).

At present there is considerable controversy as to whether fetal karyotyping should be undertaken for choroid plexus cysts found in the absence of other malformations. The possibility of isolated choroid plexus cysts being the sole abnormality in fetuses with trisomy 18 is strongly suggested by the findings of a very careful pathological study by Fitzsimons *et al.* (1989). Twelve of 14 fetuses with trisomy 18 studied at post-mortem had other structural anomalies, but bilateral choroid plexus cysts were the only abnormality in two of their fetuses. These authors suggested that the risk of finding isolated choroid plexus cysts in a fetus with trisomy 18 was higher than the risk of a 35-year-old woman having a child with trisomy 21 and, therefore, parents should be offered the option of fetal karyotyping.

Posterior fossa abnormalities

Cerebellar malformations are rare, but they may be associated with trisomy 13 and 18, hydrocephalus, spina bifida, encephalocele, or microcephaly. Cystic dilation in the area of the cisterna magna, with partial or complete agenesis of the vermis, is found in the Dandy–Walker malformation (cystic dilatation of the fourth ventricle). The aetiology of many cases of the Dandy–Walker malformation is unknown, although in some cases it may occur as a part of mendelian disorders such as Meckel syndrome. Nyberg *et al.* (1988), reported chromosomal abnormalities (trisomies 18 and 13) in two of four fetuses with cerebellar hypoplasia or the Dandy–Walker malformation.

In our series of 46 fetuses with posterior fossa cysts, 45 had additional defects, and 20 (43 per cent) had chromosomal abnormalities including trisomy 18, trisomy 13, triploidy, and partial trisomy or deletions (Table 3.1; Nicolaides *et al.* 1992*a*).

Absent corpus callosum

A small number of case reports have established an association of agenesis of the corpus callosum and trisomies 8, 13, 18, and triploidy (Comstock *et al.* 1985; Amato *et al.* 1986; Bertino *et al.* 1987). In the largest prenatal series, Bertino *et al.* (1987) found trisomy 8 in one of five fetuses.

Abnormalities of the shape of the skull

Strawberry skull

In some fetuses with trisomy 18 there is a characteristic shape of the head that is best seen in the suboccipitobregmatic view. There is flattening of the occiput and narrowing of the frontal part of the head. The most likely explanation for the narrow frontal region is hypoplasia of the face and the frontal cerebral lobes. Similarly, flattening of the occiput may be due to hypoplasia of the hindbrain. In our series of 54 fetuses with strawberry shaped head, they all had additional malformations and 44 (81 per cent) had chromosomal abnormalities (Table 3.2; Nicolaides *et al.* 1992*c*).

Brachycephaly

Brachycephaly is characterized by a relative shortening of the occipitofrontal diameter. It is found in association with chromosomal abnormalities and genetic syndromes, such as Roberts syndrome. Although in postnatal life it is well recognized that children with Down syndrome have brachycephaly, Perry *et al.* (1984) found no difference in the mean cephalic index between eight second trimester fetuses with trisomy 21 and 308 normal fetuses. Similarly, Shah *et al.* (1990*a*) found no significant difference in the biparietal diameter, occipitofrontal diameter, or cephalic index between 17 fetuses with Down syndrome at 15–23 weeks' gestation and 17 matched controls.

In our series of 114 fetuses with brachycephaly (biparietal to occipitofrontal diameter ratio above the 97.5th centile), 43 had chromosomal abnormalities, including trisomies 13, 18, and 21, triploidy and Turner syndrome (Table 3.2; Nicolaides *et al.* 1992*b*). However, it should be noted that in our total series of 69 fetuses with trisomy 21 and 231 with other chromosomal abnormalities, 90 per cent and 84 per cent, respectively, had a biparietal to occipitofrontal diameter ratio below the 97.5th centile (Fig. 3.3).

Facial defects

Facial cleft

Facial clefting, cleft lip and/or palate, is one of the commonest congenital abnormalities found in approximately 1:700 live births. Both genetic and

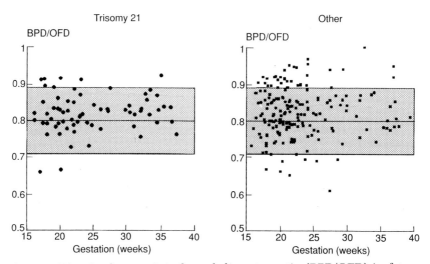

Fig. 3.3. Biparietal to occipitofrontal diameter ratio (BPD/OFD) in fetuses with trisomy 21 and other chromosomal abnormalities plotted on the reference range (mean, 5th, 95th centiles) for gestation.

environmental factors are implicated in the causation of the defect. Postnatally, chromosomal abnormalities are found in less than 1 per cent of babies with facial clefts (Pashayan 1983).

In a series of 10 fetuses with facial clefts, Saltzman *et al.* (1986) found chromosomal abnormalities in four, and they all had other detectable malformations. In our series 64 fetuses with facial cleft, 31 (48 per cent) had chromosomal abnormalities, mainly trisomy 13, or trisomy 18. However, in all 31 fetuses there were additional malformations (Table 3.2; Nicolaides *et al.* 1992*d*).

Ocular abnormalities

A variety of eye abnormalities, such as hypotelorism and cyclopia, are often seen in the presence of holoprosencephaly, and they are associated with trisomy 13 and 18 (Table 3.2; Nicolaides *et al.* 1992*d*). Although all chromosomally abnormal fetuses with holoprosencephaly have extra-craniofacial defects, the risk for chromosomal abnormalities in fetuses with holoprosencephaly is higher when facial as well as extrafacial defects are present.

Nasal defects

Nasal aplasia or hypoplasia, single nostril, or proboscis, are occasionally seen in holoprosencephaly and they are associated with trisomy 13 (Table 3.2; Nicolaides *et al.* 1992*d*).

Macroglossia

Postnatally, macroglossia is a common feature of trisomy 21. Antenatally, an enlarged tongue protruding through the open mouth can be demonstrated in the mid-sagital view of the face. In our series of 13 fetuses with macroglossia, nine had trisomy 21 and in one case of fetal karyotype was mosaic 46, XX/46, XX dup(11p) associated with Beckwith–Wiedemann syndrome (Table 3.2; Nicolaides *et al.* 1992*d*).

Micrognathia

In our series of 57 cases with sufficiently severe micrognathia to be diagnosed antenatally by ultrasonography, all had additional malformations and/or growth retardation and the condition was associated with very poor perinatal outcome. Chromosomal abnormalities, mainly trisomy 18 or triploidy, were found in 37 (65 per cent) of the cases (Table 3.2; Nicolaides *et al.* 1992*d*). Although pathological studies have demonstrated micrognathia to be present in > 80 per cent of fetuses with trisomy 18 or triploidy (Benacerraf *et al.* 1986), in our series of 83 fetuses with trisomy 18 and 42 with triploidy, micrognathia was detected by ultrasonography in only 21 (25 per cent) and 9 (21 per cent) of the cases, respectively. These findings suggest that, at present, only the most severe degrees of this defect are amenable to prenatal diagnosis.

Nuchal fluid

Nuchal cystic hygromata

Nuchal cystic hygromata are developmental abnormalities of the lymphatic system. Although they are rarely seen postnatally they are found in 0.5 per cent of spontaneously aborted fetuses (Byrne *et al.* 1984). Prenatal diagnosis by ultrasonography is based on the demonstration of a bilateral, septated, cystic structure, located in the occipitocervical region. This condition should be distinguished from nuchal oedema, which has a high association with trisomies, or unilateral cervical cysts, which are usually detected in the third trimester and have a good prognosis after postnatal surgery.

Reports on antenatally diagnosed cystic hygromata have established an association with hydrops fetalis, found in 40–100 per cent of the cases, congenital heart defects, in 0–92 per cent of the cases and chromosomal defects in 46–90 per cent of the fetuses; the commonest being Turner syndrome (Table 3.9; Chervenak *et al.* 1983; Newman and Cooperberg 1984; Redford *et al.* 1984; Marchese *et al.* 1985; Nicolaides *et al.* 1985; Pearce *et al.* 1985; Carr *et al.* 1986; Garden *et al.* 1986; Palmer *et al.* 1987; Gembruch *et al.* 1988; Hegge *et al.* 1988; Pijpers 1988; Abramowicz *et al.* 1989; Cohen *et al.* 1990; Eydoux *et al.* 1989; Miyabara *et al.* 1989; Holzgreve *et al.* 1990; Langer *et al.* 1990; Rizzo *et al.* 1990; Tannirandorn *et al.* 1990; Azar *et al.* 1991). Recently, Azar *et al.* (1991) suggested that the wide range in the reported incidence of hydrops fetalis, cardiac defects, and both the presence and types of chromosomal abnormalities may be a consequence of differences in the diagnostic criteria for cystic hygromata used in the various reports. Azar *et al.* (1991) examined only fetuses with septated, cervical, dorsal hygromata and 75 per cent had chromosomal defects; the commonest being Turner syndrome (94 per cent). Furthermore, there was a strong association between this chromosomal abnormality and decreased FL to BPD ratio (90 per cent), congenital heart defects (48 per cent), and renal abnormalities (19 per cent).

Nuchal oedema

Benacerraf *et al.* (1985, 1987) noted the association between increased soft tissue thickening on the posterior aspect of the neck and trisomy 21. In a series of 1704 consecutive amniocenteses at 15–20 weeks' gestation in which there were 11 fetuses with trisomy 21, 45 per cent of the trisomic and 0.06 per cent of the normal fetuses had nuchal thickness > 5 mm. Similarly, Lynch *et al.* (1989)

Table 3.9 Summary of reported series on antenatally diagnosed cystic hygromata providing data on the presence of associated chromosomal defects

Author	Gestation	n	Abnormal karyotype				
			Total (%)	Turner (%)	Trisomy 21 (%)	Trisomy 18 (%)	Other (%)
Chervenak et al. 1983	18–29	15	11 (73)	11 (100)			
Newman and Cooperberg 1984	16–26	3	2 (67)	1 (50)	1 (50)		
Redford et al. 1984	17–26	5	4 (80)	2 (50)	1 (25)	1 (25)	
Marchese et al. 1985	16–20	6	5 (83)	4 (80)		1 (20)	
Nicolaides et al. 1985	16–22	8	6 (75)	5 (83)	1 (17)		
Pearce et al. 1985	16–26	22	17 (77)	14 (82)	2 (12)	1 (6)	
Carr et al. 1986	17–28	5	3 (60)	2 (67)	1 (33)		
Garden et al. 1986	14–26	16	13 (81)	11 (85)		1 (8)	47XXY
Palmer et al. 1987	16–26	8	6 (75)	4 (67)	1 (17)		47XX+5p
Gembruch et al. 1988	13–26	29	17 (59)	10 (59)	6 (35)	1 (6)	
Hegge et al. 1988	15–17	4	3 (75)	2 (67)	1 (33)		
Pijpers et al. 1988	12–25	15	9 (60)	8 (89)		1 (11)	
Abramowicz et al. 1989	12–31	17	10 (59)	6 (60)	3 (30)	1 (10)	
Cohen et al. 1989	10–30	15	10 (67)	5 (50)	4 (40)	1 (10)	
Eydoux et al. 1989	12–32	41	19 (46)	14 (74)	4 (21)	1 (5)	
Miyabara et al. 1989	12–23	10	9 (90)	4 (44)		3 (33)	47XX+13; 46XX, del14p
Holzgreve et al. 1990		15	10 (67)	7 (70)	2 (20)	1 (10)	
Langer et al. 1990	12–29	17	8 (47)	7 (88)	1 (12)		
Rizzo et al. 1990	15–27	13	10 (77)	8 (80)	1 (10)	1 (10)	
Tannirandorn et al. 1990	16–23	11	7 (64)	5 (71)		1 (14)	47XX+13
Nicolaides et al. 1992e	16–26	44	33 (75)	31 (94)	1 (3)	1 (3)	
Total	12–32	319	212 (66)	161 (76)	30 (14)	16 (8)	5 (2)

who retrospectively examined the sonograms of nine pairs of discordant twins, found nuchal thickening > 5 mm in five of the nine fetuses with trisomy 21 but in none of the normal co-twins. However, Perella *et al.* (1988), retrospectively examined the sonograms of 14 fetuses with trisomy 21 and 128 normal controls and found nuchal thickening in only 21 per cent of the trisomic fetuses and in 9 per cent of the normals.

In our series of 145 fetuses with nuchal oedema ≥ 7 mm (which produces a characteristic tremor on ballotment of the fetal head), 52 (36 per cent) had chromosomal abnormalities, mainly trisomy 21, but also other trisomies, deletions or translocations, triploidy and Turner syndrome (Table 3.2; Nicolaides *et al.* 1992*e*). Furthermore, the chromosomally normal fetuses had a very poor prognosis since in many cases there was an underlying skeletal dysplasia, genetic syndrome, or cardiac defect.

Hydrops fetalis

Hydrops fetalis, with an incidence of 3–10 per 10 000 births, is characterized by generalized skin oedema and pericardial, pleural, or ascitic effusions. This is non-specific finding in a wide variety of fetal and maternal disorders, including haematological, chromosomal, cardiovascular, renal, pulmonary, gastro-intestinal, hepatic and metabolic abnormalities, congenital infection, neoplasms, and malformations of the placenta or umbilical cord (Potter 1943; Hutchison *et al.* 1982; Turkel 1982; Keeling *et al.* 1983; Nicolaides *et al.* 1985). With the widespread introduction of immunoprophylaxis and the decline in rhesus isoimmunization, non-rhesus causes have become responsible for at least 75 per cent of the cases (Giacoia 1980; Machin 1981) and make a greater contribution to perinatal mortality (Andersen *et al.* 1983). While in many instances the underlying cause may be determined by detailed ultrasound scanning, frequently the abnormality remains unexplained even after expert post-mortem examination (Keeling *et al.*1983).

In our series of 214 fetuses with non-rhesus hydrops (excluding those with cystic hygromata, mentioned above), 26 (12 per cent) had chromosomal abnormalities, mainly trisomy 21 (Table 3.2; Nicolaides *et al.* 1992*a*).

First trimester nuchal translucency

Recent publications have suggested the possible association between abnormal nuchal fluid and chromosomal abnormalities in the first trimester of pregnancy (Table 3.10; Gustavii and Edvall 1984; Dallapiccola *et al.* 1984; Reuss *et al.* 1987*a, b*; Pons *et al.* 1989; Bronshtein *et al.* 1989; Cullen *et al.* 1990; Nicolaides *et al.* 1992*f*). Although in some studies the condition was defined as multiseptated, thin-walled cystic mass similar to that seen in the second trimester, in others the term was used loosely to include nuchal thickening or

Table 3.10   Summary of reported series on first trimester fetal nuchal oedema or cystic hygromata providing data on the presence of associated chromosomal defects

Author	Gestation	n	Karyotype						
			Normal	45, X	Tr13	Tr18	Tr21	Tr22	Others
Gustavii and Edvall 1984	12	1	1						
Dallapiccola et al. 1984	12	1	1						
Reuss et al. 1987a	12	1		1					
Reuss et al. 1987b	10	1	1						
Pons et al. 1989	11–14	4	1			3			
Bronshtein et al. 1989	11–12	2		1			1		
Cullen et al. 1990	11–13	29	15	4		2	6		3*
Nicolaides et al. 1992f	10–14	51	33	0	2	4	10	1	1**
Total	10–14	90	52	6	2	9	17	1	4

*   47XY+ 15/46XX, 49XXXXY, 47XX,– 21, + der (21), t (18q; 21p)
** 47XY+ fragment

oedema. Bronshtein *et al.* (1989), in a study of eight fetuses with 'cystic hygromata' diagnosed at 9–15 weeks' gestation, classified the lesions into septated and non-septated types and suggested that the former are associated with chromosomal defects or fetal death, whereas fetuses with non-septated hygromata are chromosomally normal and often have a good outcome. In contrast, Cullen *et al.* (1990) examined 29 fetuses with 'cystic hygromata' at 10–13 weeks, and reported that neither the incidence of chromosomal defects nor the prognosis could be predicted by the ultrasonographic appearance of the lesion (septated and non-septated, posterior or lateral cervical, with or without hydrops).

In a prospective study of 827 women with singleton pregnancies undergoing first trimester fetal karyotyping because of advanced maternal age, parental anxiety, or a family history of a chromosomal abnormality in the absence of balanced parental translocation, transabdominal ultrasound examination was performed in order to obtain a sagittal section of the fetus for measurement of the maximum thickness of the subcutaneous translucency between the skin and the soft tissue overlying the cervical spine (Nicolaides *et al.* 1992f). Care was taken to distinguish between fetal skin and amnion because at this gestation both structures appear as thin membranes.

The incidence of chromosomal defects was 3 per cent (28 of 827 cases). In the 51 (6 per cent) fetuses with nuchal translucency 3–8 mm in thickness, the incidence of chromosomal defects was 35 per cent (18 cases). In contrast, only 10 of the remaining 776 (1 per cent) fetuses were chromosomally abnormal. This screening study therefore established that:

1. The incidence of fetal nuchal translucency ≥ 3 mm, detected by trans-abdominal ultrasonography, at 10–14 weeks gestation is 6 per cent.
2. The presence of fetal nuchal translucency is associated with a more than ten-fold increase and absence of translucency with a three-fold decrease in risk for chromosomal abnormality.
3. The risk of chromosomal abnormalities increases with increasing thickness of the nuchal translucency.
4. The pattern of associated chromosomal defects, trisomies rather than Turner syndrome, is similar to that observed in second trimester fetuses with nuchal oedema rather than with cystic hygromata.

Congenital diaphragmatic hernia

Congenital diaphragmatic hernia (CDH), with a birth incidence of 2–5 per 10 000, can be diagnosed by the ultrasonographic demonstration of stomach and intestines (90 per cent of the cases) or liver (50 per cent) in the thorax and the associated mediastinal shift to the opposite side. Polyhydramnios, ascites, and other malformations, predominantly craniospinal and cardiac, are often present.

Benacerraf and Adzik (1987) examined the incidence of associated malformations in cases of antenatally diagnosed CDH and found chromosomal abnormalities in four (21 per cent) and major malformations in an additional five (26 per cent) of 19 fetuses. Similarly, Thorpe-Beeston *et al.* (1989), reported chromosomal defects in 31 per cent and major malformations in an additional 17 per cent of 36 fetuses with CDH. In our extended series of 79 fetuses with CDH, 16 (20 per cent) had chromosomal defects, mainly trisomy 18 (Table 3.3; Nicolaides *et al.* 1992*a*), and in all cases, in addition to the CDH, there were other malformations such as choroid plexus cysts, facial cleft, congenital heart defects, and digital abnormalities. None of the 37 fetuses with isolated CDH had chromosomal defects.

Cardiovascular abnormalities

Gross structural abnormalities of the heart or major blood vessels which have, or potentially have, effects on the proper functioning of the heart are found in approximately 1 per cent of livebirths and 2–10 per cent of stillbirths. While some of the defects resolve spontaneously (for example ventricular septal defect) and others are easily correctable (for example patent ductus), major structural abnormalities are either inoperable (for example hypoplastic left heart) or carry high operative risks (for example truncus arteriosus). The occurrence of CHD probably depends on the interplay of multiple genetic and environmental factors (Nora and Nora 1978). Echocardiography has been applied successfully to the prenatal assessment of the fetal cardiac function and structure and has led to the prenatal diagnosis of most moderate to major cardiac abnormalities.

Nora and Nora (1978), reported that heart defects are found in more than 99 per cent of fetuses with trisomy 18, in 90 per cent of those with trisomy 13, 50 per cent of trisomy 21, 40–50 per cent of those with deletions or partial trisomies involving chromosomes 4, 5, 8, 9, 13, 14, 18, or 22 and in 35 per cent of 45X.

In two prenatal studies, of ultrasonographically detectable fetal cardiac defects, Crawford *et al.* (1988) and Copel *et al.* (1988), reported chromosomal defects in 22 per cent of 74 cases and in 32 per cent of 34 cases, respectively.

In our series of 156 fetuses with cardiac defects, 100 (64 per cent) had chromosomal abnormalities (trisomy 13, trisomy 18, trisomy 21, Turner syndrome, deletions /duplications or translocations, or triploidy). However, in 153 of the 156 cases there were additional fetal malfomations (Table 3.3; Nicolaides *et al.* 1992*a*).

Gastrointestinal tract defects

Oesophageal atresia

Oesophageal atresia is a sporadic condition found in 2–10 per 10 000 births and, in 90 per cent of the cases, there is an associated tracheoesophageal (T–E) fistula (Holder and Ashcraft 1981). Prenatally the diagnosis of oesophageal atresia is suspected when, in the presence of polyhydramnios, repeated ultrasonographic examinations fail to demonstrate the fetal stomach; other possible diagnoses include lack of fetal swallowing, due to arthrogryposis, and intrathoracic compression, due to cystic adenomatoid malformation or pleural effusion. In the presence of a T–E fistula the stomach bubble may be normal.

Other major abnormalities, mainly cardiac, are found in 50–70 per cent of the infants (Holder *et al.* 1964) and the fistula may be seen as part of the VATER association (Vertebral and Ventricular septal defects, Anal atresia, T–E fistula, Renal anomalies, Radial dysplasia and single umbilical artery) (Quan and Smith 1973). Associated chromosomal abnormalities have been reported in 3–4 per cent of live births with oesophageal atresia (German *et al.* 1976; Louhimo and Lindahl 1983).

In our series of 24 cases, there were 20 fetuses with the presumptive diagnosis of oesophageal atresia and 17 (85 per cent) of these had trisomy 18 (Table 3.3; Nicolaides *et al.* 1992*g*). Only one of these fetuses survived and the infant had a normal gastrointestinal tract. Permission for post-mortem examination was obtained from 14 of the remaining 19 parents; in 12 the diagnosis of oesophageal atresia was confirmed; in one case the gastrointestinal tract was apparently normal and in another the stomach was small but there was no oesophageal atresia. In two cases the lack of a visible stomach bubble could be attributed to no swallowing due to arthrogryposis; both these fetuses were chromosomally normal but the infants died in the neonatal period because of pulmonary hypoplasia. In an additional two cases the lack of a visible stomach could be attributed to oesophageal compression due to cystic adenomatoid malformation of the lung and pleural effusion, respectively; the former had a normal karyotype and the latter had trisomy 21.

Duodenal atresia

Duodenal atresia or stenosis has a birth incidence of 1 in 10 000 live births. In most cases the condition is sporadic, although a familial inheritance has been suggested by an autosomal recessive pattern in some families. The condition can readily be diagnosed sonographically by the characteristic 'double-bubble' appearance of the dilated stomach and proximal duodenum and the commonly associated polyhydramnios. However, obstruction due to a central web may result in only a 'single bubble' representing the fluid-filled stomach. Continuity of the duodenum with the stomach should be demonstrated to differentiate a distended duodenum from other cystic masses, including choledocal or hepatic cysts.

Approximately half the fetuses with duodenal atresia have associated malformations including: skeletal defects (vertebral and rib anomalies, sacral agenesis, radial abnormalities and talipes), gastrointestinal abnormalities (oesophageal atresia/T–E fistula, intestinal malrotation, Meckels diverticulum and anorectal atresia), cardiovascular malformations (endocardial cushion defects and ventricular septal defects), and renal defects.

Postnatally, trisomy 21 is found in 20–30 per cent of cases of duodenal atresia (Fonkalsrud *et al.* 1969; Touloukian 1978). In our series of 23 fetuses with duodenal atresia, 10 (43 per cent) had trisomy 21, and in all but one of the fetuses there were additional malformations (Table 3.3; Nicolaides *et al.* 1992*g*).

Bowel obstruction

Jejeunal and ileal obstructions are imaged as multiple fluid-filled loops of bowel in the abdomen and, in contrast to duodenal atresia, associated abnormalities are uncommon. Active peristalsis is often present and, if bowel perforation occurs, transient ascites, meconium peritonitis, and meconium pseudocysts may ensue. Another presentation of small bowel obstruction is hyperechogenicity in the fetal abdomen. Anal atresia is associated with fluid-filled loops of bowel usually seen in the lower abdomen, but is not accompanied by polyhydramnios. Anal atresia may not present any antenatally detectable sonographic features.

In a combined series of 589 infants with a total jejunoileal atresia, additional abnormalities were found in 44 per cent of cases (De Lorimier *et al.* 1969). Bowel abnormalities including malrotation of the bowel, imperforate anus, meconium peritonitis and ileus, and omphalocele or gastroschisis were present in 20 per cent of the infants. Cardiovascular or chromosomal anomalies were found in 7 per cent of cases. In cases of anorectal atresia the incidence of associated defects is 70–90 per cent. The most commonly associated defects are genitourinary and include renal agenesis or dysplasia. Vertebral, cardiovascular, and gastrointestinal anomalies have all been described.

In our series of 24 fetuses with suspected bowel obstruction (Table 3.3; Nicolaides *et al.* 1992*g*), there were 14 cases of small bowel obstruction due to an atretic segment in the jejunum or ileum, six cases of large bowel obstruction, and four cases where the dilated bowel was subsequently found to be due to megacystis–microcolon–intestinal hypoperistalsis syndrome or myotonia dystrophica. The karyotype was normal in all but one case, in which the fetus had multiple abnormalities.

Abdominal cysts

These include ovarian, mesenteric, adrenal and hepatic cysts. In our series of 25 fetuses with abdominal cysts (Table 3.11; Nicolaides *et al.* 1992*g*), there were five cases with a mesenteric cyst, five cases with an ovarian cyst, one with a hepatic cyst, and four with adrenal cysts. In two of the latter cases, the fetuses had the Beckwith–Wiedemann syndrome, and in addition to the multiple adrenal cysts, they had hepato-splenomegaly and enlarged hyperechogenic pancreas. In six cases the nature of the cysts is uncertain because they resolved antenatally and there were no pathological findings at postnatal examination. In three cases with a large central abdominal cyst, postnatal surgery demonstrated a 'hydronephrotic sac' that was excised. In another case a large tubular pre-hepatic cyst was found to be a dilated umbilical vein, and postnatally this was found to be associated with aortic valve stenosis.

In one of the fetuses with Beckwith–Wiedemann syndrome the karyotype was 46XX/46XX, dup(11p). All other fetuses had a normal karyotype.

Liver nodules

In two fetuses, referred to our unit at 21–22 weeks' gestation, there were multiple hyperechogenic nodules (2–3 mm in diameter) in the liver. In one case, there was nuchal oedema and digital abnormalities and the karyotype was trisomy 21. The pregnancy was terminated and at post-mortem examination the hepatic nodules could not be identified. In the second fetus there were no other abnormalities and the karyotype was normal; the infant was born at term and postnatal X-ray examination demonstrated areas of calcification at the origin of the right hepatic vein.

Table 3.11 Findings in 25 fetuses with abdominal cysts including maternal age (age in years), gestation at referral (GA in weeks), antenatal findings, outcome (TOP = termination of pregnancy, NND = neonatal death), gestation at delivery (GE), sex (M, male; F, female), diagnosis and comments on antenatal (AN) or postnatal (PN) treatment

Case	Age	GA	Abdominal cyst position	Septae	Size (mm)	Outcome	GE (weeks)	Sex	Diagnosis	Comment
1	20	20	central	—	16 × 21 × 29	alive	42	F	mesenteric	PN resolving at 9 months
2	31	25	central	—	44 × 47 × 52	alive	38	M	mesenteric	PN surgery
3	41	34	central	—	65 × 70 × 80	NND	35	M	mesenteric	No details available
4[1]	29	34	central	—	70 × 81 × 90	alive	38	M	mesenteric	PN surgery
5	37	20	central	—	13 × 28 × 36	alive	29	F	mesenteric	PN surgery
6	27	35	central—left	+	47 × 42 × 33	alive	36	F	ovarian	PN surgery
7	21	33	central—left	—	37 × 37 × 60	alive	37	F	ovarian	PN resolved by day 7
8	40	33	central—left	—	23 × 23 × 30	alive	38	F	ovarian	PN resolved by day 5
9	21	33	central—left	+	30 × 30 × 30	alive	37	F	ovarian	PN surgery
10	24	37	central—left	—	35 × 47 × 53	alive	37	F	ovarian	PN resolved at 6 months
11	30	37	central—right	—	22 × 23 × 35	alive	39	F	uncertain	AN resolved by 40 weeks
12	18	20	upper—anterior	+	20 × 20 × 28	alive	42	M	uncertain	AN resolved by 24 weeks
13	29	21	central	—	20 × 20 × 20	alive	39	M	uncertain	AN resolved by 32 weeks
14	26	23	central	—	20 × 20 × 25	alive	39	F	uncertain	AN resolved by 24 weeks
15	19	35	central	—	26 × 30 × 34	alive	37	F	uncertain	AN resolved by 37 weeks
16	35	38	central	+	25 × 30 × 40	alive	41	F	uncertain	AN resolved by 41 weeks
17	19	28	central	—	90 × 99 × 100	alive	39	M	left renal	PN surgery
18	28	29	central	—	65 × 70 × 100	alive	38	M	left renal	PN surgery
19	21	34	central	—	70 × 72 × 80	alive	39	M	right renal	PN surgery
20	34	23	suprarenal	+	18 × 18 × 20	alive	40	M	adrenal	PN resolved by 30 days

21	suprarenal	+	16×18×21	alive	23	26	M	adrenal	PN resolving at 7 months
22[2]	suprarenal	+	25×25×58	TOP	35	23	F*	adrenal	
23[2]	suprarenal	+	45×45×50	NND	30	30	F	adrenal	
24	hepatic	—	40×40×60	alive	23	33	F	hepatic	PN surgery
25[3]	pre-hepatic UV	—	11×24×28	NND	27	21	M	umbilical V	

* Karyotype: 46, XX/46, XX, duplication (11p 15)
1 Megacystis and bilateral hydronephrosis
2 Beckwith–Wiedemann syndrome; enlarged liver, spleen, kidneys, tongue, and echogenic pancreas
3 Nuchal oedema, aortic valve stenosis

Anterior abdominal wall defects

Exomphalos

Exomphalos has an incidence of 2–4 per 10 000 births. There is a well-recognized association with chromosomal abnormalities (Table 3.12; Nakayama *et al.* 1984; Nielson *et al.* 1985; Nicolaides *et al.* 1986*a*; Gilbert and Nicolaides 1987; Sermer *et al.* 1987; Eydoux *et al.* 1989; Hughes *et al.* 1989; Nyberg *et al.* 1989; Benacerraf *et al.* 1990*a*; Holzgreve *et al.* 1990; Rizzo *et al.* 1990; Shah *et al.* 1990*b*; Van Geijn *et al.* 1991; Nicolaides *et al.* 1992*g*), and X-linked, autosomal dominant or autosomal recessive disorders. Prenatal diagnosis is based on the demonstration of the midline anterior abdominal wall defect, the herniated sac with its visceral contents and the umbilical cord insertion at the apex of the sac.

In our series of 116 fetuses, 42 (36 per cent) had an abnormal karyotype, mainly trisomy 18 (Table 3.3; Nicolaides *et al.* 1992*g*). The karyotype was abnormal in 25 (57 per cent) of the 44 fetuses with bowel only in the exomphalos sac and in 17 (24 per cent) of the 72 with liver, heart or bladder in the sac. One (3 per cent) of the 29 fetuses with isolated exomphalos had an abnormal karyotype; in contrast, 41 (47 per cent) of the 87 fetuses with additional malformations were found to be chromosomally abnormal.

Gastroschisis

In gastroschisis, with a birth incidence of 1 per 10 000, evisceration of the intestine occurs through a small abdominal wall defect located just lateral and usually to the right of an intact umbilical cord. The loops of intestine lie uncovered in the amniotic fluid and become thickened, oedematous, and matted. Prenatal diagnosis is based on the demonstration of the normally situated umbilicus and the herniated loops of intestine, which are free-floating. The vast majority of cases are thought to be sporadic, although there are examples of familial gastroschisis suggesting the possibility of an autosomal dominant mode of inheritance, with variable expressivity. Associated chromosomal abnormalities are rare, and although other malformations are found in 10–30 per cent of the cases, these are mainly gut atresias, probably due to gut strangulation and infarction *in utero*. In our series of 26 fetuses with gastroschisis there were no chromosomal abnormalities (Table 3.3; Nicolaides *et al.* 1992*g*).

Urinary tract defects

Fetal urinary tract anomalies occur in approximately 2–3 per 1000 pregnancies. Postnatal and post-mortem studies have established that urinary tract defects are commonly found in many chromosomal abnormalities (Jones 1988). Data on antenatally diagnosed renal defects are derived from a small number of often

Table 3.12 Summary of reports on antenatally diagnosed exomphalos providing data on the relation between abnormal karyotype and the absence or presence of other malformations, contents of the exomphalos, the sex of the fetuses, and the types of chromosomal abnormalities

Author	Incidence chromosomal abnormalities			Contents		Fetal sex		Chromosomal abnormalities			
	Total	Other anomalies Absent	Present	Bowel	Liver ± Bowel	Male	Female	Tr 13	Tr 18	Tr 21	Other
Nakayama et al. 1984	1/10	1/4	0/6	0/1	1/9	0/4	1/6	—	1	—	—
Nielson et al. 1985	2/8	0/3	2/5	—	—	0/3	2/5	2	—	—	—
Nicolaides et al. 1986	8/12	1/3	7/9	—	—	7/9	1/3	—	7	—	1
Gilbert and Nicolaides 1987	19/35	1/10	18/25	—	—	17/26	2/9	—	17	—	2
Sermer et al. 1987	4/10	0/2	4/8	—	—	—	—	1	2	—	1
Eydoux et al. 1989	12/46	7/27	5/19	—	—	—	—	2	6	—	3
Hughes et al. 1989	13/30	3/8	10/22	10/10	3/20	—	—	5	4	2	2
Nyberg et al. 1989	10/26	4/17	6/9	8/8	2/18	6/11	4/15	4	4	1	1
Benacerraf et al. 1990a	4/22	0/7	4/15	4/6	0/16	—	—	2	1	—	1
Holzgreve et al. 1990	5/10	—	—	—	—	—	—	1	3	—	1
Rizzo et al. 1990	7/12	2/6	5/6	—	—	—	—	2	5	—	—
Shah et al. 1990b	2/4	—	—	—	—	—	—	—	1	—	1
Van Geijn et al. 1991	10/22	0/4	10/18	—	—	—	—	1	6	—	3
Nicolaides et al. 1992g	42/109	1/27	41/82	25/40	17/69	36/70	6/39	6	33	—	3

* Other chromosomal abnormalities = 47,XXY; 45X; 46,XY,5p–; 46,XY,14q–; 46,XY,7q–; 46,XX,i(18p); 46,XX,t(9,11)(p13,q13); 46,XY/49,XY,+2,+7,+19; 46,XY,14q–,dic(13q14q); 69,XYY; 69,XXY; 46,XX,17p–; 46,XY,3p–; 46,XY,–18+i(18q); 46,XY,–13, +der(13)t(13q18p)

unclassified 'renal defects', and the reported incidence of associated chromosomal abnormalities varies from 2–33 per cent (Table 3.13; Curry *et al.* 1984; Nicolaides *et al.* 1986a; Rizzo *et al.* 1987; Boue *et al.* 1988; Hegge *et al.* 1988; Reuss *et al.* 1988; Eydoux *et al.* 1989; Benacerraf *et al.* 1990b; Holzgreve *et al.* 1990; Rizzo *et al.* 1990; Shah *et al.* 1990b, Stoll *et al.* 1990).

Nicolaides *et al.* (1992h) examined the incidence of chromosomal abnormalities in a large series of antenatally diagnosed renal defects, including:

1. Mild hydronephrosis, where only the renal pelvis was dilated and both the bladder and amniotic fluid volume were normal.
2. Moderate to severe hydronephrosis, with varying degrees of pelvic calyceal dilatation.
3. Multicystic dysplastic, with multiple non-communicating cysts of variable size and irregular hyperechogenic stroma.
4. Renal agenesis.

The renal defects, were either unilateral or bilateral. In the fetuses with bilateral moderate/severe hydronephrosis and multicystic kidneys, the obstruction was considered to be either low (dilated bladder), or high (bladder normal or empty), and there was either oligohydramnios or the amniotic fluid volume was normal/reduced (Table 3.14).

The overall incidence of chromosomal abnormalities was 12 per cent, and the commonest defects were trisomy 13, trisomy 18, and trisomy 21. There were more than twice as many males than females, but the incidence of chromosomal defects in females was almost double (18 per cent) that in males (10 per cent). Furthermore, compared to the overall maternal age-related risk, the risk for fetal chromosomal abnormalities was three times higher when there was an isolated renal defect and 30 times higher when there were additional malformations. The risk of chromosomal abnormalities was similar for fetuses with unilateral or bilateral involvement, different types of renal defects, urethral or ureteric obstruction, and oligohydramnios or normal/reduced amniotic fluid volume. Nevertheless, the patterns of chromosomal abnormalities, and consequently that of associated malformations, were related to the different types of renal defects. Thus, in mild hydronephrosis, the commonest chromosomal abnormality was trisomy 21, whereas in moderate/severe hydronephrosis, multicystic kidneys, or renal agenesis the commonest abnormalities were trisomies 18 and 13, each with their own syndromal defects. Consequently, the patterns of associated malformations were different.

Skeletal abnormalities

There is a wide range of rare skeletal dyplasias, each with a specific recurrence risk, morphology, and implication for neonatal survival and quality of life (Jones

Table 3.13 Summary of reports on antenatally diagnosed renal anomalies with data on presence of other defects and their karyotype

Author	Renal defects	Incidence abnormal karyotype			Trisomies			Other
		Total	Isolated	Other defect	13	18	21	
Curry et al. 1984 *	mixture	3/41	0/30	3/11	—	—	1	2
Nicolaides et al. 1986a	mixture	11/45	—	—	2	6	—	3
Rizzo et al. 1987	multicystic	2/6	0/3	2/3	1	—	—	1
Boue et al. 1988	mixture	24/221	10/165	14/56	3	6	5	10
Hegge et al. 1988	mixture	1/3	—	—	—	—	—	1
Reuss et al. 1988	obstruction	5/43	2/27	3/16	2	2	1	—
Eydoux et al. 1989	mixture	12/111	1/55	11/56	3	4	2	3
Benacerraf et al. 1990b	hydronephrosis	7/210	—	—	—	—	7	—
Holzgreve et al. 1990	mixture	4/16	—	—	2	1	—	1
Rizzo et al. 1990	mixture	1/44	1/44	—	—	—	—	1
Shah et al. 1990b	mixture	3/9	—	—	1	—	1	1
Stoll et al. 1990 **	mixture	21/79	—	—	4	6	4	7
Nicolaides et al. 1992h	mixture	85/682	16/476	69/206	18	20	19	17

* Post-mortem study including 8 cases that were diagnosed antenatally
** 54.4% diagnosed antenatally; the others stillborn or liveborn up to age 5 years

Table 3.14 Abnormal karyotype in fetuses with bilateral moderate/severe hydronephrosis or multicystic kidneys in relation to the level of urinary tract obstruction (high or ureteric, and low or urethral), and to the presence or absence of amniotic fluid (AF)

	Cases	Chromosomal abnormalities Total (%)	Triploidy	Trisomies 21	18	13	Deletions	Other	Sex chromosomes 45XO	Other
High obstruction	67	6 (9)	—	1	—	—	1	1	3	—
isolated	46	— (0)	—	—	—	—	—	—	—	—
+ other	21	6 (29)	—	1	—	—	1	1	3	—
Low obstruction	156	22 (14)	2	3	9	4	1	3	—	—
isolated	114	8 (7)	2	2	—	1	1	2	—	—
+ other	42	14 (33)	—	1	9	3	—	1	—	—
AF present	103	14 (14)	1	2	7	3	1	1	—	—
isolated	65	3 (5)	1	1	—	1	—	—	—	—
+ other	38	11 (29)	—	1	7	2	—	1	—	—
AF absent	120	14 (12)	1	2	2	1	2	3	3	—
isolated	95	5 (5)	1	1	—	—	1	2	—	—
+ other	25	9 (36)	—	1	2	1	1	1	3	—

1988). Prenatal diagnosis in families at risk of such anomalies necessitates special awareness if the ultrasonographer is to be alerted to the variation in dysmorphic expression that might be encountered. Our knowledge of the expression of these syndromes *in utero* is based on a small number of case reports, and, therefore, it is often necessary to extrapolate findings from the perinatal period when attempting prenatal diagnosis of individual conditions. In the event of identification of a skeletal dysplasia during routine ultrasound screening in a pregnancy not known to be at risk of a specific syndrome, it is necessary to undertake a systematic examination in order to obtain the correct diagnosis. All four limbs must be evaluated, in terms of their length, shape, mineralization, and movement, and the possible presence of associated abnormalities, particularly in the head, thorax, and spine, should be determined. With the advent of high-resolution scanners, fetal fingers and toes can be seen and with meticulous examination abnormalities of numbers, shape, movement, and attitudes can be recognized.

Malformations of the extremities

Characteristic abnormalities in the extremities are commonly found in a wide range of chromosomal defects and the detection of abnormal hands or feet at the routine ultrasound examination should stimulate the search for other markers of chromosomal defects. Syndactyly is associated with triploidy, clinodactyly with trisomy 21, polydactyly with trisomy 13, overlapping fingers, rocker bottom feet, and talipes with trisomy 18 (Table 3.4; Nicolaides *et al.* 1992*a*).

In two series of antenatally diagnosed talipes equinovarus, Benacerraf (1986) and Jeanty *et al.* (1985) reported chromosomal abnormalities in 31 per cent and 25 per cent of 13 and 8 fetuses, respectively. All the chromosomally abnormal fetuses had multiple abnormalities. In our series of 106 fetuses with talipes, 38 (36 per cent) had chromosomal defects, mainly trisomy 18 (Table 3.4; Nicolaides *et al.* 1992*a*).

Relative shortening of the femur

Benacerraf *et al.* (1985), reported that if the ratio of the actual femur length to the expected length, based on the biparietal diameter, was ≤0.91, the sensitivity and specificity for detecting fetuses with trisomy 21 at 15–21 weeks' gestation was 68 per cent and 98 per cent, respectively. In contrast, Perella *et al.* (1988) found that although relative shortening of the femur had a positive predictive value of 3 per cent for identifying trisomy 21 in women with advanced maternal age, the predictive value decreased to 1 per cent for the general population. Lynch *et al.* (1989), in their study of nine twin pregnancies with discordant fetuses for trisomy 21, suggested that short femur was of no value in identifying the trisomic twin. Similarly, Shah *et al.* (1990*a*) found no significant difference in the mean biparietal diameter to femur length ratio in a group of 17 fetuses with Down syndrome compared to that of normal controls.

In our series of 2086 fetuses that were karyotyped for a variety of malformations or growth retardation, relative shortening of the femur was defined as head circumference to femur length ratio > 97.5th centile of our normal range. Chromosomal defects, mainly trisomies 18 and 21, triploidy and Turner syndrome, were found in 116 of the 411 (28 per cent) fetuses with short femur (Table 3.4; Nicolaides *et al.* 1992*b*).

Intrauterine growth retardation

Although low birth-weight is a common feature of many chromosomal abnormalities, the incidence of chromosomal defects in small for gestational age neonates is less than 1–2 per cent (Carr 1963; Chen *et al.* 1972; Ounsted *et al.* 1981; Khoury *et al.* 1988). However, data derived from postnatal studies may underestimate the association between chromosomal abnormalitites and growth retardation, since many pregnancies with chromosomally abnormal fetuses result in spontaneous abortion or intrauterine death. Furthermore, since the degree of growth retardation is generally more severe in the more lethal types of chromosomal abnormalities, it is expected that in antenatally diagnosed, early onset, severe growth retardation the types of chromosomal abnormalities will be different from those recognized at birth.

Snijders *et al.* (1992), examined 458 patients with severely growth retarded singleton pregnancies at 17–40 weeks' gestation, and reported that the incidence of chromosomal defects was 19 per cent. The commonest chromosomal abnormalities were triploidy, trisomies 13, 18, and 21, and deletion of the short arm of chromosome 4. The triploidies were most commonly encountered in the second trimester while the aneuploidies, deletions, and translocations appeared in the third trimester group of fetuses. These findings suggest that triploidy is associated with the most severe form of early onset growth retardation and that the majority of affected fetuses die before the third trimester of pregnancy.

The incidence of chromosomal defects was higher in:

(1) the group with malformations (40 per cent), than in those with no structural defects (3 per cent)

(2) the group with normal or increased amniotic fluid volume (40 per cent) than in those with reduced or absent amniotic fluid (7 per cent)

(3) in the group with normal waveforms from both uterine and umbilical arteries (44 per cent), than in those with abnormal waveforms from either or both vessels (40/347).

A substantial proportion of the chromosomally abnormal fetuses demonstrated the asymmetry (high head to abdomen circumference ratio), thought to be typical for fetal starvation; indeed the most severe form of asymmetrical growth retardation is found in fetuses with triploidy.

Overview

Structurally malformed or severely growth retarded fetuses are often chromosomally abnormal. Certainly the incidence of chromosomal defects for ultrasonically detectable abnormalities (300 of 2086 or 14 per cent in our series) is much higher than the incidence reported in screening studies based on advanced maternal age. Even for a 45-year-old woman the risk of any chromosomal abnormality is only 7.2 per cent (Ferguson-Smith and Yates 1984).

The ultrasound diagnosis of a marker for a specific chromosomal defect should stimulate the search for other associated malformations, and when these additional abnormalities are found the probability that the fetus is chromosomally abnormal is dramatically increased. In our series, chromosomal defects were found in 25 of the 1108 (2 per cent) fetuses with an isolated defect and in 275 of the 978 (27 per cent) with more than one malformation. The risk ratio for chromosomal defects increased from 1 for the whole group to > 60 if ≥ 8 defects were present (Table 3.15). Since karyotyping is advocated for advanced maternal age or abnormal maternal serum biochemistry where the risk is often less than 1 per cent, women with certain fetal defects, even when these are apparently isolated should also be offered the option of having fetal karyotyping since the risk of a chromosomal abnormality is often more than 1 per cent.

Table 3.15 Risk of chromosomal abnormalities with increasing number of malformations

Anomalies	Normal n	Abnormal %	n	Risk %	Ratio
≥ 1 defect	1786	100.0	300	100.0	1
≥ 2 defects	703	39.4	275	91.7	2
≥ 3 defects	250	14.0	224	74.7	5
≥ 4 defects	102	5.7	157	52.3	9
≥ 5 defects	47	2.6	94	31.3	12
≥ 6 defects	27	1.5	60	20.0	13
≥ 7 defects	7	0.4	35	11.7	30
≥ 8 defects	2	0.1	21	7.0	63

Detailed ultrasound examination should be offered to all pregnant women at 12 and 20 weeks gestation (RCOG 1990). It should be aimed at detecting both major malformations, as well as more subtle ones which may be markers of chromosomal defects. Furthermore, the examples of ventriculomegaly, exomphalos, and hydronephrosis demonstrate that for a given malformation the risk of a chromosomal defect may be inversely related to the apparent severity of the malformation.

More than 90 per cent of fetuses with trisomy 13 or 18, triploidy, and Turner syndrome have associated malformations (Jones 1988) that should be easily detectable by diligent ultrasonographic examination. However, the common malformations in trisomy 21 are more subtle (brachycephaly, relative shortening of the long bones, nuchal oedema, atrioventricular septal defect, midphalanx hypoplasia or clinodactyly in the 5th finger, sandal gap, or mild hydronephrosis), and therefore the false-positive rate for each individual feature may be unacceptably high. Nevertheless, it should be emphasized that a single ultrasound marker, such as nuchal oedema, as a risk factor for fetal karyotyping can identify 40 per cent of fetuses with trisomy 21, which compares favourably with the potential 25 per cent detection rate if the risk factor is advanced maternal age or even the 50 per cent rate if a combination of maternal age and triple biochemistry are used. Furthermore, an ultrasonographically detectable defect is not just a potentially useful marker for a chromosomal abnormality but it may also lead to the diagnosis of another significant defect, such as nuchal oedema unmasking a cardiac abnormality, or talipes leading to the diagnosis of a lethal arthrogryposis syndrome.

Although most of our patients were seen at 16–28 weeks, a substantial proportion were referred in the third trimester of pregnancy and many of the latter had chromosomally abnormal fetuses (Fig. 3.4). Therefore, fetal karyotyping should be considered even in the third trimester because knowledge of a serious chromosomal abnormality may alter the management of labour and delivery. Karyotyping should also be performed for conditions such as hydrops fetalis or severe early onset growth retardation where the risk of intrauterine death is high; autolysis may render post-mortem chromosomal studies, and therefore accurate genetic counselling for future pregnancies, impossible.

The preferred method for fetal karyotyping when a fetal malformation or growth retardation are detected by ultrasound is fetal blood sampling and cytogenetic analysis of stimulated lymphocytes. This gives accurate results within 3–4 days, compared with 2–4 weeks if the alternative method of amniocentesis is used. Rapid karyotyping reduces the duration of parental anxiety while waiting for results, allows for earlier termination of pregnancy if the fetus is affected, and makes it possible to alter perinatal management when karyotyping is undertaken late in the third trimester of pregnancy. Although placental biopsy can be undertaken throughout pregnancy (Nicolaides *et al.*

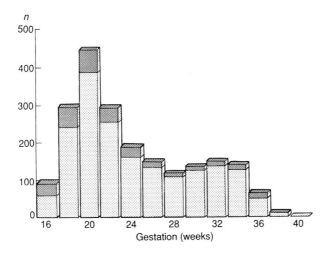

Fig. 3.4. Gestational age distribution of chromosomally normal (light shaded area) and abnormal (dark shaded area) fetuses with malformation and/or growth retardation.

1986*b*) and cytogenetic analysis from direct preparations can potentially provide results within a few hours of sampling, there is the major drawback of both false-positive and false-negative results, which are particularly high for trisomy 18, i.e. the commonest cytogenetic defect in antenatally diagnosed malformations. The additional advantage of fetal blood sampling is that it makes it possible to diagnose other causes of a given defect. For example, a series of investigations in growth-retarded fetuses have demonstrated a whole range of biochemical, endocrinological, and haematological abnormalities. Fetal blood sampling in hydrops will identify the subgroup with severe anaemia due to parvovirus infection, and the hydrops could be reversed by fetal blood transfusions. One of the causes of fetal hydrocephalus is intraventricular haemorrhage due to alloimmune thrombocytopenia; accurate diagnosis may help prevent recurrence of the problem by appropriate therapy in subsequent pregnancies.

The sensitivity of ultrasound screening for chromosomal defects in both unselected populations and in those considered to be at high risk, because of advanced maternal age or abnormal maternal serum biochemistry testing, remains to be determined. Nevertheless, present evidence suggests that ultrasonography is likely to prove the most effective method of screening for fetal chromosomal defects in addition to its role in the diagnosis of syndromal and sporadic malformations.

References

Abramowicz, J. S., Warsof, S. L., Doyle, D. L., Smith, D., and Levy, D. L. (1989). Congenital cystic hygroma of the neck diagnosed prenatally: Outcome with normal and abnormal karyotype. *Prenat. Diagn.*, **9**, 321–7.

Amato, M., Howald, H., and von Muralt, G. (1986). Fetal ventriculomegaly, agenesis of the corpus callosum and chromosomal translocation — Case report. *J. Perinat. Med.*, **14**, 271–4.

Andersen, H. M., Drew, J. H., and Beischer, N. A., Hutchison, A. A., and Fortune, D. W. (1983). Non-immune hydrops fetalis: changing contribution to perinatal mortality. *Br. J. Obstet. Gynaecol.*, **90**, 636–9.

Azar, G., Snijders, R. J. M., Gosden, C. M., and Nicolaides, K. H. (1991). Fetal nuchal cystic hygromata: associated malformations and chromosomal defects. *Fetal Diagn. Ther.*, **6**, 46–57.

Benacerraf, B. R., (1986). Antenatal sonographic diagnosis of congenital clubfoot: a possible indication for amniocentesis. *J. Clin. Ultrasound*, **14**, 703–6.

Benacerraf, B. R., and Adzick, N. S. (1987). Fetal diaphragmatic hernia: ultrasound diagnosis and clinical outcome in 19 cases. *Am. J. Obstet. Gynecol.*, **156**, 573–6.

Benacerraf, B. R., Barss, V. A., and Laboda, L. A. (1985). A sonographic sign for the detection in the second trimester of the fetus with Down's syndrome. *Am. J. Obstet. Gynecol.*, **151**, 1078–9.

Benacerraf, B. R., Frigoletto, F. D., and Green, M. F. (1986). Abnormal facial features and extremities in human trisomy syndromes: prenatal US appearance. *Radiology*, **159**, 243–6.

Benacerraf, B. R., Gelman, R., and Frigoletto, F. D. (1987). Sonographic identification of second trimester fetuses with Down's syndrome. *N. Engl. J. Med.*, **317**, 1371–6.

Benacerraf, B. R., Saltzman, D. H., Estroff, J. H., and Frigoletto, F. D. Jr. (1990a). Abnormal karyotype of fetuses with omphalcele: prediction based on omphalocele contents. *Obstet. Gynecol.*, **75**, 317–19.

Benacerraf, B. R., Mandell, J., Estroff, J. A., Harlow, B. L., and Frigoletto, F. D. (1990b). Fetal pyelectasis: A possible association with Down Syndrome. *Obstet and Gynecol.*, **976**, 59–60.

Berry, S. M., Gosden, C. M., Snijders, R. J. M., and Nicolaides, K. H. (1990). Fetal holoprosencephaly: associated malformations and chromosomal defects. *Fetal Diagn. Ther.*, **5**, 92–9.

Bertino, R. E., Nyberg, D. A., Cyr, D. R., and Mack, L. A. (1987). Prenatal diagnosis of agenesis of the corpus callosum. *J. Ultrasound Med.*, **7**, 251–60.

Boue, A., Muller, F., Briard, M. L., and Boue, J. (1988). Interest of biology in the management of pregnancies where a fetal malformation has been detected by ultrasonography. *Fetal Ther.*, **3**, 14–23.

Bronshtein, M., Rottem, S., Yoffe, N., and Blumenfeld, Z. (1989). First trimester and early second trimester diagnosis of nuchal cystic hygroma by transvaginal sonography: Diverse prognosis of the septated from the non septated lesion. *Am. J. Obstet. Gynecol.*, **161**, 78–82.

Bundy, A. L., Saltzman, D. H., Pober, B., Fine, C., Emerson, D., and Doubilet, P. M. (1986). Antenatal sonographic findings in trisomy 18. *J. Ultrasound Med.*, **5**, 361–4.

Byrne, J., Blanc, W., Warburton, D., and Wigger, J. (1984). The significance of cystic hygroma in fetuses. *Hum. Pathol.*, **15**, 61–7.

Carr, D. H. (1963). Chromosome studies in abortuses and stillborn infants. *Lancet*, **ii**, 603–6.

Carr, R. F., Ochs, R. H., Ritter, D. A., Kenny, J. D., Fridey, J. L., and Ming, P. L. (1986). Fetal cystic hygroma and Turner's Syndrome. *American Journal of Diseases of Children*, **140**, 580–3.

Chen, A. T. L., Chan, Y. K., and Falek, A. (1972). The effects of chromosomal abnormalities on birth weight in man. *Human Heredity*, **22**.

Chervenak, F. A., Isaacson, G., Blakemore, K. J., Breg, R. W., Hobbins, J. C., Berkowitz, R. L., (1983), *et al.* Fetal cystic hygroma: cause and natural history. *N. Engl. J. Med* **309**, 822–5.

Chervenak, F. A., Berkowitz, R. L., Tortora, M., and Hobbins, J. C. (1985*a*). The management of fetal hydrocephalus. *Am. J. Obstet. Gynecol.*, **151**, 933–42.

Chervenak, F. A., Isaacson, G., Hobbins, J. C., Chitkara, U., Tortora, M., and Berkowitz, R. L. (1985*b*). Diagnosis and management of fetal holoprosencephaly. *Obstet. Gynecol.*, **66**, 322–6.

Chitkara, U., Cogswell, C., Norton, K., Wilkins, I. A., Mehalek, K., and Berkowitz, R. L. (1988). Choroid plexus cysts in the fetus: a benign anatomic variant or pathologic entity? Report of 41 cases and review of the literature. *Obstet. Gynecol.*, **72**, 185–9.

Chudleigh, P., Pearce, J. M., and Campbell, S. (1984). The prenatal diagnosis of transient cysts of the fetal choroid plexus. *Prenatal. Diagnosis*, **4**, 135.

Cochrane, D. D., Myles, S. T., Nimrod, C., Still, D. K., Sugarman, R. G., and Wittmann, B. K. (1984). Intrauterine hydrocephalus and ventriculomegaly: associated abnormalities and fetal outcome. *Can. J. Neurol. Sci.*, **12**, 51–9.

Cohen, M. M., Schwartz, S., Schwartz, M. F., Blitzer, M. G., Raffel, L. J., Mullins-Keene, C. L., *et al.* (1989). Antenatal detection of cystic hygroma. *Obstet. Gynecol. Surv.*, **44**, 481–90.

Comstock, C., Culp, D., Gonzalez, J. and Boal, D. B. (1985). Agenesis of the corpus callosum in the fetus: its evolution and significance. *J. Ultrasound Med.*, **4**, 613–16.

Copel, J. A., Cullen, M., Green, J. J., Mahoney, M. J., Hobbins, J. C., and Kleinman, C. S. (1988). The frequency of aneuploidy in prenatally diagnosed congenital heart disease: an indication for fetal karyotyping. *Am. J. Obstet. Gynecol.*, **158**, 409–13.

Crawford, D. C., Chita, S. K., and Allan, L. D. (1988). Prenatal detection of congenital heart disease: factors affecting obstetric management and survival. *Am. J. Obstet. Gynecol.*, **159**, 352–6.

Cullen, M. T., Gabrielli, S., Green, J. J., Rizzo, N., Mahoney, M. J., Salafia, C., *et al.* (1990). Diagnosis and significance of cystic hygroma in the first trimester. *Prenat. Diagn.*, **10**, 643–51.

Curry, C. J. R., Jensen, K., Holland, J., Miller, L., and Hall, B.D. (1984). The Potter sequence: A clinical analysis of 80 cases. *Am. J. Med. Genet.*, **19**, 679–702.

Dallapiccola, B., Zelante, L., Perla, G., and Villani, G. (1984). Prenatal diagnosis of recurrence of cystic hygroma with normal chromosomes. *Prenat. Diagn.*, **4**, 383–6.

De Lorimier, A. A., Fonkalsrud, E. W., and Hays, D. M. (1969). Congenital atresia and stenosis of the jejunum and ileum. *Surgery*, **65**, 819–27.

Drugan, A., Krause, B., Canady, A., Zador, I. E., Sacks, A. J., and Evens, M. I. (1989). The natural history of prenatally diagnosed cerebral ventriculomegaly. *Journal of the American Medical Association*, **261**, 1785–8.

Eydoux, P., Choiset, A., Le Porrier, N., Thepot, F., Szpiro-tapia, S., Alliet, J., *et al.* (1989). Chromosomal prenatal diagnosis: Study of 936 cases of intrauterine abnormalities after ultrasound assessment. *Prenat. Diagn.*, **9**, 255–68.

Ferguson-Smith, M. A. and Yates, J. R. W. (1984). Maternal age specific rates for chromosome aberrations and factors influencing them: Report of a collaborative European study on 52, 965 amniocenteses. *Prenat. Diagn.*, **4**, 5–44.

Filly, R. A., Chin, D. H., and Callen, P. W. (1984). Alobar holoprosencephaly: ultrasonographic prenatal diagnosis. *Radiology*, **151**, 455–9.

Fitzsimons, J., Wilson, D., Pascoe-Mason, J., Mei Shaw, C., Cyr, D. R., and Mack, L. A. (1989). Choroid plexus cysts in fetuses with trisomy 18. *Obstet. Gynecol.*, **73**, 257–60.

Fonkalsrud, E. W., DeLorimier, A. A., and Hays, D. M. (1969). Congenital atresia and stenosis of the duodenum. A review compiled from the members of the Surgical Section of the American Academy of Pediatrics. *Pediatrics*, **43**, 79–83.

Furness, M. E. (1987). Choroid plexus cysts and trisomy 18. *Lancet*, **ii**, 693.

Gabrielli, S, Reece, A. R., Perolo, A., Rizzo, N., Bovicelli, L., *et al.* (1989). The significance of prenatally diagnosed choroid plexus cysts. *Am. J. Obstet. Gynecol.*, **160**, 1207–10.

Garden, A. S., Benzie, R. J., Miskin, M., and Gardner, H. A. (1986). Fetal cystic hygroma colli: Antenatal diagnosis, significance, and management. *Am. J. Obstet. Gynecol.*, **154**, 221–5.

Gembruch, U., Hansmann, M., Bald, R., Zerres, K., Schwanitz, G., and Fodisch, H. J. (1988). Prenatal diagnosis and management in fetuses with cystic hygroma colli. *Eur. J. Obstet. Gynecol. Reprod. Biol.*, **29**, 241–55.

German, J. C., Mahour, G. H., and Wooley, M. M. (1976). Esophageal atresia and associated anomalies. *J. Pediatr. Surg.*, **11**, 299–306.

Giacoia, G. P. (1980). Hydrops fetalis (fetal oedema). A survey. *Clin. Pediatr.*, **19**, 334.

Gilbert, W. M. and Nicolaides, K. H. (1987). Fetal omphalocele: associated malformations and chromosomal defects. *Obstet. Gynecol.*, **70**, 633–5.

Gustavii, B. and Edvall, H. (1984). First-trimester diagnosis of cystic nuchal hygroma. *Acta Obstet. Gynecol. Scand*, **63**, 377–8.

Hegge, F. N., Prescott, G. H., and Watson, P. T. (1988). Sonography at the time of genetic amniocentesis to screen for fetal malformations. *Obstet. Gynecol.*, **71**, 522–5.

Holder, T. M., Cloud, D. T., and Lewis, J. E. (1964). Esophageal atresia and tracheoesophageal fistula. A survey of its members by the surgical section of the American Academy of Pediatrics. *Pediatrics*, **34**, 542–9.

Holder, T. M. and Ashcraft, K. W. (1981). Developments in the care of patients with esophageal atresia and tracheoesophageal fistula. *Surg. Clin. N. Am.*, **61**, 1051.

Holzgreve, W., Miny, P., Gerlach, B., Westendrop, A., Ahlert, D., and Horst, J. (1990). Benefits of placental biopsies for rapid karyotyping in the second and third trimesters (late chorionic villus sampling) in high-risk pregnancies. *Am. J. Obstet. Gynecol.*, **162**, 1188–92.

Hudgins, R. J., Edwards, M. S. B., Goldstein, R., Callen, P. W., Harrison, M.R., Filly, R.A., *et al.* (1988). Natural history of fetal ventriculomegaly. *Pediatrics*, **82**, 692–7.

Hughes, M., Nyberg, D. H., Mack, L. H., and Pretorius, D. H. (1989). Fetal omphalocele: prenatal US detection of concurrent anomalies and other predictors of outcome. *Radiology*, **173**, 371–6.

Hutchison, A. A., Drew, J. H., Yu, V. Y. H., Williams, M. L., Fortune, D. W., and Beisher, N. A. (1982). Non-immunologic hydrops fetalis: a review of 61 cases. *Obstet. Gynecol.*, **59**, 347–52.

Jeanty, P., Romero, R., d'Alton, M., Venus, I., and Hobbins, J. C. (1985). *In utero* sonographic detection of hand and foot deformities. *J. Ultrasound Med.*, **4**, 595–601.

Jones, K. L. (1988). *Smith's recognizable patterns of human malformation.* 4th edn. W. B. Saunders, London.

Keeling, J. W., Gough, D. J., and Iliff, P. J. (1983). The pathology of non-rhesus hydrops. *Diagn. Histopathol.*, **6**, 89–111.

Khoury, M. J., Erickson, J. D., Cordero, J. F., and McCarthy, B. J. (1988). Congenital malformations and intrauterine growth retardation: a population study. *Pediatrics*, **82**, 163–72.

Khouzam, M. N. and Hooker, J. G. (1989). The significance of prenatal diagnosis of choroid plexus cysts. *Prenat. Diagn.*, **9**, 213–16.

Langer, J. C., Fitzgerald, P. G., Desa, D., Filly, R. A., Golbus, M. S., Adzick, N. S., *et al.* (1990). Cervical cystic hygroma in the fetus: Clinical spectrum and outcome. *J. Pediatr. Surg.*, **25**, 58–62.

Louhimo, I. and Lindahl, H. (1983). Esophageal atresia: primary results of 500 consecutively treated patients. *J. Pediatr. Surg.*, **18**, 217–29.

Lynch, L., Berkowitz, G. S., Chitkara, U., Wilkins, I. A., Mehalek, K. E., and Berkowitz, R. L. (1989). Ultrasound detection of Down syndrome: is it really possible? *Obstet. Gynecol.*, **73**, 267–70.

Machin, G. A. (1981). Differential diagnosis of hydrops fetalis. *Am. J. Med. Genet*, **9**, 341.

Marchese, C., Savin, E., Dragone, E., Carozzi, F., De Marchi, M., Campogrande, M. *et al.* (1985). Cystic hygroma: Prenatal diagnosis and genetic counselling. *Prenat. Diagn.*, **5**, 221–7.

Miyabara, S., Sugihara, H., Maehara, N., Shouno, H., Tasaki, H., Yoshida, K., *et al.* (1989). Significance of cardiovascular malformations in cystic hygroma: A new interpretation of the pathogenesis. *Am. J. Med. Genet.*, **34**, 489–501.

Nakayama, D. K., Harrison, M. K., Gross, B. H., Callen, P. W., Filly R. H., Golbus, M. S., *et al.* (1984). Management of the fetus with an abdominal wall defect. *J. Pediatr. Surg.*, **19**, 408–13.

Newman, D. E. and Cooperberg, P. I. (1984). Genetics of sonographically detected intrauterine fetal cystic hygromas. *Can. Med. Assoc. J.*, **35**, 77–9.

Nicolaides, K. H., Rodeck, C. H., Lange, I., Watson, J., Gosden, C. M., Miller, D., *et al.* (1985). Fetoscopy in the assessment of unexplained fetal hydrops. *Br. J. Obstet. Gynaecol.*, **92**, 671–9.

Nicolaides, K. H., Rodeck, C. H., and Gosden, C. M. (1986*a*). Rapid karyotyping in non-lethal fetal malformations. *Lancet*, **i**, 283–6.

Nicolaides, K. H., Soothill, P. W., Rodeck, C. H., Warren, R., and Gosden, C. M. (1986*b*). Why confine chorionic villus (placental) biopsy to the first trimester. *Lancet*, **ii**, 543–4.

Nicolaides, K. H., Berry, S., Snijders, R. J. M., Thorpe-Beeston, J. G., and Gosden, C. M. (1990). Fetal lateral cerebral ventriculomegaly: associated malformations and chromosomal defects. *Fetal Diagn. Ther.*, **5**, 5–14.

Nicolaides, K. H., Snijders, R. J. M., and Gosden, C. M. (1992*a*). Ultrasound markers of chromosomal abnormalities in 2086 fetuses. *Lancet,* **340**, 704–7.

Nicolaides, K. H., Snijders, R. J. M., and Gosden, C. M. (1992*b*). Fetal biometry and chromosomal abnormalities in 2086 fetuses. *Fetal Diagn. Ther.* (In press).

Nicolaides, K. H., Salvesen, D., Snijders, R. J. M., and Gosden C. M. (1992*c*). Strawberry shaped skull: associated malformations and chromosomal defects. *Fetal Diagn. Ther.* **7**, 132–7.

Nicolaides, K. H., Salvesen, D., Snijders, R. J. M., and Gosden, C. M. (1992*d*). Facial defects: associated malformations and chromosomal defects. *Fetal Diagn. Ther.*, (In press).

Nicolaides, K. H., Azar, G., Snijders, R. J. M., and Gosden, C. M. (1992*e*). Fetal nuchal edema: associated malformations and chromosomal defects. *Fetal Diagn. Ther.*, (In press).

Nicolaides, K. H., Azar, G. B., Byrne, D., and Marks, K. (1992*f*). Fetal nuchal translucency: ultrasound screening for chromosomal defects in the first trimester of pregnancy. *Brit Med. J.* 304: 867–9

Nicolaides, K. H., Snijders, R. J. M., Cheng, H., and Gosden, C. M. (1992*g*). Fetal abdominal wall and gastrointestinal tract defects: associated malformations and chromosomal defects. *Fetal Diagn. Ther.* 7; 102–15.

Nicolaides, K. H., Cheng, H., Snijders, R. J. M., and Gosden, C. M. (1992*h*). Fetal renal defects: associated malformations and chromosomal defects. *Fetal Diagn. Ther.* 7; 1–11.

Nielson, L. B., Bang, J. and Norgaard-Pedersen, B. (1985). Prenatal diagnosis of omphalocele and gastrochisis by ultrasonography. *Prenat. Diagn.*, **5**, 381–92.

Nora, J. J., and Nora, A. H. (1978). The evolution of specific genetic and environmental counselling in congenital heart disease. *Circulation*, **57**, 205.

Nyberg, D. A., Mack, L. A., Hirsch, J., Pagon, R., and Shepard, T.H. (1987*a*). Fetal hydrocephalus: sonographic detection and clinical significance of associated anomalies. *Radiology*, **163**, 187–91.

Nyberg, D. A., Mack, L. A., Bronstein, A., Hirsch, J., and Pagon, R. A. (1987*b*). Holoprosencephaly: prenatal sonographic diagnosis. *AJR*, **149**, 1051–8.

Nyberg, D. A., Cyr, D. R., Mack, L. A., Fitzsimmons, J., Hickok, D., and Mahony, B. S. (1988). The Dandy-Walker malformation: prenatal sonographic diagnosis and its clinical significance. *J. Ultrasound Med.*, **7**, 65–71.

Nyberg, D. H., Fitzsimmons, J., Mack, L. H., Hughes, M., Pretorius, D. H., Hickok, D., *et al.* (1989). Chromosomal abnormalities in fetuses with omphalocele. Significance of omphalocele contents. *J. Ultrasound Med.*, **8**, 299–308.

Ostlere, S. J., Irving, H. C., and Lilford, R. J. (1989). A prospective study of the incidence and significance of fetal choroid plexus cysts. *Prenat. Diagn.*, **9**, 205–11.

Ounsted, M., Moar, V., and Scott, A. (1981). Perinatal morbidity and mortality in small-for-dates babies: the relative importance of some maternal factors. *Early Human Development*, **5**, 367–75.

Palmer, C. G., Miles, J. H., Howard-Peebles, P. N., Magenis, R. E., Patil, S., and Friedman, J. M. (1987). Fetal karyotype following ascertainment of fetal anomalies by ultrasound. *Prenat. Diagn.*, **7**, 551–5.

Pashayan, H. M. (1983). What else to look for in a child born with a cleft of the lip or palate. *Cleft Palate J.*, **20**, 54–82.

Pearce, M. J., Griffin, D., and Campbell, S. (1985). The differential prenatal diagnosis of cystic hygromata and encephalocele by ultrasound examination. *J. Clin. Ultrasound*, **13**, 317–20.

Perella, R., Duerinckx, A. J., Grant, E. G., Tessler, F., Tach, K., and Crandall, B. F. (1988). Second trimester sonographic diagnosis of Down syndrome: role of femur length shortening and nuchal-fold thickening. *AJR*, **151**, 981–5.

Perry, T. B., Benzie, R. J., Cassar, N., *et al.* (1984). Fetal cephalometry by ultrasound as a screening procedure for the prenatal detection of Down syndrome. *Brit. J. Obstet. Gynaecol.*, **91**, 138–43.

Pijpers, L., Reuss, A., Stewart, P. A., Wladimiroff, J. W., and Sachs, E. S. (1988). Fetal cystic hygroma: Prenatal diagnosis and management. *Obstet. Gynecol.*, **72**, 223–4.

Pilu, G., Rizzo, N., Orsini, L. F., and Bovicelli, L. (1986). Antenatal recognition of cerebral anomalies. *Ultrasound in Med. and Biol.*, **12**, 319–26.

Pons, J. C., Diallo, A. A., Eydoux, P., Rais, S., Doumerc, S., Frydman, R., *et al.* (1989). Chorionic villus sampling after first trimester diagnosis of fetal cystic hygroma colli. *Eur. J. Obstet, Gynecol. Reprod. Biol.*, **33**, 141–6.

Potter, E. L. (1943). Universal oedema of the fetus unassociated with erythroblastosis. *Am. J. Obstet, Gynecol.*, **46**, 130–4.

Pretorius, D. H., Davis, K., Manco-Johnson, M. L., Manchester, D., Meier, P. R., and Clewell, W. H. (1985). Clinical course of fetal hydrocephalus: 40 cases. *AJR*, **144**, 827–31.

Quan, L. and Smith, D. W. (1973). The VATER association, Vertebral defects, Anal atresia, T–E fistula with oesophageal atresia, Radial and Renal dysplasia. *J. Paediatr.*, **82**, 104.

RCOG Study Group (1990). *The antenatal diagnosis of fetal abnormalities.* (ed. J. O. Drife and D, Donnai). Springer Verlag, London.

Redford, D. H. A., Mcnay, M. B., Ferguson-Smith, M. E., and Jamieson, M. E. (1984). Aneuploidy and cystic hygroma detectable by ultrasound. *Prenat. Diagn.*, **4**, 377–82.

Reuss, A., Pijpers, L., Schampers, P. T. F. M., Wladimiroff, J. W., and Sachs, E. S. (1987*a*). The importance of chorionic villus sampling after first trimester diagnosis of cystic hygroma. *Prenat. Diagn.*, **7**, 299–301.

Reuss, A., Pijpers, L., van Swaaij, E., Jahoda, M. G. J., and Wladimiroff, J. W. (1987b). First-trimester diagnosis of recurrence of cystic hygroma using a transvaginal ultrasound transducer. Case report. *Eur. J. Obstet. Gynecol. Reprod. Biol.*, **26**, 271–3.

Reuss, A., Wladimiroff, J. W., Stewart, P. A., and Scholtmeijer, R. J. (1988). Non-invasive management of fetal obstructive uropathy. *Lancet*, **ii**, 949–51.

Ricketts, N. E. M., Lowe, E. M., and Patel N. B. (1987). Prenatal diagnosis of choroid plexus cysts. *Lancet*, **i**, 213–14.

Rizzo, N., Gabrielli, S., Pilu, G., Perolo, A., Cacciari, A., Domini, R., *et al.* (1987). Prenatal diagnosis and obstetrical management of multicystic dysplastic kidney disease. *Prenat. Diagn.*, **7**, 109–118.

Rizzo, N., Pitalis, M. C., Pilu, G., Orsini, L. F., Perolo, A., and Bovicelli, L. (1990). Prenatal karyotyping in malformed fetuses. *Prenat. Diagn.*, **10**, 17–23.

Saltzman, D. H., Benacerraf, B. R., and Frigoletto, F. D. (1986). Diagnosis and management of fetal facial clefts. *Am. J. Obstet. Gynecol.*, **155**, 377–9.

Serlo, W., Kirkinen, P., Jouppila, P., and Herva, R. (1986). Prognostic signs of fetal hydrocephalus. *Childs Nerv. Syst.*, **2**, 93–7.

Sermer, M., Benzie, R. J., Pitson, L., Carr, M. and Skidmore, M. (1987). Prenatal diagnosis and management of congenital defects of the anterior abdominal wall. *Am. J. Obstet. Gynecol*, **156**, 308–12.

Shah, Y. G., Eckl, C. J. Stinson, S. K., and Woods, J. R. (1990*a*). Biparietal diameter/femur length ratio, cephalic index, and femur length measurements: not reliable screening techniques for Down syndrome. *Obstet. Gynecol.*, **75**, 186–8.

Shah, D. M., Roussis, P., Ulm, J., Jeanty, P. and Boehm, F. H. (1990b). Cordocentesis for rapid karyotyping. *Am. J. Obstet. Gynecol.*, **162**, 1548–50.

Snijders, R. J. M., Sherrod, C., Gosden, C. M., and Nicolaides, K. H. Severe fetal growth retardation: associated malformations and chromosomal abnormalities. *Am. J. Obstet. Gynecol.* (submittcd).

Stoll, C., Alembik, Y., Roth, M. P., Dott, B., and Sauvage, P. (1990). Risk factors in internal urinary system malformations. *Pediatr. Nephrol.*, **4**, 319–23.

Tannirandorn, Y., Nicolini, U., Nicolaidis, P., Fisk, N. M., Arulkumaran, S., and Rodeck, C. H. (1990). Fetal cystic hygromata: insights gained from fetal blood sampling. *Prenat. Diagn.*, **10**, 189–93.

Thorpe-Beeston, G., Gosden, C. M., and Nicolaides, K. H. (1989) Congenital diaphragmatic hernia: associated malformations and chromosomal defects. *Fetal Ther.*, **4**, 21–8.

Thorpe-Beeston, G., Gosden, C. M., and Nicolaides, K. H. (1990). Choroid plexus cysts and chromosomal defects. *Brit. J. Radiol*, **63**, 783–6.

Touloukian, R. J. (1978). Intestinal atresia. *Clin. Perinatol.*, **5**, 3–18.

Turkel, S. B. (1982). Conditions associated with non-immune hydrops fetalis. *Clin. Perinatol.*, **9**, 613–25.

Vintzileos, A. M., Campbell, W. A., Weinbaum, P. J., and Nochimson, D. J. (1987). Perinatal management and outcome of fetal ventriculomegaly. *Obstet. Gynecol.*, **69**, 5–11.

Van den Hof, M. C., Nicolaides, K. H., Campbell, J., and Campbell, S. (1990). Evaluation of the lemon and banana signs in one hundred thirty fetuses with open spina bifida. *Am. J. Obstet. Gynecol.*, **162**, 322–7.

Van Geijn, E. J., van Vugt, Sollie, J. E., and van Geijn, H. P. Ultrasonographic diagnosis and perinatal management of fetal abdominal wall defects. *Fetal Diagn. Ther.*, **6**, 2–10.

Wald, N. J., Cuckle, N. S., Densem, J. W., *et al.* (1988). Maternal serum screening for Down's syndrome in early pregnancy. *Brit. Med. J.*, **276**, 883–7.

4
The fetal lung
David A. Nyberg

Introduction

The fetal lung is not evaluated as a specific organ system during routine prenatal sonography. Nevertheless, the lung is invariably included on views of the fetal heart, so that potentially important information regrading it can be obtained during standard obstetric sonography. The number of published studies and case reports attests to the fact that a variety of lung abnormalities can now be identified with prenatal sonography.

In the following chapter, normal and abnormal development of the fetal lung are reviewed. Prenatal sonographic findings are emphasized, with particular emphasis placed on recent advances in our understanding of fetal lung abnormalities. Because fetal lung abnormalities are encountered infrequently at any one centre, this discussion is based on the accumulative experience of available literature.

Normal lung development and function

Development of the bronchial tree can be categorized into four overlapping stages with a gradual transition from one stage to the next (Bucher and Reid 1961):

(1) the embryonic period (conception until the fifth week)

(2) the pseudoglandular period (5–17 weeks)

(3) the cannicular phase (17–24 weeks)

(4) the alveolar phase (24 weeks to term).

Alveoli continue to develop even after birth, increasing in number until at least eight years of age, and increasing in size with growth of the chest wall.

Lung maturity, defined as the ability to sustain independent respiratory function after birth, depends on a number of factors including lung development, growth, and the development of normal surfactant lining the alveoli. Sonographic determination of gestational age based on a first-trimester sonogram is perhaps the most useful finding in predicting lung maturity, since the lungs are usually mature at 36 weeks and can be confidently considered mature at 38 weeks. Although the echo pattern of the lung varies with gestational age, clinically this has not proven to be useful for predicting lung maturity (Fried *et al.* 1985). In addition, no other sonographic finding has proved useful in reliably predicting lung maturity *in utero*.

Fluid motion can be identified within the trachea or through the nose with colour flow Doppler or duplex Doppler (Utsu *et al.* 1983; Chiba *et al.* 1985; Birnholz 1990). Normal blood flow within the pulmonary vessels can also be demonstrated with sensitive colour flow Doppler systems (Emerson *et al.* 1990). However, the clinical significance of these observations has not yet been realized.

The lungs are known to be important sites of both amniotic fluid production and resorption. Polyhydramnios and hydrops are also common complications of lung abnormalities (Hilpert and Pretorius 1990). Compression of the systemic veins, mediastinum, and oesophagus are commonly cited as causative factors, although it seems more likely the polyhydramnios develops from alterations in normal fluid dynamics. Development of polyhydramnios could result from either inhibition of fluid resorption or increased fluid production. Increased 'leakiness' would help to explain the occasional association of elevated maternal serum alpha-fetoprotein (MS-AFP) levels with various lung masses

Lung abnormalities

A variety of lung abnormalities can be detected with prenatal sonography (Table 4.1) (Hilpert and Pretorius 1990). The most common abnormalities identified sonographically include hydrothorax, diaphragmatic hernia, cystic adenomatoid malformation of the lung (CAML), sequestration, and bronchogenic or duplication cysts. Uncommon lung and thoracic masses that can be identified include neuroblastoma, vascular malformations, hamartoma, haemangioma, and lymphangioma. Pulmonary hypoplasia can also be assessed, usually in the setting of oligohydramnios.

Table 4.1   Major aetiologies for an intra-thoracic mass

1. Diaphragmatic hernia or eventration
2. Cystic adenomatoid malformation
3. Bronchopulmonary sequestration
4. Bronchogenic cyst or duplication cyst
5. Bronchial, laryngeal atresia
6. Pericardial teratoma
7. Chest wall hamartoma
8. Neuroblastoma

Selected specific abnormalities are discussed in the following sections. A discussion of spontaneously resolving thoracic masses is also presented at the end of this chapter.

Pulmonary hypoplasia

Pulmonary hypoplasia has been defined as an absolute decrease in lung volume and weight for gestational age or as a decreased ratio of lung-weight to body-weight. It occurs in 1.4 per cent of all live births and 6.7 per cent of all stillbirths. The severity of pulmonary hypoplasia depends upon the gestational age at onset, duration of the inciting conditions, and severity of the insult.

Factors contributing to normal lung growth are:

(1) adequate intrathoracic space to allow pulmonary parenchymal growth and development

(2) adequate intrauterine space (sufficient amniotic fluid) to allow thoracic growth and motion

(3) normal balance of fluid volume and pressure within the trachea and airspaces

(4) normal fetal breathing movements.

Abnormalities of any of these factors may result in pulmonary hypoplasia.

Sonographic evaluation of pulmonary hypoplasia is most commonly assessed in the setting of severe oligohydramnios, or in association with certain disorders, such as short-limb skeletal dysplasias. A thoracic circumference less than the 5th percentile or an abnormal ratio relating thoracic circumference to another biometric parameter can suggest pulmonary hypoplasia (Johnson *et al.* 1987; Songster *et al.* 1989; Vintzileos 1989). Unfortunately, measurements of the thorax are of little use when a pleural effusion or other intrathoracic mass is present. For example, diaphragmatic hernia is invariably associated with some degree of pulmonary hypoplasia, even though the thoracic measurement is either normal, or large.

In an effort to define normal lung size and better identify pulmonary hypoplasia, some authors have recently defined normal lung size by direct measurement of the lung itself. Decreased lung length (Roberts and Mitchell 1990) has been found to correlate with pulmonary hypoplasia, but can be difficult to determine because overlying ribs often obscure the upper lung. Others (Musa *et al.* 1990) have measured the lung circumference and diameter at the level of the heart. However, this measurement is also difficult due to the complex lung shape. Determination of lung volume might be helpful, but such calculations are very complex and so are impractical.

A possible role for therapeutic amniofusion has been suggested in an attempt to prevent lethal pulmonary hypoplasia among pregnancies presenting with oligohydramnios (Fisk *et al.* 1991). Fisk *et al.* (1991) reported some degree of pulmonary hypoplasia in only two of nine pregnancies (22 per cent) complicated by severe oligohydramnios and treated before 22 weeks, compared with 60 per cent of pregnancies treated at 28 weeks. However, only a small number of patients could potentially benefit from this treatment.

Hydrothorax

Hydrothorax (pleural effusion) may result from various causes. Excluding hydrops, the most common cause of pleural effusion (hydrothorax) is chylothorax. Hydrothorax may also accompany any thoracic masses such as sequestration (Thomas *et al.* 1986; Hernanz-Schulman *et al.* 1991) or cardiac tumours and these should be excluded.

Chylothorax probably results from a malformation of, or a rent in, the fetal thoracic duct. Because of the anatomical course of the thoracic duct, leakage from the lower portion more often results in a right pleural effusion, and leakage from the upper portion produces a left pleural effusion. Chylothorax may occur as an isolated finding, but can also be seen in a variety of syndromes including trisomy 21 (Fig. 4.1), monosomy X (Turner syndrome), trisomy 13, and syndromes involving lymphatic or vascular abnormalities (Hilpert and Pretorius 1990; Petrikovsky *et al.* 1991). Right pleural effusion may also be the primary clue to right diaphragmatic hernia (Gilsanz *et al.* 1986).

Prior to oral milk feeding, the fluid appears clear and colorless due to the absence of chylomicrons. Lipoprotein electrophoresis of pleural fluid obtained by fetal thoracentesis may show typical predominance of high density lipo-protein and allow a confident diagnosis of chylothorax *in utero* (Benacerraf *et al.* 1986). Pleural fluid lymphocyte counts alone have been reported to be unreliable in establishing the diagnosis of chylothorax *in utero* (Eddleman *et al.* 1991).

Hydrothorax of any cause has an overall perinatal mortality of more than 50 per cent, with a higher mortality rate in fetuses who have hydrops than in fetuses for whom the effusion is an isolated finding. The outcome of a fetus with an abnormal pleural fluid collection depends upon the underlying cause of the effusion and the degree of associated pulmonary hypoplasia.

Prenatal thoracentesis or the placement of indwelling pleuro-amniotic catheters (Rodeck *et al.* 1988) has been advocated for treatment of large pleural effusions. Drainage of the fetal thorax can occasionally reverse polyhydramnios and hydrops (Longaker *et al.* 1989). However, other authorities (Pijpers *et al.* 1989) advocate conservative management with monitoring alone. If interven-tional procedures are considered, the karyotype should be determined and a thorough sonographic examination should be performed.

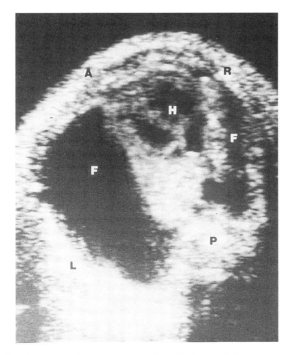

Fig. 4.1. Hydrothorax and trisomy 21. Axial view of the thorax at 31 weeks shows a large left pleural effusion and a smaller right pleural effusion. Serial thoracentesis were performed *in utero*. The fetus proved to have trisomy 21 (Down syndrome) after birth. F, pleural effusion; H, heart; A, anterior; P, posterior; L, left; R, right. (Reprinted with permission from Hilpert P. L. and Pretorius D. H., 1990.)

Diaphragmatic hernia

Congenital diaphragmatic hernia (CDH) occurs in approximately one in 2000–3000 births. CDH occurs as a sporadic malformation, although CDH is a prominent feature of some inheritable syndromes (Norio *et al.* 1984; Bocian *et al.* 1986). Bochladek hernias comprise more than 90 per cent of all diaphragmatic abnormalities affecting the fetus. It characteristically occurs posterolaterally and on the left side.

Concurrent anomalies and the degree of pulmonary hypoplasia correlate directly with the outcome (Benjamin *et al.* 1988). The overall mortality rate of CDH detected prenatally is approximately 75 per cent. This decreases to 66 per cent when CDH is an isolated anomaly, but increases to 93 per cent when additional anomalies are present. The protean clinical manifestations of CDH reflect variations in associated structural or chromosomal abnormalities and in the size, location, and chronicity of the mass effect.

Sonographically, CDH is suspected when the stomach, liver, or bowel are found in the thorax (Fig. 4.2). Typically, the stomach is identified in the left thorax and there is a secondary mediastinal shift. Compression of the left ventricle and left atrium may be demonstrated from the adjacent mass effect (Fig. 4.2). This should not be interpreted as a structural cardiac anomaly, although it may be a poor prognostic factor due to the significant mass effect.

Eventration may be difficult to distinguish from diaphragmatic hernia (Seeds *et al.* 1984; Jurcak-Zaleski *et al.* 1990; Thiagarajah *et al.* 1990), but can be

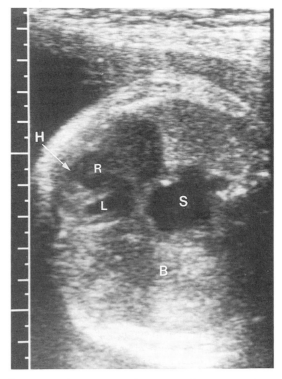

Fig. 4.2. Diaphragmatic hernia. Axial view of the thorax shows a large mass effect in the left hemithorax with secondary displacement of the heart (H) to the right. The stomach (S) is seen as a fluid-filled structure posterior and to the left of the heart. The remainder of the left hemithorax is occupied by bowel (B) which has a similar echo pattern to lung. Note relative hypoplasia of the left cardiac ventricle (L) compared to the right ventricle (R) from the mass effect. Following delivery, the infant died despite surgical correction of the defect.

suggested by visualizing the diaphragm superior to a mass near the base of the lungs.

Detection of additional anomalies carries a poor outcome in fetuses with diaphragmatic hernia. Other sonographic indicators (Adzick *et al.* 1985a; Harrison *et al.* 1985) of a poor prognosis include:

(1) marked mediastinal shift;

(2) presence of the liver within the thorax

(3) intrauterine growth retardation

(4) polyhydramnios

(5) hydrops fetalis

(6) detection prior to 25 weeks.

Despite the number of potential prognostic findings, prediction of outcome in an individual fetus with diaphragmatic hernia should be approached cautiously.

In a postnatal series (Burge *et al.* 1989), demonstration of the stomach within the thorax has been associated with a worse outcome than have diaphragmatic hernias without stomach displacement. However, this observation carries little significance for prenatal sonography since most affected fetuses are recognized precisely because the stomach is displaced into the thorax.

A major problem contributing to neonatal mortality is the development of pulmonary hypertension due to vasconstriction, typically after a 'honeymoon' period of 12–48 hours. Factors contributing to pulmonary hypertension include hypoxia, hypercarbia, acidosis, and possibly altered respiratory mechanics following repair of the defect (Molenaar *et al.* 1991).

Early surgical repair has traditionally been employed in infants identified with CDH. However, this approach does not help the pre-existing pulmonary hypoplasia and associated pulmonary hypertension. A number of investigators have now found that delayed repair of CDH after medical stabilization results in similar survival rates as immediate repair (Breaux 1991; Langer *et al.* 1988). Postponing surgical repair of CDH until resolution of the pulmonary hypertension may even improve the survival rate (Haugen *et al.* 1991).

Prenatal correction of diaphragmatic hernia has generated interest (Harrison *et al.* 1990). This approach may be most appropriate in fetuses identified with CDH before 24 weeks since the prognosis is known to be poor in this group, and surgical repair at this time has the greatest potential to circumvent development of pulmonary hypoplasia. Prenatal sonography can monitor the effect of surgical correction *in utero* (Fig. 4.3).

Extracorporeal Membrane Oxygenation (ECMO) has been used to treat a variety of respiratory conditions in the neonatal period. By circumventing the infants own pulmonary circulation, ECMO helps to reverse the vicious cycle of pulmonary hypertension and iatrogenic lung damage in infants who can

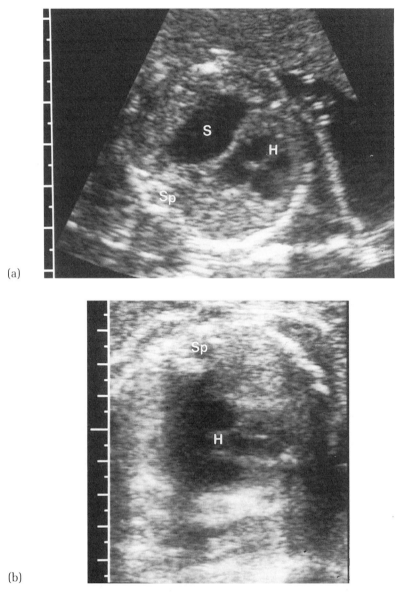

(a)

(b)

Fig. 4.3. Diaphragmatic hernia, repaired *in utero*. (a) Axial view of the thorax at 24 weeks shows characteristic findings of diaphragmatic hernia with the fluid-filled stomach (S) in the left thorax and displacement of heart (H) to the right thorax. Sp, spine. (b) Following *in utero* surgical repair of the hernia the patient is seen on follow up at 34 weeks. There is no mass effect and the heart (H) is seen in its normal position. An echogenic patch was identified at the level of the diaphragm. This fetus was the second successful case of diaphragmatic hernia corrected *in utero* as reported by the San Francisco surgical group (Harrison *et al.* 1990). Sp, spine.

subsequently sustain respiratory function. The overall survival rate using ECMO is 60 per cent (Newman *et al.* 1990; O'Rourke 1991).

Cystic adenomatoid malformation

Cystic adenomatoid malformation of the lung (CAML) is thought to result from arrested cellular development at an early stage. Proliferation of polypoid glandular tissue without normal alveolar differentiation produces the 'adenomatoid' histology.

Three subtypes have been defined based upon clinical gross and histological features (Stocker *et al.* 1977). Type I CAML may produce either a single cyst or, more commonly, multiple large cysts (>2 cm) within the hemithorax (Fig. 4.4). These cysts often involve an entire pulmonary lobe. The multiple large cysts distinguish this entity from a bronchogenic cyst which is typically small, solitary, and near the midline. Macrocystic type II CAML creates a mass with small cysts (Fig. 4.5). A confident distinction from other types of hemithoracic masses may be difficult. Microcystic type III CAML produces a homogeneously echogenic mass without discernible individual cysts. The echogenic mass may closely resemble pulmonary sequestration or intrathoracic bowel from a diaphragmatic hernia.

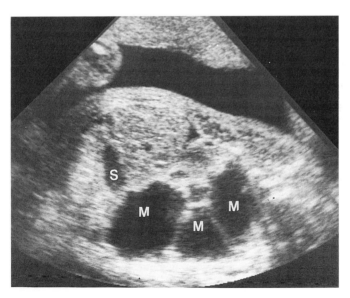

Fig. 4.4. Cystic adenomatoid malformation, type I. Longitudinal view shows a large cystic mass (M) occupying the left hemithorax. The mass was mistaken for a diaphragmatic hernia at a referring facility. However, the left hemidiaphragm is displaced inferiorly and the stomach (S) is seen beneath the diaphgragm.

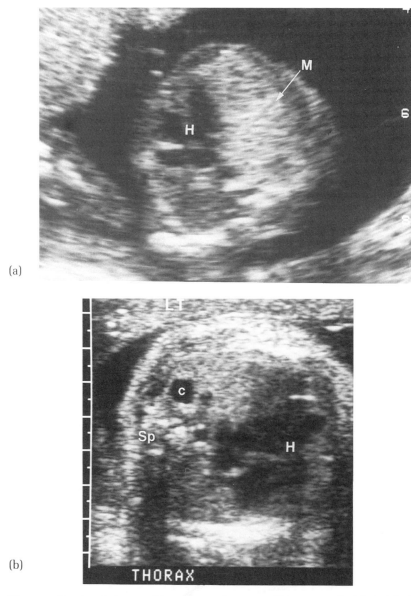

(a)

(b)

Fig. 4.5. Cystic adenomatoid malformation, type II (presumed). (a) Axial view of the thorax at 21 weeks shows an echogenic mass (M) occupying the left hemithorax and causing marked displacement the heart (H) to the right. (b) Follow up sonogram 10 weeks later shows significant less mass effect although a small cystic area (c) is identified in the left lung base. The heart (H) is now in its normal position. Serial scans showed nearly complete resolution of the mass by the time of delivery. Sp, spine; LT, left.

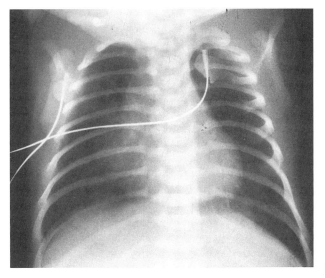

(c)

Fig. 4.5. Cystic adenomatoid malformation, type II (presumed). (c) Postnatal chest radiograph shows no evidence of mass. However, a CT scan showed a small mass at the left lung base. The infant remains asymptomatic at 9 months of age.

The earliest reported case of CAML has been at 20 weeks' gestation. Polyhydramnios has been observed in two-thirds of prenatal cases (Adzick *et al.* 1985*b*). Some masses may be associated with elevated levels of maternal serum alpha-fetoprotein, presumably due to leaking of the protein across the alveolar membrane (Petit *et al.* 1987; Albright and Katz 1989; Johnston *et al.* 1988).

The presence of hydrops carries a poor prognosis; all fetuses with CAML and hydrops detected prenatally have died or were electively terminated. CAML may occasionally improve or resolve spontaneously *in utero*. Type III CAML has a poor prognosis with reports of only a few surviving fetuses (Neilson *et al.* 1991).

Bronchopulmonary sequestration

Bronchopulmonary sequestration is a congenital pulmonary malformation in which a portion of the bronchopulmonary mass is separated from the normal bronchial system. Sequestration is closely related to CAML and other foregut anomalies, both developmentally and histologically (Morin *et al.* 1989).

Bronchopulmonary sequestration is subcategorized into intralobar and extralobar types based upon the pleural covering. Both types occur most often in the lower lobes, particularly the posterior basal segments. Intralobar sequestration occurs with equal frequency on the right and left sides, whereas 80 per cent of extralobar sequestrations occur in the left hemithorax. Approximately 5 per cent of sequestrations occur below the diaphragm. Males and females are affected with equal frequency.

Associated anomalies are found in approximately 60 per cent of fetuses with extralobar sequestration and 14 per cent of fetuses with intralobar sequestration. Hydrops and pleural effusion may complicate extralobar sequestration.

Sonographically, sequestration typically produces a well-defined, homogeneous, highly echogenic mass (Maulik 1987). The solid mass of bronchopulmonary sequestration may closely resemble other echogenic masses, especially CAML type III. Because sequestration may also contain cysts, the sonographic appearance may also resemble cystic forms of CAML (types I and II).

Hydrothorax may dominate some cases of extralobar sequestration (Thomas *et al.* 1986). Hernanz-Schulman *et al.* (1991) suggest that the fluid develops from torsion of the sequestered segment with occlusion of the efferent venous and lymphatic channels.

Recognition of a vascular bundle supplying a lung mass may be an important clue to lung sequestration. Sauerbrei (1991) diagnosed a fetus with lung sequestration at 19 weeks using Duplex Doppler. Arterial flow was demonstrated from the abdomen into the mass and venous flow in the opposite direction towards the abdomen. Similar observations have been made on postnatal sonography of sequestration (Kaude and Laurin 1984; West *et al.* 1989; Hernanz-Schulman *et al.* 1991). These features are considered to be diagnostic of sequestration.

Extrathoracic extralobar sequestration typically produces a well-defined mass above the kidneys (Mariona *et al.* 1986; Weinbaum 1989; Stern *et al.* 1990); this can be mistaken for neuroblastoma or other tumour. Biopsy of the mass can establish the correct diagnosis (Davies *et al.* 1989).

Other masses

Bronchogenic cysts result from abnormal budding of the ventral foregut diverticulum between 26 and 40 days of embryogenesis. Typically, the cyst does not communicate with the tracheobronchial tree and is an incidental radiographical finding during childhood.

Bronchogenic cysts have been diagnosed prenatally as a small (1.5–2.5 cm), well-defined, unilocular intrathoracic cystic lesion adjacent to the mediastinum (Newnham *et al.* 1984; Lebrun *et al.* 1985). They may be associated with elevated maternal serum alpha-fetoprotein level, or other anomalies (Albright *et al.* 1988). Bronchogenic cysts may also produce obstruction of the adjacent bronchus (Young *et al.* 1989). Other lung masses include duplication or neurenteric cysts.

Neuroblastoma has been reported prenatally at 37 weeks in one fetus (De Filippi *et al.* 1986). The mass showed an echogenic margin and a more hypoechoic centre. Slight posterior shadowing was noted.

Airway obstruction

Airway obstruction *in utero* produces accumulation of fluid and accelerated lung development in both experimental and natural conditions (Wigglesorth *et al.* 1987; Silver *et al.* 1988; Wigglesworth and Desai 1979; Didier *et al.* 1990). In the fetal rabbit, tracheal ligation has been shown to prevent the lung hypoplasia that normally follows cervical cord transection. Human fetuses with both laryngeal atresia and renal agenesis show a marked increase in lung volume and hyperplasia and polyhydramnios, even though renal agenesis would be expected to cause pulmonary hypoplasia and oligohydramnios.

Various forms of airway atresia have been diagnosed by prenatal sonography. Bronchial atresia has been detected as an echogenic mass involving one lung (McAlister *et al.* 1987). Laryngeal atresia has been described as showing markedly enlarged echogenic lungs that compressed the central mediastinum and heart (Arizawa *et al.* 1989; Watson *et al.* 1990). Both cases reported prenatally have been associated with hydrops. In one case, the patient had a normal ultrasound examination at 18 weeks, but developed echogenic lungs and ascites at 22 weeks. Anechoic areas were present representing dilated mucus-filled bronchi.

Siffring *et al.* (1989) described a case of bronchopulmonary foregut malformation the produced obstruction of the affected bronchial segment. The obstructed lung segment appeared as a large echogenic mass in the right hemithorax. The bronchus was remarkable in that the epithelium was respiratory, but the underlying structure was alimentary. These histological findings were considered characteristic of a bronchopulmonary foregut malformation.

Spontaneous resolution of lung masses

Some lung masses may resolve spontaneously without apparent clinical sequelae (Figs 4.5 and 4.6). Resolution of hydrops or ascites in association with lung masses has also been demonstrated (Meizner *et al.* 1990). It is important to consider these observations when counselling women suspected of carrying a fetus with a lung abnormality, since even large masses have been observed to resolve on serial examinations.

Spontaneous resolution of fetal lung masses appears most likely when the mass appears solid and echogenic; nearly all reported cases have shown this pattern. Some of the masses have represented CAML (Saltzman *et al.* 1988; Fine *et al.* 1988), whereas in other cases the aetiology of the mass has remained

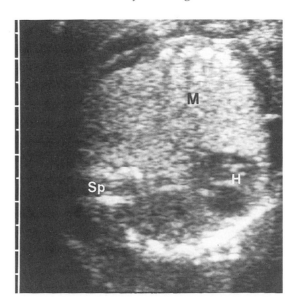

Fig. 4.6. Resolution of lung mass. Axial view of the thorax at 30 weeks shows a large echogenic mass (M) occupying the left hemithorax and displacing the heart (H) to the right. Compare the echogenic left lung to the right lung. Serial scans showed progressive resolution of the mass by 36 weeks. The infant was asymptomatic and the chest radiograph was normal at birth. Sp, spine.

undocumented (Sonek *et al.* 1991). Obtaining adequate follow-up after birth in such cases may be very difficult, especially when the infant is asymptomatic and the chest radiograph is nearly normal.

Although the explanation for resolving lung masses remains speculative at this time, available information suggests to this author that the masses may represent obstructed lung segments. Improvement in obstruction could then cause resolution of the 'mass'. The cause for the obstruction can then be categorized as: 1. intrinsic to the bronchi, 2. a transient obstruction, or 3. extrinsic to the bronchi.

In the case of an intrinsic bronchial obstruction, one can suggest that an atretic or hypoplastic bronchial branch would cause distal obstruction. Broncho-pulmonary foregut duplication might be present, as exhibited in the case of Siffring *et al.* (1989). Expansion of the adjacent normal lung and progressive collapse of the affected segment would result in normal aeration and a normal chest radiograph after delivery. Documentation of an atretic or hypoplastic bronchus would then be very difficult without bronchoscopy or bronchography.

In the case of transient bronchial obstruction, one must speculate that a plug of mucus could cause a transient obstruction. As the bronchi enlarge, the mass would cause incomplete obstruction and eventually dislodge. Some credence for the possibility of mucous plug obstruction *in utero* comes from an observation of transient segmental echogenic lung in a fetus who eventually proved to have cystic fibrosis (Dr James Crane, St Louis, MO, personal communication).

In the case of extrinsic obstruction, transient bronchial obstruction might result from a small but critically placed mass near the bronchus. The obstruction might then resolve as the bronchus enlarges and strengthens. This appears to be the operative mechanism in a fetus reported by Young *et al.* (1989), this fetus had a small cyst near the hilum with secondary obstruction of the lung. This mechanism would also help to explain the apparent improvement in the mass effect of some fetuses with CAML diagnosed prenatally (Saltzman *et al.* 1988; Fine *et al.* 1988).

Summary

Sonography is important in the evaluation of lung masses, hydrothorax, and suspected pulmonary hypoplasia. Prenatal sonography can not only detect these abnormalities, but also provide important prognostic information regarding them.

References

Adzick, N. S., Harrison, M. R., Glick, P. L., Nakayama, D. K., Manning, F. A., and deLorimier, A. A. (1985*a*). Diaphragmatic hernia in the fetus: Prenatal diagnosis and outcome in 94 cases. *J. Pediatr. Surg*, **20**, 357–61.

Adzick, N. S., Harrison, M. R., Glick, P. L., *et al.* (1985*b*). Fetal cystic adenomatoid malformation: prenatal diagnosis and natural history. *J. Pediatr. Surg.* **20**, 483–8.

Albright, E. B., Crane, J. P. and Shackelford, G. D. (1988). Prenatal diagnosis of a bronchogenic cyst. *J. Ultrasound Med*, **7**, 90–5.

Albright, S. G. and Katz, V. L. (1989). Alpha fetoprotein findings in a cases of cystic adenomatoid malformation of the lung. *Clin. Genet.*, **35**, 75–6.

Arizawa, M., Imai, S., Suehara, N. and Nakayama, M. (1989). Prenatal diagnosis of laryngeal atresia (Translation). *Nippon Sanka Fijinka Gakkai Zasshi*, **41**, 907–10.

Benacerraf, B. R., Frigoletto, F. D. Jr, and Wilson, M. (1986). Successful midtrimester thoracentesis with analysis of the lymphocyte population in the pleural effusion. *Am. J. Obstet. Gynecol.*, **155**, 398–9.

Benjamin, D. R., Juul, S., and Siebert, J. R. (1988). Congenital posterolateral diaphragmatic hernia: Associated malformations. *J. Pediatr. Surg.*, **23**(10), 899–903.

Birnholz, J. C. (1990). Fetal nose breathing patterns. Presented to the 35th Annual Convention of the American Institute of Ultrasound in Medicine. *J. Ultrasound Med*, **10**, s19.

Bocian, M., Spence, M. A., Marazita, M. L. *et al.* (1986). Familial diaphragmatic defects: early prenatal diagnosis and evidence for major gene inheritance. *Am. J. Med. Genet.* (Suppl.), **2**, 163–76.

Breaux, C. W. Jr, Rouse, T. M., Cain, W. S., and Georgeson K. E. (1991). Improvement in survival of patients with congenital diaphragmatic hernia utilizing a strategy of delayed repair after medical and/or extracorporeal membrane oxygenation stabilization. *J. Pediatr. Surg*, **26**(3), 333–8.

Bucher, U. and Reid, L. (1961). Development of the intrasegmental bronchial tree: the pattern of branching and development of cartilage at various stages of intra-uterine life. *Thorax*, **16**, 207–18.

Burge, D. M., Atwell, J. D., and Freeman, N. V. (1989). Could the stomach site help predict outcome in babies with left sided congenital diaphragmatic hernia diagnosed antenatally? *J. Pediatr. Surg.*, **24**, 567–9.

Chiba,Y., Utsu, M., Kanzaki, T. *et al.* (1985). Changes in venous flow and intratracheal flow in fetal breathing movements. *Ultrasound Med. Biol.*, **11**, 43–9.

Davies, R. P., Ford W. D., Lequesne, G. W. *et al.* (1989). Ultrasonic detection of subdiaphragmatic pulmonary sequestration *in utero* and postnatal diagnosis by fine needle aspiration biopsy. *J. Ultrasound med.*, **8**, 47–9.

De Filippi, G., Canestri, G., Bosio, U., *et al.* (1986). Thoracic neuroblastoma: antenatal demonstration in a case with unusual postnatal radiographic findings. *Br. J. Radiology*, **59**, 704–6.

Didier, F., Droulle, R., and Marchal, C. (1990). Apropos of prenatal screening of tracheal and laryngeal atresia (letter) *Arch. Fr. Pediatr*, **47**(5), 396–7.

Eddleman, K. A., Levine, A. B., Chitkara, U., and Berkowitz, R. L. (1991). Reliability of pleural fluid lymphocyte counts in the antenatal diagnosis of congenital chylothorax. *Obstet. Gynecol.*, **78**, 530–2.

Emerson, D. S., Cartier, M. S., DeVore, G. R., Altieri, L. A., Felker, R. E., and Smith, W. C. (1990). Distal pulmonary artery branches in the fetus: new observations with color flow and pulsed Doppler. Presented to the 35th Annual Convention of the American Institute of Ultrasound in Medicine. *J. Ultrasound Med.*, **10**, s19.

Fine, C., Adzick, N. S., and Doubilet, P. M. (1988). Decreasing size of congenital cystic adenomatoid malformation *in utero*. *J. Ultrasound Med*, **7**, 405–8.

Fisk, N. M., Ronderos-Dumit, D., Soliani A. *et al.* (1991). Diagnostic and therapeutic transabdominal amnioinfusion in oligohydramnios. *Obstet. Gynecol*, **78**, 270–8.

Fried, A. M., Loh, F. K., Umer, M. A., *et al.* (1985). Echogenicity of fetal lung: relation to fetal age and maturity. *American Journal of Roengenology*, **145**, 591–4.

Gilsanz, V., Emons, D., Hansmann, M., *et al.* (1986). Hydrothorax, ascites, and right diaphragmatic hernia. *Radiology*, **158**, 243–6.

Harrison, M. R., Adzick, N. S., Nakayama, D. K., and deLorimier, A. A. (1985). Fetal diaphragmatic hernia: fatal but fixable. *Seminars Perinatol*, **9**(2), 103–12.

Harrison, M. R., Adzick, N. S., Longaker, M. T., *et al.* (1990). Successful repair *in utero* of a fetal diaphragmatic hernia after removal of herniated viscera from the left thorax. *N. Engl. J. Med.*, **322**(22), 1582–4.

Haugen, S. E., Linde, D., Eik-Nes, S.. *et al.* (1991). Congenital diaphragmatic hernia: determination of the optimal time for operation by echocardiographic monitoring of the pulmonary arterial pressure. *J. Pediatr. Surg.*, **26**(5), 560–2.

Hernanz-Schulman, M., Stein, S., Neblett, W. W., *et al.* (1991). Pulmonary sequestration: diagnosis with color Doppler sonography and a new theory of associated hydrothorax. *Radiology*, **180**, 817–21.

Hilpert, P. L. and Pretorius, D. H. (1990). The thorax. In *Diagnostic Ultrasound of Fetal Anomalies*, ed. D. A. Nyberg, B. S. Mahony and D. H. Pretorius pp. 262–99, Year Book Publishers, Chicago.

Johnson, A., Callan, N. A., Bhutani, V. K., Colmorgen, G. H. C., Weiner, S., and Bolognese R. J. (1987). Ultrasonic ratio of fetal thoracic to abdominal circumference: An association with fetal pulmonary hypoplasia. *Am. J. Obstet. Gynecol.*, **157**, 764–9.

Johnston, R. J., McGahan, J. P., Hanson, F. W. *et al.* (1988). Type III congenital cystic adenomatoid malformation associated with elevated maternal serum alpha fetoprotein. *J. Perinatol.*, **8**, 222–4.

Jurcak-Zaleski, S., Comstock, C. H. and Kirk, J. S. (1990). Eventration of the diaphragm. *J. Ultrasound Med.*, **9**, 351–4.

Kaude, J. V. and Laurin, S. (1984). Ultrasonographic demonstration of systemic artery feeding extrapulmonary sequestration. *Pediatr. Radiol.*, **14**, 226–7.

Langer, J. C., Filler, R. M., Bohn, D. J., *et al.* (1988). Timing of surgery for congenital diaphgragmatic hernia: Is emergency operation necessary? *J. Pediatr. Surg.*, **23**, 731–4.

Lebrun, D., Avni, E. F., Goolaerts, J. P., *et al.* (1985). Prenatal diagnosis of a pulmonary cyst by ultrasonography. *Eur. J. Pediatr.*, **144**, 399–402.

Longaker, M. T., Laberge, J. M., Dansereau, J., *et al.* (1989). Primary fetal hydrothorax: Nautral history and management. *J. Pediatr. Surg.*, **24**, 573–6.

McAlister, W. H., Wright, J. R., and Crane, J. P. (1987). Main stem bronchial atresia: intrauterine sonographic diagnosis. *American Journal of Roentgenology*, **148**, 364–6

Mariona, F., McAlpin, G., Zador, I., *et al.* (1986). Sonographic detection of fetal extrathoracic pulmonary sequestration. *J. Ultrasound Med.*, **5**, 283–5.

Maulik, D., Robinson, L., Dailey, D. K., *et al.* (1987). Prenatal sonographic depiction of intralobar pulmonary sequestration. *J. Ultrasound Med.*, **6**, 703–6.

Meizner, I., Carmi, R., Mares, A. J., *et al.* (1990). Spontaneous resolution of isolated fetal ascites associated with extralobar lung sequestration *J. Clin Ultrasound*, **18**, 57–60.

Molenaar, J. C., Bos, A. P., Hazebroek, F. W. J., and Tibboel, D. (1991). Congenital diaphragmatic hernia, what defect? *J. Pediatr. Surg.*, **26**(3), 248–54.

Morin, C., Filiatrault, D., and Russo P. (1989). Pulmonary sequestration with histologic changes of cystic adenomatoid malformation. *Pediatr. Radiol.*, **19**, 130–2.

Musa, A. A., Hata, T., Hata, K., Aoki, S., Makihara, K., and Kitao, M. (1990). Ultrasonographic measurement of fetal lung. *Gynecol. Obstet. Invest.*, **30**, 139–42.

Neilson, I. R., Laberge, J. M., Filiatrault, D., *et al.* (1991). Congenital adenomatoid malformation of the lung: current management and prognosis. *J. Pediatr. Surg*, **26**(8), 975–81.

Newman, K. D., Anderson, K., Van Meurs, K., Parson, S., Loe, W., and Short, B. (1990). Extracorporeal membrane oxygenation and congenital diaphragmatic hernia: should any infant be included? *J. Pediatr. Surg.*, **10**, 1048–53.

Newnham, J. P., Crues, J. V. 3d, Vinstein, A. L,. *et al.* (1984). Sonographic diagnosis of thoracic gastroenteric cyst *in utero*. *Prenat. Diagn*, **4**, 467–71.

Norio, R., Kaariainen, H., Rapola, J., *et al.* (1984). Familial congenital diaphragmatic defects: aspects of etiology, prenatal diagnosis, and treatment. *Am. J. Med. Genet.*, **17**, 471–83.

O'Rourke, P. P., Lillehei, C. W., Crone, R. K., and Vacanti, J. P. (1991). The effect of extracorporeal membrane oxygenation on the survival of neonates with high-risk congenital diaphragmatic hernia: 45 cases from a single institution. *J. Pediatr. Surg.*, **26**(2), 147–52.

Petit, P., Bossens, M., Thomas, D., *et al.* (1987). Type III congenital cystic adenomatoid malformation of the lung: another cause of elevated alpha fetoprotein? *Clin. Genet.*, **32**, 172–4.

Petrikovsky, B. M., Shmoys, S. M., Baker, D. A., and Monheit, A. G. (1991). Pleural effusion in aneuploidy. *Am. J. Perinatol.*, **8**(3), 214–16.

Pijpers, L., Reuss, A., Stewart, P. A., and Wladimiroff, J. W. (1989). Noninvasive management of isolated bilateral fetal hydrothorax. *Am. J. Obstet. Gynecol.*, **161**, 330–2.

Roberts, A. B. and Mitchell, J. M. (1990). Direct ultrasonographic measurement of fetal lung length in normal pregnancies and pregnancies complicated by prolonged rupture of membranes. *Am. J. Obstet. Gynecol.*, **163**, 1560–6.

Rodeck, C. H., Fisk, N. M., Fraser, D. F., and Nicolini, U. (1988). Long-term *in utero* drainage of fetal hydrothorax. *N. Engl. J. Med.*, **310**, 1135–8.

Saltzman, D. H., Adzick, N. S., and Benacerraf, B. R. (1988). Fetal cystic adenomatoid malformation of the lung: apparent improvement *in utero*. *Obstet. Gynecol*, **71**, 1000–2.

Sauerbrei, E. (1991). Lung sequestration. Duplex Doppler diagnosis at 19 weeks gestation. *J. Ultrasound Med.*, **10**, 101–5.

Seeds, J. W., Cefalo, R. C., Lies, S. C., *et al.* (1984). Early prenatal sonographic appearance of rare thoraco abdominal eventration. *Prenat. Diagn.*, **4**, 437–41.

Siffring, P. A., Forrest, T. S., Hill, W. C., and Frick, M. P. (1989). Prenatal sonographic diagnosis of bronchopulmonary foregut malformation. *J. Ultrasound Med.*, **8**, 277–80.

Silver, M. M., Thurston, W. A., and Patrick, J. E. (1988). Perinatal pulmonary hyperplasia due to laryngeal atresia. *Hum. Pathol.*, **19**, 110–13.

Sonek, J. D., Foley, M. R., and Iams, J. D. (1991). Spontaneous regression of a large intrathoracic fetal lesion before birth. *Am. J. Perinatol.*, **8**(1), 41–3.

Songster, G. S., Gray, D. L., and Crane, J. P. (1989). Prenatal prediction of lethal pulmonary hypoplasia using ultrasonic fetal chest circumference. *Obstet. Gynecol.*, **73**, 261–6.

Stern, E., Brill, P. W., Winchester, P., *et al.* (1990). Imaging of prenatally detected intra-abdominal extralobar pulmonary sequestration. *Clin. Imag.*, **12**, 152–6.

Stocker, S. T., Madewell, J. E., and Drake, R. M. (1977). Congenital cystic adenomatoid malformation of the lung. *Hum. Pathol.*, **8**, 155–71.

Thiagarajah, S., Abbitt, P. L., Hogge, W. A., *et al.* (1990). Prenatal diagnosis of eventration of the diaphragm *Journal of Clinical Ultrasound*, **18**, 46–9.

Thomas, C. S., Leopold, G. R., Hilton, S., *et al.* (1986). Fetal hydrops associated with extralobar pulmonary sequestration. *J. Ultrasound Med.*, **5**, 668–71.

Utsu, M., Sakakibara, S., Ishida, T., *et al.* (1983). Dynamics of tracheal fluid flow in the human fetus, studied with pulsed Doppler ultrasound. *Nippon Sanka Fujinka Gakkai Zasshi*, **35**, 2017–18.

Vintzileos, A. M., Campbell, W. A., Rodis, J. F., *et al.* (1989). Comparison of six different ultrasonographic methods for predicting lethal pulmonary hypoplasia. *Am. J. Obstet. Gynecol.*, **161**, 606–12.

Watson, W. J., Thorp, J. M. Jr, Miller, R. C., *et al.* (1990). Prenatal diagnosis of laryngeal atresia. *Am. J. Obstet. Gynecol*, **163**, 1456–67.

Weinbaum, P. J., Bors Koefoed, R., Green, K. W., *et al.* (1989). Antenatal sonographic findings in a case of intra abdominal pulmonary sequestration. *Obstet. Gynecol*, **73**, 860–2.

West, M. S., Donaldson, J. S., and Shkolnik, A. (1989). Pulmonary sequestration: diagnosis by ultrasound. *J. Ultrasound Med*, **8**, 125–9.

Wigglesworth, J. S. and Desai, R. (1979). Effect on lung growth of cervical cord section in the rabbit fetus. *Early Hum. Dev.*, **3**, 51–65.

Wigglesworth, J. S., Desai, R., and Hislop A. A. (1987). Fetal lung growth in congenital laryngeal atresia. *Pediatr. Pathol.*, **7**, 515–25.

Young, G., L'Heureux, P. R., Krueckeberg, S. T., *et al.* (1989). Mediastinal bronchogenic cyst: prenatal sonographic diagnosis. *American Journal of Roengenology*, **152**, 125–7.

5

The dilated fetal renal tract: imaging and prenatal management

T. Wheeler and Philippe Jeanty

Introduction

The dilated fetal urinary tract is a frequent ultrasound finding and is associated with a wide range of prognoses. Mild disease typically remains stable or resolves entirely, but is unlikely to result in adverse consequences for the neonate. More severe degrees of dilation, however, are associated with partial or complete urinary tract obstruction that may lead to neonatal renal failure. An accurate assessment of fetal renal function and the extent to which it can be expected to deteriorate is essential for management plans, which may include serial surveillance, early delivery for operative management, or *in utero* intervention measures.

Ultrasonography is the most useful method available for the initial assessment of these disorders. Portions of the fetal genitourinary tract may be delineated as early as 15 weeks' gestation. Obstructive lesions are common and constitute the majority of neonatal abdominal masses. Careful sonographic evaluation of the fetal abdomen should detect these fluid-filled lesions and decrease the likelihood that a significant lesion will be missed if not palpated on the postnatal physical exam.

Definition

Dilation of the urinary tract frequently, but not necessarily, signifies obstruction (Arger *et al.* 1985). It is also possible for a fetus to have obstructive uropathy in the absence of urinary tract dilation. In either case, after 20 weeks gestation, measurement of the anteroposterior diameter of the fetal renal pelvis (PD), the diameter of the kidney (RD), and an assessment of the degree of calyceal dilatation provide important clinical information (Fig. 5.1(a), (b)).

Parameters:

(1) renal pelvic diameter greater than 10 mm in the AP dimension

(2) pelvis/kidney ratio greater than 30 per cent

(3) ability to visualize the ureters

(4) rounded calyces

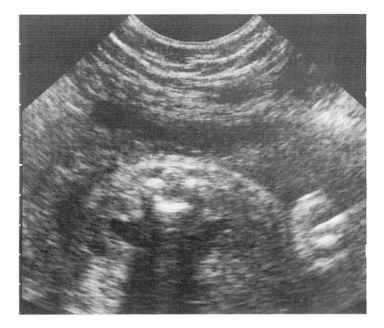

a

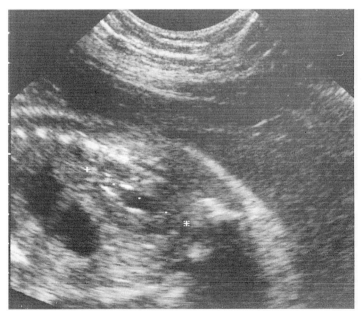

b

Fig. 5.1 (a) Transverse section of the kidney. (b) Longitudinal section of the kidney. A small degree of distension of the collecting system is noted. The renal pelvis is partially extrarenal. This is probably still within the upper limit of normal.

Recent studies have indicated that minimal degrees of hydronephrosis are common in fetuses older than 24 weeks' gestation (Arger *et al.* 1985; Mahony *et al.* 1988). Transient vesicoureteral reflux has also been implicated in mild hydronephrosis (Blane 1983). The aetiology of this finding is uncertain, but its relative frequency suggests a large range of normality. Knowledge of the range of normality in fetal urinary tract dilatation may limit unnecessary and expensive over-investigation of this physiologic event, but the tendency not to follow these cases may also result in missed pathology. It is reasonable to assume that most cases of moderate and severe hydronephrosis once passed through a stage of ultrasonographic-appearing mild hydronephrosis. This dilemma necessitates follow-up examinations on many fetuses within the range of normal

Diagnosis

Indication for study:
In many centres, ultrasonography is routinely performed in all pregnancies to assess gestational age and to survey for malformations. More specific indications for antenatal study of the fetal genitourinary tract include:

(1) fetal size less than expected for gestational age

(2) oligohydramnios

(3) family history of renal anomaly

(4) elevated maternal serum alpha-fetoprotein

Due to the natural history of this disorder, it may be difficult to detect abnormal dilatation early enough to intervene. Populations who routinely receive mid-trimester evaluation have experienced minimal success with early diagnosis. A recently reported series of 12 000 pregnancies with routine evaluations performed at 17 and 33 weeks detected only three urinary tract anomalies during the initial examination (Helin and Persson 1986). During the follow-up examination at 33 weeks' gestation, however, 30 fetuses with renal anomalies were detected. Sixty per cent of these fetuses had findings consistent with hydronephrosis, but went undetected on initial examination.

Pocock *et al.* (1985) recently reported a series of 28 infants with a prenatal diagnosis of a genitourinary tract anomaly. Seventeen of these infants (60 per cent) survived the neonatal course. It is notable that 15 of the survivors (88 per cent) had sonograms prior to 24 weeks' gestation; however, the abnormality was found in only one fetus. They concluded that if the anomaly was not sonographically present before 24 weeks' gestation, then a good outcome could be anticipated. Factors associated with the 11 non-survivors include bilateral disease, associated extrarenal anomalies, and severe oligohydramnios.

When routine examinations are not employed, initial evaluations are often prompted by a clinical discrepancy between uterine size and gestational age. The mean gestational age at the time of suspicion is around 28 weeks (Quinlan 1986). This clinical sign is insensitive, as referral is typically made beyond the critical period in which irreversible pulmonary hypoplasia is thought to occur, and renal function is irretrievably lost (Golbus 1985).

Oligohydramnios is probably the most significant criterion for determining the eventual outcome (Manning 1989). This finding represents a longstanding absence of fetal urine production and is most consistent with either bilateral disease, complete obstruction, or with renal agenesis/dysgenesis. Transudate from the fetal skin, lung, and umbilical cord may contribute to the amniotic fluid volume prior to 16 weeks' gestation. After this, keratinization begins; however, significant decreases in amniotic fluid production are the result of renal disease.

In most cases, the mechanism of death in fetuses with severe renal anomalies is not renal but rather pulmonary (Manning *et al.* 1986). The relationship between absent urine flow and pulmonary hypoplasia is well established. At least 80 per cent of the neonatal deaths with obstructive uropathies are due to proximate pulmonary complications (Manning *et al.* 1986). The absence of amniotic fluid may allow for the collapse of the bronchial tree or compression of the fetal chest wall against the uterus, preventing development of the alveoli.

An ultrasound screen of the genitourinary tract should include a thorough assessment of the extrarenal organs. Some series report up to 50 per cent of cases of subvesical obstruction and cystic kidney disease to be associated with significant extrarenal defects (Grignon *et al.* 1986). Chromosomal abnormalities are also prevalent, as some series report an incidence as high as 23 per cent in fetuses with known urinary tract abnormalities (Nicolaides *et al.* 1986). These anomalies are typically associated with bilateral disease; however, the literature includes descriptions of various trisomic, partial deletion, and duplication syndromes associated with unilateral disease as well (Temple and Shapira 1981).

True obstructive uropathy is an indication for the need of cytogenetic studies for counselling, with respect to the risk of recurrence or prior to undertaking any therapeutic intervention. Rapid karyotype may be obtained through percutaneous umbilical blood sampling (PUBS) or chorionic villus sampling. Routine amniocentesis may be difficult with oligohydramnios, but culture of cells obtained from fetal urine in the bladder or dilated kidney should yield cytogenetic results in 2–3 weeks.

Associated anomalies

Detection of certain urinary tract abnormalities often indicates the presence of other abnormalities or syndromes.

1. Down syndrome — Benacerraf *et al.* (1990) published a series of cases demonstrating a significant association between fetal hydronephrosis and the presence of trisomy 21. Their data demonstrates a 3.3 per cent incidence of trisomy 21 in the presence of fetal renal pyelectasis. When fetal pyelectasis is demonstrated, the risk of Down syndrome is considerably higher than the risk associated with advanced maternal age or a low serum alpha-fetoprotein.

2. Meckel–Gruber syndrome — Polycystic kidneys with encephalocele, club-foot, and polydactyly.

3. VACTERL — Association of anomalies Vertebral, Anal, Cardiac, Tracheo–Esophageal, Renal and Limb abnormalities.

4. Zellwager syndrome — (cerebrohepatorenal syndrome) — Small renal cysts with hepatomegaly and hypothermia.

Prognosis

The majority of fetuses with a genitourinary anomaly will do well postnatally (Callan *et al.* 1990). Better prognoses have been noted for fetuses with an antenatal diagnosis of hydronephrosis allowing for antibiotic prophylaxis and immediate surgical intervention. The spectrum of the fetal response to urinary tract obstruction is primarily determined by the gestational age at the onset of the obstruction.

In 1971, Beck (1971) published data showing that if ureteral obstruction occurs prior to 70 days of gestation in the sheep fetus (term is 150 days), there will be resulting renal dysplasia with large amounts of undifferentiated mesenchymal stroma, reduced glomeruli, and cystic dilation of Bowman's capsule. If the obstruction occurs after 80 days' gestation, the renal architecture remains well preserved despite the consequent hydronephrosis. Harrison *et al.* (1983) have reported comparable findings in a more recent study. This group noted that early and complete obstruction precipitated renal dysplasia and secondary pulmonary hypoplasia. When obstruction occurs at a later gestational age, hydronephrosis and oligohydramnios may result (Fig. 5.2(a), (b)), but recovery of some renal function is still possible (Beck 1971).

Assessment of unilaterality, or bilaterality, and of symmetry of urinary tract involvement may also help in the diagnosis and prognosis of obstructive anomalies (Fig. 5.3). Unilateral disease occurs at, or proximal to, the ureteral bud and should have a good prognosis (Mahony 1988). Bilateral asymmetric disease implies involvement at the level of the urethra and has a more variable outcome. Bilateral symmetric disease often reflects a genetic abnormality with a poor prognosis:

(1) autosomal recessive polycystic kidney disease

(2) bilateral multicystic dysplastic kidneys

(3) renal agenesis

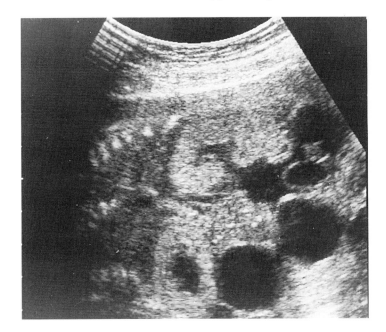

(a)

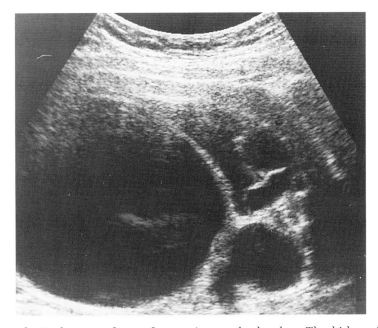

(b)

Fig. 5.2a, b: Early onset form of posterior urethral valve. The kidney is dysplastic (echogenic) and a markedly distended ureter and bladder are visible.

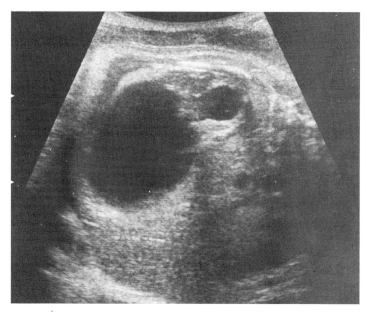

Fig. 5.3. Duplicated kidney. The lower pole is obstructed and distended. The large renal pelvis of the inferior portion of the kidney compresses the ureter of the upper pole, producing some moderate secondary upper pole hydronephrosis.

Differential diagnosis

The sonographic findings consistent with obstructive uropathy include fetal bladder enlargement, hydroureter, and hydronephrosis with or without dysplastic degeneration (Hobbins *et al.* 1984). Frequently, a reduction in amniotic fluid is an associated finding. Obstructive uropathy is identified as unilateral or bilateral and can be divided according to anatomical level.

High: Dilated renal pelvis only
          Ureteropelvic junction obstruction (UPJ) (Fig. 5.4) or ureteral atresia

Mid: Ureteral dilation with or without a dilated renal pelvis
          Ureterovesical junction obstruction (Figs 5.5–7), bladder atresia, transient hydroureter

Low: Dilated bladder and proximal urinary tract
          Posterior urethral valves or urethral atresia

The true obstructive uropathies of the lower GU tract are almost always due to one of three conditions:

1. *Posterior urethral valve syndrome*: disease isolated to male fetuses resulting from mucosal folds or valves that occlude the proximal portion of the

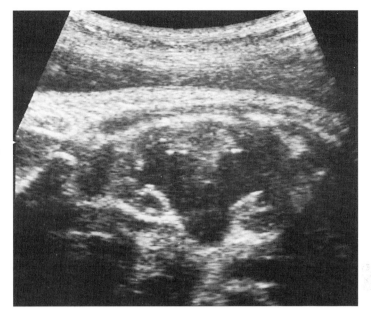

Fig. 5.4. Moderate distension in a ureteropelvic junction obstruction.

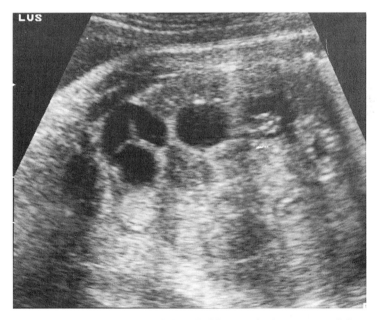

Fig. 5.5. Absence of distension of the bladder, with distension of the ureter and moderate distension of the kidney. These are the typical findings of ureterovesical junction obstruction.

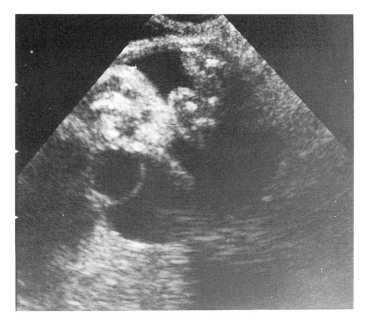

Fig. 5.6. The thin membrane inside the bladder represents a ureterocele. Those detected prenatally often result in bilateral hydronephrosis by prolapsing in the bladder neck.

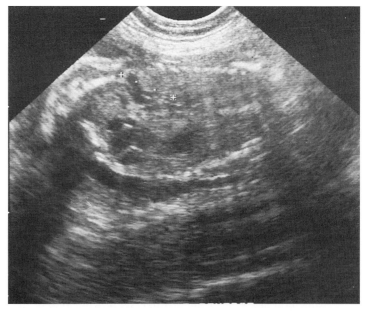

Fig. 5.7. Isolated distension of ureter.

posterior urethra. The proximal posterior urethra will dilate up to the point of the obstruction, and the fetal bladder will become initially hypertrophied, and ultimately distended and thin-walled. The ureters may become dilated and tortuous, and hydronephrosis is observed. Oligohydramnios may be present in 50 per cent of cases and is considered a poor prognostic sign (Mahony 1988).

2. *Urethral atresia*: this disorder results from the failure of canalization of the urethra. It affects both sexes equally and is likely to progress to multicystic parenchymal disease.

3. *Persistent cloacal syndrome*: this is more common in female fetuses and is characterized by the development of a cystic pelvic mass, ambiguous genitalia, and progressive hydronephrosis.

There are at lease three non-obstructive anomalies of the genitourinary tract which may present with ultrasound features similar to those of obstructive uropathy. Differentiation may be difficult, but it is important because *in utero* intervention is not indicated for non-obstructive disorders:

1. *Massive bilateral ureteral reflux* (Fig. 5.8): may cause hydroureter and hydronephrosis. The fetal bladder size is usually normal, though hypertrophy may occur. Amniotic fluid volume is typically within normal limits (Blane *et al.* 1983).

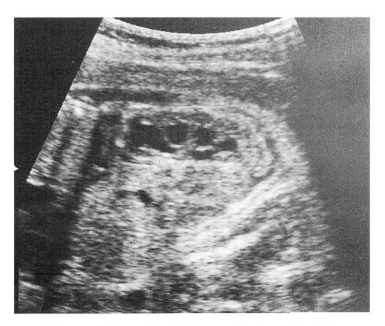

Fig. 5.8. Hydronephrosis due to reflux in a little girl.

2. *The megacystis microcolon-intestinal hyperperistalsis syndrome (MMIH)*: this is a rare, uniformly lethal disorder of smooth muscle development. Ultrasound features include megacystis, hydroureter, and bilateral hydronephrosis. Amniotic fluid volume is typically normal.

3. *Prune-belly syndrome*: a condition characterized by megacystis, hydroureter, variable degrees of hydronephrosis, and the absence of abdominal wall musculature.

Pathogenesis

Isolated hydronephrosis results from a functional stricture in the immediate proximal portion of the ureter (Kleiner 1987). Ureteropelvic junction (UPJ) is the most common congenital urinary tract lesion and accounts for up to 40 per cent of the recognized anomalies in this organ system (Duval 1985). A functional disturbance in either the initiation or the propagation of the normal peristaltic activity within the ureter creates an obstruction and leads to proximal dilation of the renal pelvis. The renal parenchyma typically is not affected, and decreased urine production is an unusual finding. The disease process is usually unilateral, and no hereditary basis has been identified (Duval 1985). Appropriate management includes monthly sonograms and attentive postnatal follow-up.

Primary renal anomalies may involve the glomerulus or the collecting system within the kidney. If the glomerulus unit is functioning, then the sonogram will reflect an abnormal accumulation of urine. When the glomerulus is not functioning, however, findings include a non-filling bladder and consequent oligohydramnios (Manning 1989). Segmental anomalies of the glomerulus are characterized by the absence of communication between the glomerulus and the collecting system. The attendant pathology may range from complete absence, agenesis, to various degrees of disorganization, dysgenesis.

Renal dysgenesis is characterized by disorganized epithelial structures, abundant fibrous tissue, and cortical cysts. Current belief holds that renal dysplasia results from prolonged obstruction to urine passage (Beck 1971; Harrison *et al.* 1983). The level of the urinary tract obstruction does not uniquely determine the extent of the pathology, as severe renal dysplasia may occur with proximal intraparenchymal lesions or more distal urethral or urethral obstruction.

It is possible to differentiate renal dysplasia from hydronephrosis, however, these two lesions are not exclusive of each other. Depending on the timing and completeness of the urinary tract obstruction, irreversible dysplasia may coexist with remediable hydronephrosis in the same or contralateral kidney (Mahony 1988). Attempts are made to predict histological renal dysplasia among fetuses with obstructive uropathy based on ultrasound criteria. The presence of renal cortical cysts, increased echogenicity of the renal parenchyma, and extreme pelvocalyceal dilation have all been associated with renal dysplasia.

Demonstration of renal cysts in a fetus with known obstructive uropathy is a sensitive indication of dysplasia as early as 21 weeks' gestation (Mahony 1988). Assessment of renal echogenicity and pelvocalyceal dilation, however, are comparatively less sensitive predictions of irreversible renal damage.

Therapy

Diagnostic and management challenges begin with the recognition of a 'true' obstructive uropathy and then quickly focus on the aetiology and pathophysiology of the obstruction. A decade of research suggests that relief of the obstruction during the most active phase of nephrogenesis (20–30 weeks' gestation) may negate further damage and allow renal and pulmonary development to proceed normally (Golbus *et al.* 1985). Anecdotal experiences and data from the Fetal Surgery Registry catalogue about 80 cases of fetal intervention in the form of fetal surgery and chronic *in utero* urinary diversion (Manning *et al.* 1986). The overall survival rate has been no more than 30 per cent; however, the more recent outcomes have improved as the selection process for intervention candidates has become more stringent.

The proper selection of those fetuses with bilateral hydronephrosis who might be candidates for intervention is difficult to achieve in a non-invasive manner. Sonographic evaluation of the fetal kidneys provides prognostic information if cystic or increased echogenicity are noted, but dysplasia is not excluded in their absence (Mahony 1988). Similarly, amniotic fluid volume is predictive only in extremes; normal volumes suggest adequate urine output, while oligohydramnios suggests chronic renal insufficiency (Glick *et al.* 1984).

Attempts have been made to develop more accurate assessments of the degree of understanding of normal fetal urine biochemistry and its variations with compromised situations. Data derived by transabdominal percutaneous intrauterine suprapubic bladder shunting by Golbus *et al.* (1985) suggest that fetuses with isosthenuria do poorly, while fetuses with dilute urine have better prognoses. This theory suggests that non-functioning kidneys essentially act like a sieve with respect to filtration of serum. Functioning kidneys, however, will display normal selective tubular reabsorption of sodium and chloride.

Temporary external drainage of the fetal bladder facilitates accurate measurement of fetal urine production rates, estimates of fetal GFR by creatinine or iothalamate excretion, and urine electrolyte composition. In the fetus with intact renal function, the urinary sodium is always less than 100 mEq/dl, the chloride less than 90 mEq/dl, and the osmolality less than 200 mOsm/L (Glick 1983). Urinary levels of B_2 macroglobulin may also be a sensitive indicator, with parameters varying with gestational age (Evans *et al.* 1991).

Recent studies have challenged these fetal urine parameters as an accurate predictor of neonatal renal function (Wilkins *et al.* 1987). Critics also question whether the aspiration of obstructed urine from the fetal bladder reflects 'current' renal function and whether serial aspirations reflect changes consistent with a post-obstructive diuresis. Evans *et al.* (1991) recently published data suggesting that relief of the urinary obstruction may help improve the urine chemistry over time. Fetuses with dilute urine on initial aspirations generally had good outcomes while those with persistent isosthenuria on serial aspirations had poor outcomes. There was a subpopulation of fetuses, however, whose values improved with serial aspiration. This group appears to be the best candidate for intervention therapy in the form of a chronic indwelling vesico amniotic shunt (Evans *et al.* 1991).

Most intrauterine fetal shunting procedures have used ultrasound-guided percutaneous placement of a vesicoamniotic catheter. Correct placement of the catheter is verified by a decrease in the size of the fetal bladder and the reaccumulation of amniotic fluid. Weekly evaluation of amniotic fluid volume, urinary tract dilation, and catheter placement are necessary, as it is not uncommon for the shunts to become obstructed or displaced (Manning 1989).

The efficacy of intervention therapy has been demonstrated in fetuses with a diagnosis of posterior urethral valve syndrome. This lesion is not associated with other karyotypic or structural anomalies, but produces bilateral renal disease, and it is typically associated with oligohydramnios. The International Fetal Surgery Registry recently reported a series of 73 treated cases in which 21 had an unequivocal diagnosis of posterior urethral values (Manning *et al.* 1986). The survival rate for this subset of treated patients was 76.2 per cent. The 16 survivors were free of respiratory insufficiency, and only one infant subsequently developed chronic renal failure.

The anticipated outcome for similar, but non-treated, fetuses is difficult to evaluate. Many of these infants must survive, because paediatric specialists have been imaging these neonates long before intervention was a reality. Nakayama *et al.* (1986) recently identified 11 neonates in whom the diagnosis of posterior urethral valves was made at birth. Five of these infants, all of whom demonstrated extreme oligohydramnios *in utero*, succumbed to pulmonary hypoplasia. Small series are difficult to compare, in terms of significant differences in therapeutic efficacy, but the data of similar fetuses treated *in utero* demonstrated a two-fold difference in mortality.

Conclusion

The combination of sonographic and physiologic criteria facilitates the selection of those fetuses with progressive bilateral disease most likely to benefit from therapeutic intervention. Rigid selection criteria are necessary because significant risks of pre-term labour, abdominal wall defects, and chorioamnionitis are highly associated with intervention (Glick *et al.* 1983). Fetuses of sufficient maturity for extrauterine survival should not be considered as candidates.

Thirty-two weeks' gestation is often mentioned as a cut-off point. Fetuses with karyotypic abnormalities or significant structural abnormalities are also poor candidates for interventive procedures. Even with these rigid exclusion criteria, the presence of amniotic fluid reaccumulation, normalized renal parenchyma, and appropriate urinary electrolytes, there is no guarantee of normal neonatal renal and pulmonary function.

Review of the data indicates that there is still a significant 'learning curve' in the intervention treatment of fetuses with a dilated urinary tract. Difficult ethical scenarios may result from potential maternal and fetal infections as well as the sequelae of extreme prematurity. An additional consequence of fetal therapy may be the survival of a neonate who otherwise would have died from pulmonary hypoplasia, but whose survival is accompanied by severe renal insufficiency. Renal insufficiency can be managed postnatally in some capacity, but the long-term outlook for these neonates remains suspect.

The concept of 'fetus as patient' creates a new legal and bioethical dilemma concerning the accuracy of diagnosis, the acceptability of late second and third trimester terminations, and the expected risks and benefits of intervention therapy. Intervention techniques have continued to improve, and indications for procedures will become more apparent in time. It is hoped that a proposed randomized clinical study comparing antenatal intervention with aggressive postnatal management will further delineate the standard of care. Such a study has been proposed by the International Fetal Medicine and Surgery Society and is eagerly awaited.

References

Arger, P. H., Coleman, B. G., Mintz, M. C., *et al.* (1985). Routine fetal genitourinary tract screening. *Radiology*, **156**, 485–9.

Beck, D. A. (1971). Effect of intrauterine urinary obstruction upon development of the fetal kidney. *Journal of Urology*, **105**, 784.

Benacerraf, B. R., Mandell, J., Estroff, J., Harlow, B. L., and Frigoletto, F. D. (1990). Fetal pyelectasis: a possible association with Down Syndrome. *Obstetrics and Gynecology*, **76**, 58–60.

Blane, C. E., Koff, S. A., Bowerman, R. A., and Barr, M. J. (1983). Nonobstructive fetal hydronephrosis: Sonographic recognition and therapeutic implications. *Radiology*, **147**, 95–9.

Callan, N. A., Blakemore, K., Park, J., Snaders, R. C., Jeffs, R. D., and Gearhart, J. P. (1990). Fetal genitourinary tract anomalies: Evaluation, operative correction, and follow up. *Obstetrics and Gynecology*, **75**, 67–74.

Duval, J. M., Milan, J., and Coadou, Y. (1985). Ultrasonographic anatomy and diagnosis of fetal uropathies affecting the upper urinary tract. I. Obstructive uropathics. *Anatomy Clinics*, **7**, 301.

Evans, M., Sacks, A., Johnson, M., Robichaux, A., May, M., and Moghissi, K. (1991). Sequential invasive assessment of fetal renal function and intrauterine treatment of fetal obstructive uropathies. *Obstetrics and Gynecology*, **77**, 545–50.

Glick, P. L., Harrison, M. R., and Golbus, M. S. (1983). Management of the fetus with congenital hydronephrosis II. Prognostic criteria and selection for treatment. *Journal of Pediatric Surgery*, **20**, 76.

Glick, P. L., Harrison, M. L., and Adzick, N. S. (1984). Correction of congenital hydronephrosis *in utero* IV: *In utero* decompression prevents renal dysplasia. *Journal of Pediatric Surgery*, **19**, 149.

Golbus, M. S., Filly, R. A., Callan, P. W., Glick, P. L., Harrison, M. R., and Anderson, R. L. (1985). Fetal urinary tract obstruction: Management and selection for treatment. *Seminars in Perinatology*, **9**, 91.

Grignon, A., Filion, R., Filiatrault, D., Rabitaille, P., Humsy, Y., and Boutin, H. (1986). Urinary tract dilatation *in utero*: Classification and clinical applications. *Radiology*, **160**, 645–7.

Harrison, M. R., Ross, N., Noall, R., and de Lorimier, A., (1983). Correction of congenital hydronephrosis *in utero* I. Fetal urethral obstruction produces hydronephrosis and pulmonary hypoplasia in fetal lambs. *Journal of Pediatric Surgery*, **18**, 247–56.

Helin, I., and Persson, P. H. (1986). Prenatal diagnosis of urinary tract abnormalities by ultrasound. *Pediatrics*, **78**, 879–83.

Hobbins, J. C., Romero, R., Grannum, P., Berkowitz, R., Cullen, M., and Mahoney, M., (1984). Antenatal diagnosis of renal anomalies with ultrasound. *American Journal of Obstetrics and Gynecology*, **148**, 868–75.

Kleiner, B., Callen, P. W., and Filly, R. A. (1987). Sonographic analysis of the fetus with ureteropelvic junction obstruction. *Am. J. Roentgenol.*, **148**, 359–63.

Mahony, B. S., (1988). The genitourinary system. In *Ultrasonography in obstetrics and gynecology* (ed. P. Callan), pp. 254–276. W. B. Saunders, London.

Manning, F. (1989). Common fetal urinary tract anomalies. In *Clinics in diagnostic ultrasound* (ed. J. Hobbins and B. Benacerraf), pp. 139–61. Churchill Livingstone, London.

Manning, F., Harrison, M., and Rodeck, C., (1986). Catheter shunts for fetal hydronephrosis and hydrocephalus. Report of the International Fetal Surgery Registry. *New England Journal of Medicine*, **315**, 336–41.

Nakayama, D. K., Harrison, M. R., and de Lorimier, A. (1986). Prognosis of posterior urethral valve syndrome presenting at birth. *Journal of Pediatric Surgery*, **21**, 43–8.

Nicolaides, K. H., Rodeck, C. H., and Gosden, C. M. (1986). Rapid karyotyping in non-lethal fetal malformations. *Lancet*, **i**, 283–5.

Pocock, R. D., Witcombe, J. B., Andrews, H. S., Berry, P. J., and Frank, J. (1985). The outcome of antenatally diagnosed urologic abnormalities. *British Journal of Urology*, **57**, 788–92.

Quinlan, W., Cruz, A., and Huddleston, J., (1986). Sonographic detection of fetal urinary tract anomalies. *Obstetrics and Gynecology*, **67**, 658–65.

Temple J. K., and Shapira, E., (1981). Genetic determinants of renal disease in neonates. *Clinics in Perinatology*, **8**, 361–73.

Wilkins, I., Chitkara, U., Lynch, L., Goldberg, J., Mehaler, K., and Berkowitz, R. (1987). The nonpredictive value of fetal urinary electrolytes: Preliminary report of outcomes and correlations with pathologic diagnosis. *American Journal of Obstetrics and Gynecology*, **157**, 694–8.

6

Symposium: Fetal infections

A   Clinical problems and laboratory diagnosis
S. Wesselingh and D. L. Gordon

Introduction

A diverse range of viral, parasitic, and bacterial microorganisms may result in infections of the fetus. Many of these are preventable and some are amenable to treatment. To the obstetrician, the greatest clinical problem is to determine the presence of maternal infection, to subsequently estimate the risk of infection in the fetus, and the likely sequelae, so that appropriate advice and counselling can be given to the parents. This may be a difficult task as frequently the maternal infection is asymptomatic despite still posing a risk to the fetus; unless gross fetal abnormalities are present, there may still be great difficulties in defining if fetal infection has occurred. In addition, many variables influence maternal–fetal

Table 6.1 Factors that may affect risk of maternal–fetal transmission and the sequelae*

Characteristics of pathogen
   Strain and virulence
   Inoculum
Maternal factors
   Gestation
   Coexisting infections or illness
   Immune status
      — humoral
      — cellular
      — primary versus secondary infection
   Placental abnormalities or inflammation
   Viraemia, parasitaemia, or bacteraemia
Fetal factors
   Gestational age
   Immune response

*Based in part on McGregor 1991

transmission of microorganisms (McGregor 1991) (Table 6.1). More invasive techniques, such as cordocentesis and embryoscopy, now allow direct sampling of fetal blood or visualization of the fetus (Copel *et al.* 1990; Hoskins 1991) and appear to be useful in the diagnosis of some congenital infections. However, these procedures are not without risks and limitations. Serological diagnosis by fetal IgM is not possible until 19–23 weeks' gestation, and highly sensitive techniques such as polymerase chain reaction (PCR) may detect minute maternal contamination. In this chapter we will briefly review congenital infections of greatest concern to the obstetrician/ultrasonographer, rather than the equally important microorganisms that are associated primarily with perinatal infection (for example Group B *Streptococci*) but which are unlikely to result in ultrasound abnormalities. Where possible, estimates of risk to the fetus and the possible sequelae will be discussed, and approaches to laboratory diagnosis will be reviewed.

Viral infections

Viral infections during pregnancy pose a number of clinical problems and create anxieties for both the parents and the clinician. Maternal viral infections are very common and the clinical presentation is usually non-specific; it is, therefore, often difficult to distinguish clinically between the presentation of a benign infection from one that may generate morbidity or mortality. There are, however, a number of general principles which apply to most maternal viral infections and which can guide the clinician:

1. Primary maternal viral infections are much more likely to lead to fetal infection than secondary infections.
2. Primary infections are also more likely to lead to fetal morbidity and mortality.
3. The gestational age determines the pathology generated. Infections during the first 8–12 weeks, when organogenesis is occurring, often lead to major congenital abnormalities, whereas maternal infections late in pregnancy may lead to prematurity and neonatal infections, and the problems associated with the viral infections of very young infants.

Once the diagnosis of a 'significant' viral infection has been made the risk to fetus must be calculated, based on the stage of the pregnancy and the immune status of the mother.

There is unfortunately a sparsity of good, quick confirmatory investigations. Recently, however, a number of technological advances have shown promise in this area. These include rapid viral culture, polymerase chain reaction, and cordocentesis (Copel *et al.* 1990).

The management of maternal viral infections consists mainly of counselling and of supportive measures. There are increasing numbers of antiviral drugs becoming available and some of these may prove useful during pregnancy, but there is still limited information on their efficacy and safety. In addition, there are a number of prophylactic measures for the prevention and amelioration of specific viral infections.

In this section we will review the common viral pathogens that may be encountered during pregnancy, and discuss important aspects of diagnosis and management. Due to limitations of space, this review will not be all encompassing but rather highlight issues that relate to specific viruses.

The following viruses will be discussed; rubella, cytomegalovirus (CMV), herpes simplex virus (HSV), human immunodeficiency virus (HIV), hepatitis B and C, enteroviruses, varicella–zoster virus (chickenpox and shingles), measles and mumps, parvovirus, and influenza A and B.

Rubella

Maternal rubella infection has become much less frequent with the extensive use of vaccine. The mainstay of laboratory diagnosis of maternal infection is serology, a positive diagnosis being based on the presence of rubella specific IgM, or a significant rise in rubella specific IgG titres between acute and convalescent sera.

Women who have responded to vaccination or who have had a natural infection are protected. Difficulties may arise in women of unknown vaccination status but this can usually be resolved by careful serology.

In view of the risk of late sequelae of congenital rubella infection, it is important to try to make a definitive diagnosis in the neonate. This is usually achieved by direct culture techniques of samples from the nasopharynx or, less commonly, from conjunctivae or cerebrospinal fluid.

There is up to an 80 per cent risk of fetal infection after first trimester maternal infection (Table 6.2) and although the fetus is at risk throughout

Table 6.2 Risk of congenital rubella during primary maternal infection

Gestation (weeks)	% Risk of congenital infection
1–12	> 80
13 14	54
15–20	25
> 20	Negligible

(Based in part on Miller *et al.* 1982)

pregnancy, the later risk is very small (Miller *et al.* 1982). Reinfection, or infection after vaccination, usually cause no problem, although very rare cases of congenital infection after maternal reinfection have been reported.

There is approximately a 70 per cent congenital abnormality rate after maternal infection in the first trimester, the risk being highest (90 per cent) after maternal infection before the eleventh week (Miller *et al.* 1982). There is also an increased risk of miscarriage and stillbirth. The most common congenital defects involve the heart, eyes and ears, and central nervous system. Congenital heart disease occurs in at least 40 per cent of children infected in the first 12 weeks, with common lesions being patent ductus arteriosus, pulmonary artery stenosis, and pulmonary valvular stenosis.

Some defects may not be apparent until the first or second years of life, particularly insulin-dependent diabetes mellitus, thyroid disease, deafness, and progressive central nervous system disease.

The most difficult clinical situation is one of a positive diagnosis of rubella infection in a pregnant woman. Clearly the most expert counselling available should be sought. In general terms, the risk to the fetus should be estimated based on the timing of maternal infection and the immune status of the mother. The risk of major fetal abnormalities is much higher in the first eight weeks, the period during which organogenesis occurs but, as mentioned, congenital abnormalities can result from infection during any time in the pregnancy. In addition, it is important to note that the risk of infection in a previously immune mother is extremely low as is the risk of fetal abnormality.

Cytomegalovirus

Cytomegalovirus is the most common viral infection transmitted to the fetus *in utero* affecting approximately 1 per cent of all live births in the United States (Stagno 1990).

Cytomegalovirus infection commonly presents in a way similar to 'flu' or 'glandular fever', with fever, lymphadenopathy, and often a rash, which is difficult to differentiate clinically from Epstein–Barr virus and toxoplasma infection. Alternatively, it may present as a non-specific viral infection. The fetus can develop central nervous system defects: hydrocephaly, microcephaly, intracerebral calcification, and chorioretinitis. However, neonatal developmental delay and deafness, are probably the most common defects (Alford *et al.* 1990). Petechiae, hepatosplenomegaly, jaundice, pneumonitis, intra-uterine growth retardation, and prematurity are also seen.

Diagnosis by serology is based on a four-fold rise in CMV IgG titre or positive CMV IgM. It is important to be particularly wary of making a diagnosis based purely on positive CMV IgM, as false-positives are common, for example, induced by rheumatoid factor. Most laboratories will now have rapid CMV culture techniques available, with results available in 3–4 days. A positive blood culture is diagnostic of a primary infection. As discussed in the following chapter, the culture of amniotic fluid (Grose and Weiner 1990) or a combination of ultrasonography, amniocentesis, and fetal blood sampling (Lynch *et al.* 1991) may be useful in confirming infection.

CMV culture of urine and throat swabs from the neonate is also particularly important in the confirmation of congenital infection, as serology may be difficult to interpret. The development of PCR techniques may also allow the rapid diagnosis of infection.

In order to counsel a pregnant women with a positive diagnosis of CMV infection, the risk to the fetus must be assessed (Table 6.3). During primary CMV infection, there is 40 per cent transmission to the fetus with 10 per cent of these babies developing clinical disease; 90 per cent of these develop significant sequelae. Of the 90 per cent of fetuses that develop asymptomatic infection, approximately 5–15 per cent will develop late sequelae (Alford *et al.* 1990). In summary, there is an approximately 4 per cent risk of significant fetal abnormality following a primary maternal CMV infection. It should be noted that secondary or recurrent infection is very rare, and sequelae are generally mild.

An antiviral drug directed at CMV has been developed (Ganciclovir), but its role in pregnancy and neonatal infection is still to be established.

Herpes simplex virus

Aside from HIV, herpes simplex infections create most anxiety in both the parents and the clinician. Ironically, anxiety arises in situations in which the risk of neonatal infection is almost the lowest. The majority of cases of neonatal herpes infection occur when there is no history of maternal genital herpes infection. In addition, the risk of transmission and consequent fetal disease is much higher if the pregnant woman is suffering from her first or primary genital herpes infection as compared to a recurrent infection (Prober *et*

Table 6.3 Risk and sequelae of congenital CMV during primary maternal infection

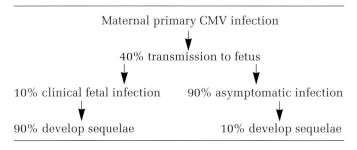

al. 1987; Brown *et al.* 1991). The reasons for this are probably the high titres of virus that are shed during primary infection, the length of time virus is shed (i.e. 5–7 days in a primary infection as compared to 1–2 days in a recurrent infection), and the presence of passively transferred maternal antibody after recurrent infection.

Neonatal infection, when it does occur, is usually severe and can either be localized to the skin, eyes and mouth, or to the central nervous system (encephalitis), or be disseminated. Intrauterine infection may also occur during primary infections leading to vesicles and scarring, ventricular dilatation, microcephaly, hydranencephaly, and chorioretinitis, particularly with primary infections in the first trimester.

The diagnosis of herpes infections in both the mother and the neonate can generally be made clinically and be confirmed by direct viral antigen detection and viral culture. Regular surveillance for viral shedding has no place in the modern management of herpes infections in pregnancy. Serology is also not particularly useful due to cross reaction between HSV 1 and 2 in most commercial kits.

Human immunodeficiency virus

In the short space of 10 years HIV, has, on a global scale, become the congenital infection generating most morbidity and mortality.

The stage at which HIV infects the fetus or neonate is not precisely known, however current evidence support intra-uterine infection rather than infection at the time of labour, i.e. there appears to be no increased rate of fetal infection associated with vaginal delivery. The risk of fetal infection is not precisely known, current estimates range from 13 per cent to 39 per cent (Hira *et al.* 1989; Goedert *et al.* 1989; European Collaborative Study 1991). The risk of fetal infection may depend on the stage of the maternal disease, particularly the CD4 count and the presence of viraemia and perhaps other factors, such as the presence of chorioamnionitis (Holmes 1991).

An embryopathy associated with maternal HIV infection has been described, but further studies have not confirmed this description (European Collaborative Study 1991). No definitive findings on ultrasound have been described. Clinical presentation in the child may include symptoms from opportunistic infections, encephalopathy, interstitial lung disease, and failure to thrive.

The early diagnosis of neonatal HIV infection is difficult due to the confounding effects of the passive transfer of maternal antibodies and the technical difficulties of viral culture. Further development of PCR and serology (i.e. HIV-IgA levels) is needed. In practice, diagnosis is made by carefully watching the infant's clinical state, performing sequential serology, and monitoring immune parameters.

The use of AZT (HIV antiviral agent) during pregnancy is controversial. No good clinical trials have yet been published.

Hepatitis viruses B (HBV) and C

Vertical transmission (from mother to baby) is one of the major forms of transmission of HBV, particularly in the developing world. This leads to very high rates of chronic hepatitis B carriage, and consequently to a high incidence of chronic liver disease and hepatocellular carcinoma. Transmission of HBV occurs most commonly at the time of delivery or transplacentally very late in pregnancy. It has, therefore, been possible to develop protocols to limit the rate of transmission (Beasley *et al.* 1981). These protocols necessitate performing HBV serology on all pregnant women. The infants of HBV surface antigen positive mothers are given HBV hyperimmune gamma-globulin and HBV vaccine immediately after delivery. They are then followed both to determine their sero-status and also to ensure the completion of the HBV vaccine course. There is no conclusive evidence to support advising HBV surface antigen positive mothers not to breast feed or to undergo elective caesarean section. Mothers who are HBV e antigen positive are at increased risk of transmitting the virus to their infants.

Hepatitis C, a flavivirus-like agent is the probable cause of 80 per cent of what was previously called Non-A, Non-B hepatitis. There is no doubt that it is transmitted via blood products; the possibility of vertical transmission is still under study. A major problem is that the only diagnostic test available measures antibodies which develop several months after infection. Currently, there is no measure of acute infection or of infectivity. Consequently, at present there is no consensus on the use of immunoprophylaxis for infants born to mothers who are hepatitis C positive.

Enteroviruses: polio, coxsackievirus, echovirus

Enteroviruses are a common cause of non-specific viral illness, but in addition cause a number of easily recognizable clinical syndromes, such as aseptic meningitis, pleurodynia, herpangina, pericarditis, and myocarditis.

Transplacental infection probably occurs with all enteroviruses. An increased risk of abortion with naturally occurring acute polio infection, but not with polio vaccines, has been reported (Siegel and Greenberg 1956). Coxsackievirus infection in the first trimester has been thought to be associated with congenital abnormalities of the central nervous system (Gauntt *et al.* 1985).

Significant infection with all of the enteroviruses has been associated with prematurity and stillbirth. Neonatal infection is the most commonly diagnosed sequela to maternal enteroviral infection — leading from subclinical infection to a range of clinical syndromes from mild disorder to severe septic like illness.

The diagnosis is generally a clinical one, since good quick diagnostic laboratory investigations are not available. Diagnosis can be made by culture, but this often takes a number of weeks.

Clinical clues are the season (summer and autumn) and a maternal history of a recent febrile illness or definitive syndrome, such aseptic meningitis, pleuro-dynia, herpangina, pericarditis, or myocarditis, as well as a neonate who appears septic but doesn't respond to antibiotics. The infants often require cardio-vascular and respiratory support, and unfortunately there is no specific antiviral agent currently available. Steroids are not indicated.

Varicella–zoster virus: chickenpox and shingles

Maternal VZV infection or maternal contact with chickenpox is a very common reason for enquiry to obstetric departments, and with the widespread use of the measles, mumps, and rubella vaccine, HZV infection is now more common in pregnancy than measles or mumps.

It is controversial whether chickenpox during pregnancy is more severe than in the non-pregnant women, however the development of varicella pneumonia is always of particular concern.

Transplacental spread and fetal infection has been well documented, resulting in congenital malformation, particularly skin scarring, limb hypoplasia, and eye and central nervous system damage (Alkalay *et al.* 1987). This usually occurs if the mother is infected during the first 20 weeks. If maternal infection occurs close to the time of labour, neonatal chickenpox commonly results; which, if untreated, carries a significant morbidity and mortality (Rubin *et al.* 1986).

Management involves the treatment of significant HZV infections with high dose acyclovir in both the mother and the neonate, the use of varicella–zoster hyperimmune gammaglobulin (VZIG) to prevent or ameliorate maternal and fetal disease, and the counselling of parents when maternal infection has occurred during the first trimester. The latter is most difficult, as there are no good data on the incidence of fetal abnormalities following first trimester maternal infection. Current estimates for the incidence of congenital varicella syndrome range between 2 per cent and 6.5 per cent (Preblud *et al.* 1986), although a recent prospective study of 40 patients with first trimester varicella infection revealed no cases of congenital varicella syndrome (Balducci *et al.* 1991).

There is very low risk to the fetus from maternal zoster, although rare instances of malformations have been reported (Webster and Smith 1977).

Measles and mumps

The incidence of measles and mumps infection in pregnancy has decreased since the widespread use of the measles, mumps, and rubella vaccine.

Neither virus has been definitively associated with congenital abnormalities although there is some evidence to link first trimester maternal mumps infection with fetal endocardial fibroelastosis (Noren *et al.* 1963). Both viruses have, however, been associated with increased rates of prematurity and abortion (Siegel 1973).

Parvovirus

Recently a human parvovirus, 'B19' has been shown to be the aetiological agent of erythema infectiosum, and to cause aplastic crises in patients with chronic haemolytic anaemias. Intrauterine infection has also been well documented. Maternal infection is associated with an approximately 33 per cent trans-placental transmission and a fetal loss rate of 9 per cent (Public Health Service Laboratories Working Party on Fifth Disease 1990). Fetal loss is usually due to fetal anaemia and cardiac failure, most often in the second trimester.

It is, however, critical to note that although maternal infection is associated with increased fetal loss it is not associated with an increased rate of congenital malformations. Therapeutic abortion is, therefore, not indicated (Levy and Read 1990).

Sero-epidemiological studies indicate that more than 65 per cent of adult women have serum antibody to B19; it is, therefore, a relatively uncommon infection in pregnancy. It should nevertheless be suspected in any pregnant woman with a febrile illness associated with a rash (particularly on the face), adenopathy, arthralgia, or arthritis. Diagnosis is generally a clinical one as serological tests (B19-IgM) are not yet generally available and, although invasive procedures such as cordocentesis and amniocentesis can be helpful, the risks associated with these procedures probably do not justify their use (Peters and Nicolaides 1990). The fetus can, however, be monitored by repeated ultra-sound examination to look for signs of hydrops (see Furness and Chambers, Chapter 6B this volume). Increased levels of maternal serum alpha-fetoprotein suggest a fetal aplastic crisis (Levy and Read 1990).

Influenza A and B

In some studies, first trimester maternal influenza infections have been associated with congenital abnormalities — particularly of the central nervous system. In all studies, it was of very low frequency and there is some suggestion that it may have been due to increased drug use during the febrile illness rather than to the viruses themselves (Hakosalo and Saxen 1971).

Parasitic infections

With the exception of toxoplasmosis, parasitic infections are rarely encountered by most obstetricians in non-endemic areas. It is important to remember, however, that parasitic infections may pose a threat to the developing fetus and they should be considered, in particular, in immigrants or travellers from endemic areas. The life cycle of many parasites is confined to localized areas such as the skin (for example louse, scabies) or gastrointestinal tract (for example giardia), and apart from indirect effects, such as malnutrition, they will not affect fetal development. Intestinal nematodes such a *Strongyloides stercoralis* may cause similar effects but, in addition, the immunosuppression associated with pregnancy may rarely result in disseminated infection. Parasites with persistent hematogenous phases (for example Trypanosoma, malaria, filarial parasites) may cause placental and fetal infection. Finally, large inflammatory masses in the pelvis (produced by, for example, echinococcus (hydatid) or schistosomiasis) may have adverse mechanical effects (Lee 1988). The laboratory diagnosis of these diverse infections may require one or more of the following: stool examination, blood smears, serology, or histopathology, and should occur in consultation with local experts. Only toxoplasmosis and malaria will be discussed in more detail here.

Toxoplasmosis

Toxoplasma gondii is a widely distributed intracellular protozoan parasite. Sexual reproduction occurs in the intestines of the definitive host, i.e. cats, which sheds oocysts in their faeces. Oocysts are ingested by many animals and cysts then form in tissues of these intermediate hosts. The life cycle is completed when the cat eats infected animal flesh (McCarthy 1983).

Human infection occurs either following ingestion of oocysts from contact with cat faeces or direct ingestion of tissue cysts in inadequately cooked meat. In the normal host, infection is usually subclinical, but it may result in a self-limiting illness with fever, malaise, and lymphadenopathy. Reactivation of primary infection in immunosuppressed patients, particularly with the Acquired Immune Deficiency Syndrome, is now frequently seen and typically presents as encephalitis.

The prevalence of toxoplasma antibody varies in different geographical locations, but is usually 30–50 per cent. In France, up to 85 per cent of the population in some areas have evidence of a previous infection. Women with pre-existing toxoplasma IgG antibody do not transmit toxoplasma to their fetuses, and congenital infection *only* occurs in non-immune mothers with a primary infection during pregnancy. Thus, in most areas 50–70 per cent of the pregnant population may be susceptible to toxoplasmosis, and although reliable figures are not available, overall it is estimated that congenital toxoplasmosis occurs in 1:1000 — 1:2000 pregnancies.

Transmission of infection to the fetus during a maternal primary infection can occur at any stage of pregnancy. However, the risk of congenital infection and clinical manifestations vary considerably. In the first trimester, congenital infection is less likely but when it does occur it tends to be severe, often resulting in fetal loss, or the classic triad of hydrocephalus, intracranial calcification, and chorioretinitis. Conversely, congenital infection is more likely in the third trimester but is usually asymptomatic (Table 6.4). However, many of these clinically unaffected infants at birth may subsequently develop neurological problems or chorioretinitis.

Prevention of congenital toxoplasmosis is difficult since there is no effective vaccine and most maternal infections are asymptomatic. Some countries have established serological screening programmes of susceptible women throughout pregnancy to detect recent infections, with administration of the macrolide antibiotic spiramycin for acute infections (Daffos *et al.* 1988). This approach, combined with treatment of confirmed fetal infections with pyrimethamine and sulphonamides appears to reduce the severity of clinical manifestations (Daffos *et al.* 1988; Hohlfeld *et al.* 1989). However, others have questioned the benefits of routine screening in pregnancy and note that controlled studies of spiramycin in pregnancy have not been performed (Jeannel *et al.* 1990; Klapper and Morris 1990).

For the obstetrician or ultrasonographer the usual clinical problem is to determine if the mother has acute toxoplasmosis and, if so, if there is evidence of fetal infection. Evidence of maternal infection is best obtained by demonstrating a rise in toxoplasma IgG, and by the presence of specific IgM. Later in pregnancy, comparison with serum obtained in the first trimester is particularly valuable. Thus all laboratories should store samples obtained at the first antenatal visit for at least 9–12 months. Reliance on IgM tests alone should be avoided since false-positive results may occur and with newer, more sensitive tests, specific IgM may be found to persist for years after primary infection. If any doubt exists, specimens should be tested by several methods in a reference

Table 6.4 Risk and sequelae of congenital toxoplasmosis during untreated primary maternal infection

Trimester	% Risk of transmission	Sequelae
1st	15	Serious infection frequent Severe neurological sequelae Fetal loss Growth retardation
2nd	30	Intermediate severity
3rd	60	Usually asymptomatic at birth Later sequelae common — chorioretinitis — learning difficulty — neurological problems

laboratory. Additional tests such as the polymerase chain reaction (PCR) may be useful in the future (Ho-Yen and Joss 1991).

The first successful attempts at the prenatal diagnosis of congenital toxoplasmosis involved fetal blood sampling for IgM antibody and isolation, in mice, of the parasite from fetal blood or amniotic fluid (Desmonts *et al.* 1985). However, this approach is limited by the late appearance of specific IgM in the fetus, and the prolonged time required and limited availability of animal inoculation (Grose *et al.* 1989). Chorionic villus sampling and early amniotic fluid culture may permit earlier diagnosis (Foulon *et al.* 1990), but rapid techniques of antigen detection in amniotic fluid by PCR appear promising (Grover *et al.* 1990) and should be more useful clinically in permitting the earlier diagnosis and treatment of infected fetuses.

Malaria

In endemic areas, where partial maternal immunity to malaria has been acquired, congenital malaria is uncommon, even in the face of maternal parasitaemia. Non-immune mothers are more likely to develop severe malaria, resulting in placental infection and intrauterine growth retardation, prematurity, abortion, or fetal death (Lee 1988). Diagnosis of an acute attack can generally be made by examining blood smears, but congenital malaria can occur in the absence of maternal symptoms or detectable maternal parasitaemia.

Bacterial infections

The developing fetus is relatively well protected from maternal bacteraemia, apart from some organisms such as *Treponema pallidum* or *Listeria monocytogenes* which more readily establish placental and subsequent fetal infection. Thus, abnormalities detected on ultrasound examination will more likely be associated with viral or parasitic infections. The introduction of bacterial microorganisms into the uterine cavity after ascent from the vagina and cervix may produce amnionitis; this may be subclinical but it can also result in premature labour, with or without concurrent fetal infection. Ultrasonographic abnormalities will not be present. Amniotic fluid may be collected for microbiological analysis. To facilitate isolation of fastidious or anaerobic organisms, material is best transported directly to the laboratory in the syringe used for aspiration.

Syphilis

In many areas in recent years there has been an alarming increase in the number of reported cases of syphilis which has resulted in parallel increases in congenital syphilis. This largely preventable condition is occurring in women without antenatal care and screening, and when infection occurs late in pregnancy (Dorfman and Glasser 1990). The aetiological agent of syphilis, *Treponema pallidum*, can cross the placenta at any stage of pregnancy. The risk of fetal infection (Fiumara *et al.* 1952) is shown in Table 6.5. Although approximately one-third of untreated affected fetuses are stillborn, 50 per cent of liveborn neonates with congenital syphilis are asymptomatic, particularly if infection has been acquired during the third trimester (Wendel 1989). Signs of congenital syphilis may subsequently occur, months to years later, if untreated. Perhaps because of early fetal immunoincompetence, clinical manifestations of congenital syphilis do not occur before 16–18 weeks gestation. When signs of syphilis occur during pregnancy serological diagnosis is usually straightforward. Maternal serum is tested by a non-treponemal test, such as the rapid plasma reagin (RPR) or Venereal Disease Research Laboratory (VDRL), which are subsequently used to monitor disease activity. Positive results are confirmed by a specific treponemal test such as the fluorescent treponemal antibody (FTA-ABS) or haemagglutination assays (TPHA, MHA-TP). Serological tests may be negative early in primary infection but are virtually always positive with follow-up testing and in secondary syphilis. Patients with HIV infection and syphilis occasionally also have negative syphilis serology (Musher *et al.* 1990).

Evaluation of neonates to determine the presence of infection or response to antenatal treatment is more complex and may require serial monitoring of non-treponemal tests, FTA-ABS IgM, direct examination of skin lesions, nasal discharge, cerebrospinal fluid, placenta and cord for treponemes, and radiological examinations. When doubt exists, treatment for congenital syphilis is justified and in all cases, careful follow-up is mandatory.

Listeria monocytogenes

Listerial infection should be considered whenever a pregnant women presents with chills and rigors, particularly if they are associated with back pain and negative urine cultures. Blood cultures are diagnostic, but are often not done.

Table 6.5 Risk of congenital syphilis in untreated maternal syphilis

Stage of maternal infection	% Risk of fetal infection
Primary or secondary	95–100
Early latent	40
Late latent	6–14

The outcome is variable. Premature labour may occur, or there may be transplacental transmission and development of granulomatosis infantiseptica. If the diagnosis is made during pregnancy, the women should be treated aggressively with ampicillin or penicillin (or erythromycin if she is allergic to penicillin). If premature labour is avoided, a good outcome is possible. The incidence and severity of listeria infections may be greater in pregnant women with additional immunosuppression, for example AIDS (Fan *et al.* 1989).

References

Alford, C. A., Stagno, S., Pass, R. F., and Britt, W. J. (1990). Congenital and perinatal cytomegalovirus infection. *Reviews of Infectious Disease*, **12**, 7, s745–53.

Alkalay, A. L., Pomerance, J. J., and Rimoin, D. L. (1987). Fetal varicella syndrome. *Journal of Pediatrics*, **111**, 320–3.

Babbott, F. L., Jr. and Gordon, J. E. (1954). Modern measles. *American Journal of Medical Science*, **228**, 334.

Balducci, F., Rodis, J., Rosengren, S., Vintzileos, A., Davis, G., and Vosseller, C. (1991). Neonatal outcome after first trimester varicella infection. (abstract) *American Journal of Obstetrics and Gynecology*, **164**, 298.

Beasley, R. P., Hwang, L., Lin, C. C., *et al.* (1981). Hepatitis B immune globulin (HBIG) efficacy in the interruption of perinatal transmission of hepatitis B virus carrier state. Initial report of randomized double-blind placebo controlled trial. *Lancet*, **ii**, 388–93.

Brown, Z. A., Benedetti, J., Ashley, R., *et al.* (1991). Neonatal herpes simplex infection in relation to asymptomatic maternal infection at the time of labour. *New England Journal of Medicine*, **324**, 1247–52.

Copel, J. A., Cullen, M. T., Grannum, P. A., and Hobbins, J. C. (1990). Invasive fetal assessment in the antepartum period. *Obstetrics and Gynecology Clinics of North America*, **17**, 201–21.

Daffos, F., Forestier, F., Capella-Pavlovsky, M., Thulliez, P., Aufrant, C., Valenti, D., *et al.* (1988). Prenatal management of 746 pregnancies at risk for congenital toxoplasmosis. *The New England Journal of Medicine*, **318**, 271–5.

Desmonts. G., Daffos, F., Forestier, F., Capella-Pavlovsky, M., Thulliez, Ph., and Chartier, M. (1985). Prenatal diagnosis of congenital toxoplasmosis. *Lancet*, March 2, 500–4.

Dorfman, D. H. and Glaser, J. H. (1990). Congenital syphilis presenting in infants after the newborn period. *New England Journal of Medicine*, **323**, 1299–302.

European Collaborative Study (1991). Children born to women with HIV-1 infection: natural history and risk of transmission. *Lancet* **337**, 253–60.

Fan, Y. D., Pastorek, J. G., Janney, F. A., and Sanders, C. V. (1989). Listeriosis as an obstetric complication in an immunocompromised patient. *Southern Medical Journal*, **82**, 1044–5.

Fiumara, N. J., Fleming, W. L., Downing, J. G., and Good, F. L. (1952). The incidence of prenatal syphilis at the Boston City Hospital. *New England Journal of Medicine*, **247**, 48–52.

Foulon, W., Naessens, A., Catte, L. de, and Amy, J. J. (1990). Detection of congenital toxoplasmosis by chorionic villus sampling and early amniocentesis. *American Journal of Obstetrics and Gynecology*, **163**, 1511–13.

Gauntt, C. J., Gudvangen, R. J., Brans, Y. W., *et al.* (1985). Coxsackievirus group B antibodies in ventricular fluid of infants with severe anatomic defects in the central nervous system. *Pediatrics*, **76**, 64.

Goedert, J. J., Mendez, H., Drummond, J. E., *et al.* (1989). Mother to infant transmission of human immunodefiency virus type 1: association with prematurity or low anti-gp 120. *Lancet*, **2**, 1351–4.

Grose, C. and Weiner, C.P. (1990). Prenatal diagnosis of congenital cytomegalovirus infection: two decades later. *American Journal of Obstetrics and Gynecology*, **163**, 447–50

Grose C., Itani, O., and Weiner, C. P. (1989). Prenatal diagnosis of fetal infection: advances from amniocentesis to cordocentesis — congenital toxoplasmosis, rubella, cytomegalovirus, varicella virus, parvovirus and human immunodeficiency virus. *Pediatric Infectious Diseases Journal*, **8**, 459–68.

Grover, C. M., Thulliez, P., Remington, J. S., and Boothroyd, J. C. (1990). Rapid prenatal diagnosis of congenital toxoplasma infection by using polymerase chain reaction and amniotic fluid. *Journal of Clinical Microbiology*, **28**, 2297–301.

Hakosalo, J. and Saxen, L. (1971). Influenza epidemic and congenital defects. *Lancet*, **ii**, 1346.

Hira, S. K., Kamanga, J., Bhat G. J., *et al.* (1989). Perinatal transmission of HIV-1 in Zambia. *British Medical Journal*, **299**, 1250–2.

Hohlfeld, P., Daffos, F., Thulliez, P., Aufrant, C., Couvreur, J., MacAleese, J., *et al.* (1989). Fetal toxoplasmosis: Outcome of pregnancy and infant follow-up after *in utero* treatment. *Fetal and Neonatal Medicine*, **115**, 765–9.

Holmes, W. (1991) Vertical transmission of HIV (letter). *Lancet*, **337**, 794–5.

Hoskins, I. A. (1991). Cordocentesis in isoimmunization and fetal physiological measurement, infection, and karyotyping. *Current Opinion in Obstetrics and Gynecology*, **3**, 266–71.

Ho-Yen, D. O., and Joss, A. W. L. (1991). Toxoplasma and cytomegalovirus infections in pregnancy. *Current Obstetrics and Gynecology*, **1**, 62–6.

Jeannel, D., Costagliola, D., Niel, G., Hubert, B., and Danis, M. (1990). What is known about the prevention of congenital toxoplasmosis? *Lancet*, **336**, 359–61.

Klapper, P. E. and Morris, D. J. (1990). Screening for viral and protozoal infections in pregnancy. A review. *British Journal of Obstetrics and Gynaecology*, **97**, 974–83.

Lee, R. V. (1988). Parasites and pregnancy: The problems of malaria and toxoplasmosis. *Clinics in Perinatology*, **15**, 351–63.

Levy, M. and Read, S. E. (1990). Erythema infectiosum and pregnancy-related complications. *Canadian Medical Association Journal*, **1439**, 849–58.

Lynch, L., Daffos, F., Emanuel, D., *et al.* (1991). Prenatal diagnosis of cytomegalovirus infection. *American Journal of Obstetrics and Gynecology*, **165**; 714–18.

McCarthy, M. (1983) Of cats and women. *British Medical Journal*, **287**, 445–6.

McGregor, J. A. (1991). Maternal and fetal infection. *Current Opinion in Obstetrics and Gynecology*, **3**, 15–23.

Miller, E., Cradock-Watson, J. E., and Pollock, T. M. (1982). Consequences of confirmed maternal rubella at successive stages of pregnancy. *Lancet*, **ii**, 781.

Musher, D. M., Hamill, R. J., and Baughn, R. E. (1990). Effect of human immuno-deficiency virus (HIV) infection on the course of syphilis and on the response to treatment. *Annals of Internal Medicine*, **113**, 872–81.

Noren, G. R., Adams, P. Jr., and Anderson, R. C. (1963). Positive skin reactivity to mumps virus antigen in endocardial fibroelastosis. *Journal of Pediatrics*, **62**, 604.

Peters, M. T. and Nicolaides, K. H. (1990). Cordocentesis for the diagnosis and treatment of human fetal parvovirus infection. *Obstetrics and Gynecology*, **75**, 501–4.

Preblud, S., Cochi, S., and Orenstein, W. (1986). Varicella–zoster infection in pregnancy. *New England Journal of Medicine*, **315**, 1415.

Prober, C. G., Sullender, C. A., Yasukawa, L. L., *et al.* (1987). Low risk of herpes simplex infections in neonates exposed to the virus at the time of delivery to mothers with recurrent genital herpes simplex virus infection. *New England Journal of Medicine*, **316**, 240.

Public Health Laboratory Service Working Party on Fifth Disease (1990). Prospective study of human parvovirus (B19) infection on pregnancy. *British Medical Journal*, **300**, 1166–70.

Rubin, L., Leggiadro, R., Elie, M.T., *et al.* (1986). Disseminated varicella in a neonate: implications for immunoprophylaxis of neonates postnatally exposed to varicella. *Pediatric Infectious Diseases*, **5**, 100.

Siegel, M. (1973). Congenital malformations following chickenpox, measles, mumps, and hepatitis. Results of a cohort study. *Journal of the American Medical Association*, **226**, 1521.

Siegel, M. and Greenberg, M. (1956). Poliomyelitis in pregnancy. Effect on fetus and newborn infant. *Journal of Pediatrics*, **49**, 280.

Skinner *et al.* 1989.

Stagno, S. (1990). Cytomegalovirus. In *Infectious diseases of the fetus and the newborn infant*, (ed. J. S. Remington and J. O. Klein), pp. 241–81. W. B. Saunders, Philadelphia.

Webster, M. H. and Smith, C. S. (1977). Congenital abnormalities and maternal herpes zoster. *British Medical Journal*, **4**, 1193.

Wendel, G. D., Jr. (1989). Early and congenital syphilis. *Obstetrics and Gynecology Clinics of North America*, **16**, 479–94.

6
Symposium: Fetal infections
B Ultrasound imaging
M. E. Furness and H. M. Chambers

Introduction

As described in the previous chapter, the possibility of fetal infection opens up many areas of uncertainty, which make counselling the parents very difficult. The sonographic abnormalities resulting from infection are non-specific, although particular combinations of findings raise the suspicion of infection, or of a particular organism. When maternal infection is known to have occurred, ultrasound is limited in its ability to diagnose whether or not the fetus has also become infected. (At present, antenatal ultrasound scans are unable to recognize one of the commonest markers of congenital infection, chorioretinitis.) Nor can ultrasound reliably predict whether an infected fetus will be affected, for example by cytomegalovirus (CMV), in which a proportion of infected fetuses are unharmed. Even an infection which is subclinical at birth is potentially damaging; 5–15 per cent of asymptomatic neonates with CMV (Alford *et al.* 1990), 33 per cent of those with rubella (Dickinson and Gonik 1990), and almost all with untreated toxoplasmosis (Ho-Yen and Joss 1991) will ultimately manifest evidence of developmental injury. The so-called benign form of treated toxoplasmosis with asymptomatic intracranial calcification must have the potential to cause epilepsy.

Diagnosis of infection by immunological or microbiological methods is also limited. It is important to remember that a single negative test cannot exclude infection, and that diagnosis of infection may require a combination of tests. Specific IgM is not produced by the fetus until 19–23 weeks, and commonly is not detectable at all for some infections. Furthermore, chronic maternal infection may result in transmission of organisms to the fetus after the time of testing. Even minimal maternal contamination of fetal blood cells at cordocentesis may give false-positive results in tests involving polymerase chain reaction (PCR) enhancement.

The extent to which a particular pregnancy should be investigated is debatable; it is influenced by local endemic infections, the resources and skills available, and, increasingly, by the medico-legal environment. Fetal infection severe enough to produce abnormalities on ultrasound scanning has a very poor prognosis, and termination of pregnancy without further antenatal investigation may be appropriate. For continuing pregnancies, there is a need to document the diagnosis and progression in order to increase our knowledge of the natural history of these conditions. Registries of the common infections will be important. Invasive investigation, however, is potentially hazardous. The infected fetus commonly has thrombocytopenia, and is at risk of prolonged bleeding after cordocentesis. The impressive low complication rates reported by world leaders in cordocentesis are not likely to be achieved by units on the learning curve, or those with a small workload. Clinical and laboratory staff need to be aware of their own risks from maternal and fetal fluids and tissues.

Similarly, treatment of fetal infections is not clear-cut. Spiramycin has not been proven to prevent transplacental passage of toxoplasmosis; a randomized trial has been suggested, but would be difficult to achieve in the face of consumer politics (Jeannel *et al.* 1990). Transfusion of fetuses with parvovirus infection has been suggested, but may not be necessary in all cases, since spontaneous resolution of parvovirus-induced hydrops has been documented (Morey *et al.* 1991). Furthermore, it is not known whether it is prudent to salvage such fetuses, in view of the teratogenic effects of animal parvoviruses. Ganciclovir has been suggested as a possible future treatment of fetal CMV, but it is marrow-toxic and can cause permanent infertility in adults. The best treatment for fetal infection at present lies in prevention, via education of the public about measures to decrease the hazards (Ho-Yen and Joss 1991).

What is certain, however, is that fetuses aborted because ultrasound showed abnormalities should be submitted for examination by a specialized perinatal pathologist; this examination must include a full morphological evaluation of the fetus, photographs and X-rays, and where indicated, microbiological and cytogenetic assessment (Members of the Joint Study Group on Fetal Abnormalities 1989). If invasive prenatal diagnostic procedures have been performed, pathological examination of the fetus, placenta, cord, and membranes is imperative in order to document any complications. It is these examinations which provide the quality control essential for the practice of diagnostic fetal ultrasound.

General pathology of fetal infections

Most infections reach the fetus by the transplacental route from the maternal circulation with invasion of placental villous vascular endothelium. The permeability of the placental barrier to blood-borne infection varies with the gestational age and with the organism. Maternal non-polio enterovirus infections rarely involve the fetus (Amstey *et al.* 1988), whereas the transmission rate of rubella from mother to fetus is high, especially in the first trimester and the last month of pregnancy (Grose *et al.* 1989). There remains an unexplained variability in infectivity — antenatal toxoplasmosis, for example, has been described in only one of dichorionic twins (Hohlfield *et al.* 1991*a*). In general, the earlier fetal infection occurs, the more severe its impact. Syphilis, however, although it can cross the placenta as early as 6 weeks' gestation, does not cause injury until the fetus becomes able to mount an immune response, at around 18 weeks (Wendel 1989). Thereafter it produces disseminated disease.

The mechanisms for tissue damage differ with the infection, with some mechanisms common to several diseases. Some agents exert an overall inhibitory effect on somatic growth (CMV, rubella), or on the development of a particular organ at a critical stage (for example the effect of rubella infection on the embryonic heart). Acute inflammation may cause not only tissue necrosis but also changes in tissue maturation. In the brain this leads to delayed neuronal migration and microcephaly (CMV, rubella). The vasculitis accompanying acute inflammation may be followed by thrombosis and localized ischaemic tissue injury. Dystrophic calcification of necrotic tissue, especially in the brain and liver, is common in many fetal infections. The reparative sequelae of acute inflammation in the brain may cause obstructive hydrocephalus. Acute inflammatory change may compromise specific organ function. Infection of the developing nervous system by varicella–zoster virus leads to scarring in a dermatome distribution and to peripheral limb reduction defects, thought to reflect denervation at the dorsal-root ganglia during embryogenesis (Alkalay *et al.* 1987). Myocarditis can cause cardiac failure. Agents that affect the haemopoietic system and cause anaemia may present as hydrops. They may also cause haemorrhage, since thrombocytopenia is a major feature of the common congenital infections.

Hydrops in fetal infection is usually due to a combination of causes (Nyberg *et al.* 1990). Myocarditis, with or without arrhythmias, may cause cardiac failure. Hepatitis can cause not only hepatic congestion, leading to portal hypertension, but also decreased albumin and protein production, leading to decreased colloid oncotic pressure. Chronic anaemia can cause similar liver dysfunction by replacement of liver parenchyma with haemopoietic tissue, and can also cause high-output cardiac failure. Generalized endothelial damage, with increased capillary permeability, is a further possibility.

Toxoplasma has a particular affinity for the central nervous system (CNS) and the eye. The parasite invades fetal vessels, with inflammation and thrombosis, leading to vessel rupture with haemorrhage, and to ischaemic necrosis. Toxoplasma pseudocysts are released from macrophages in areas of damaged tissue, producing a vicious cycle of further inflammation and vasculitis. Acute inflammatory, granulomatous and chronic lesions may thus be present all at the same time. In the CNS, toxoplasmosis causes random parenchymal liquefaction and subsequent calcification; porencephalic cysts, ventricular dilatation, or hydranencephaly may occur. Focal micropolygyria has been described, presumably due to localized scar formation.

Cytomegalovirus and rubella cause cellular injury either by direct viral cytolysis, or by a non-cytocidal suppression of cell proliferation and retardation of growth. Both mechanisms may give rise to delayed brain growth. Large areas of tissue damage are not common in the brain, in contradistinction to toxoplasmosis, but have been described. An indirect tissue effect is also said to occur through immuno complex vasculitis (Ben-Ami *et al.* 1990).

Parvovirus attacks its target organ, the erythroblast, as soon as it appears, at 6 weeks. In the first half of pregnancy it involves the liver; later it has more impact on bone marrow. It also can cause myocarditis, which may contribute to hydrops (Morey *et al.* 1991).

Sonographic findings suspicious of infection

General

Hydrops refers to excess body fluid in at least two sites. Isolated ascites or pleural effusion appear to have different causes and usually a better prognosis, but they may also be early signs of generalized hydrops. It has been suggested that hydrops consisting of a dilated heart with tense ascites, but little oedema or pleural fluid, is likely to reflect anaemia (Peters and Nicolaides 1990).

Some infections are common causes of hydrops, while others are rare. The relative incidence depends on local endemic and epidemic infections; whether the commonest infective cause of hydrops is parvovirus or syphilis depends on whether you practise in Scotland or New York. These local variations probably account for the wide variation in reports of the proportion of hydrops which is caused by infection. Infections which are convincing causes of hydrops include CMV, coxsackievirus, parvovirus, syphilis, and toxoplasmosis. Associations (not necessarily causative) have been described with adenovirus[1], Chagas' disease hepatitis B, herpes simplex type 1, influenza B, leptospirosis, listeriosis, respiratory syncytial virus, rubella, and varicella–zoster.

Intra-uterine growth reduction (IUGR) is common after fetal infection (CMV, rubella; rarely parvovirus, varicella–zoster), but is too non-specific and frequent a finding to warrant investigation for infection, unless there are other suspicious findings or a suggestive history. Abnormal Doppler studies are likewise non-specific.

Substantially raised maternal serum alpha-fetoprotein, in the absence of demonstrable fetal abnormality or a maternal source, may be a marker for fetal hepatitis.

Multiple abnormal findings on ultrasound examination are suspicious of infection (among other things), especially if they include scattered calcification, hydrops, hydrocephalus, and a bulky placenta.

---

[1] We have seen adenovirus infection early in the second trimester cause progessive hydrops, hepatic necrosis and progessive hydrocephalus.

Fetal akinesia deformation sequence (Figs 6.1 and 6.2) refers to a number of conditions (Pena–Shokeir type 1, multiple pterygium syndrome, congenital arthrogryposis) whose abnormalities are considered to result from a lack of fetal movement. Ultrasound findings include non-visualization of the stomach, with polyhydramnios (lack of swallowing), small thorax and pulmonary hypoplasia (lack of fetal breathing), multiple joint deformities (lack of limb movements), short umbilical cord (lack of trunk movements), scoliosis and micrognathia. Although an association with fetal infection has not been recognized, there have been isolated reports of infection co-existing with pseudoparalysis (syphilis), arthrogryposis (CMV, rubella, Venezuelan equine encephalitis virus), pulmonary hypoplasia despite polyhydramnios (CMV) (Grose *et al.* 1989; Drose *et al.* 1991), hypotonia, and reduced fetal movement. It is conceivable than an infected fetus with profound neurological damage could present in this way. In view of the 1991 outbreak of poliomyelitis in Bulgaria, it is worth recalling that polio can cause fetal paralysis, and that the spontaneous abortion rate has been reported as 13–24 per cent (Dickinson and Gonik 1990).

Head

Intracranial abnormality is common in the common fetal infections, but visualization in the fetus may be impaired by a reverberation artefact, especially

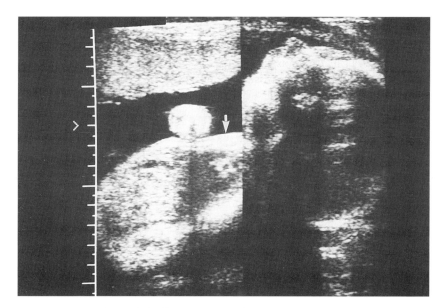

Fig. 6.1. 29 weeks, polyhydramnios. Fetal akinesia, not related to infection. Sagittal scan of fetal trunk and head, caudal to the left, showing small thorax (arrow) and micrognathia.

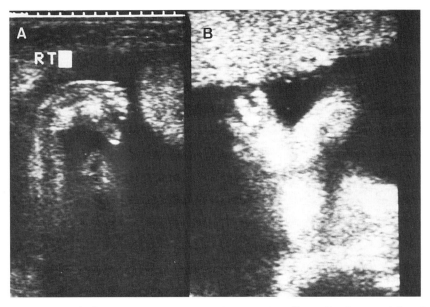

Fig. 6.2. Fetal akinesia, same case as Fig. 6.1. A, talipes. B, abnormal hand posture.

in the third trimester or in the presence of microcephaly. We have included some features which we would not expect to be able to identify antenatally at present, but which may become detectable with further improvements in equipment. If intracranial abnormality is suspected, trans-fontanellar views should be sought, if necessary by trans-vaginal scanning.

1. Ventricular dilatation may be due to obstruction, most commonly at the aqueduct, by organizing ependymitis following either infective inflammation or haemorrhage (Fig. 6.3). It is most commonly seen with toxoplasma infection, but has also been described with adenovirus, influenza, and varicella–zoster. Aqueduct stenosis is known to follow infection with CMV, mumps, and syphilis in animals (Romero *et al.* 1988). Obstructive hydrocephalus can develop very rapidly (Hohlfield *et al.* 1991*a*), but in the fetus enlargement of the head is a late finding.

2. Ventricular dilatation may also reflect loss of parenchyma ('*hydrocephalus ex vacuo*'), usually with microcephaly; widening of the subarachnoid space may also be visible (Fig. 6.4).

3. Microcephaly is one of the conditions which is preferable to under-diagnose rather than overdiagnose if it is an isolated finding, in view of the severe emotional stress to the parents caused by a false-positive diagnosis. However, if ventricular dilatation and/or intracranial calcification are present, infection is a strong possibility. This is the central nervous system abnormality

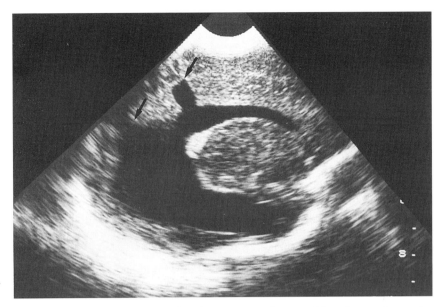

Fig. 6.3. Neonate day 1, large head. Parasagittal scan of head, anterior to the right. Porencephaly (arrow) and hydrocephalus. Focal calcifications were seen on other views. Proven toxoplasmosis.

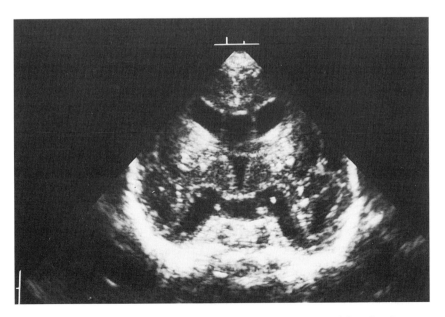

Fig. 6.4. Neonate day 1, microcephaly. Coronal scan of head, showing dilatation of ventricles and subarachnoid space, and periventricular hyperechoic areas. Proven CMV.

commonly caused by CMV and rubella; rare causes include coxsackievirus, Epstein–Barr virus, herpes simplex, toxoplasmosis and varicella–zoster.

4. Focal parenchymal loss may lead to parenchymal or porencephalic cysts (Fig. 6.3), (toxoplasmosis, rarely CMV). In extreme cases, hydranencephaly has been described (toxoplasmosis, herpes simplex), presumably due to infarction of both internal carotid territories.

5. Focal hyperechoic areas can reflect brain necrosis without calcification (Hohlfield *et al.* 1991*a*). Dystrophic calcification can follow tissue necrosis from any cause, but may not be sufficiently dense to produce shadowing. CMV is traditionally described as producing periventricular calcification, and toxoplasmosis, random calcific foci. This distinction may be less clear-cut in the fetus and neonate. Calcification may be harder to recognize antenatally than in the neonate (Fig. 6.5). Herpes simplex and varicella–zoster viruses can both cause intracranial calcification, microcephaly, and ventricular dilatation (Dickinson and Gonik 1990).

6. Haemorrhage, although not often recognized antenatally, is at least a theoretical possibility, since thrombocytopenia is a common feature of fetal infections.

7. Subependymal cysts/intraventricular adhesions are well-known non-specific markers of intrauterine infection in the neonate (Fig. 6.6). They may follow infection or haemorrhage. They should not be confused with the choroid cysts seen in the second trimester.

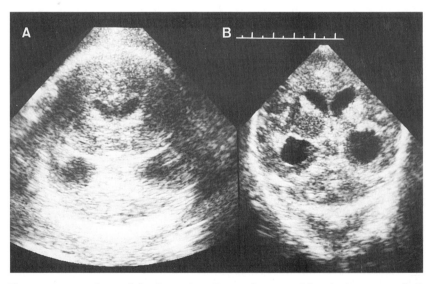

Fig. 6.5. 38 weeks, polyhydramnios. Coronal scans of head. A, antenatal; B, postnatal, 1 day later, showing focal hyperechoic areas and ventricular dilatation. Proven toxoplasmosis.

8. Echogenic streaks in the basal ganglia are known to occur in the neonate with CMV, herpes simplex, rubella, and syphilis (also with trisomy 13 and maternal drug abuse). They are thought to reflect a mineralizing vasculopathy of the lenticulostriate arteries, and may be related to deposition of immune complexes (Ben-Ami *et al.* 1990).

9. The eyes may be affected. Microphthalmia is a late finding in some infections (Epstein–Barr virus, herpes simplex, rubella, and varicella–zoster) (Dickinson and Gonik 1990). Cataracts, which can also follow infections, have been recognized on antenatal ultrasound (Shapiro *et al.* 1991). In contrast to the known teratogenicity of animal parvoviruses, there has been only one case report to date of a teratogenic effect of human parvovirus, (Hartwig *et al.* 1989) with features like rubella. A single case has been described of cyclopia-holoprosencephaly in a neonate with histological evidence of CMV.

Thorax

Non-specific markers of infection include:

1. Pleural or pericardial effusions, oedema, usually as components of generalized hydrops.

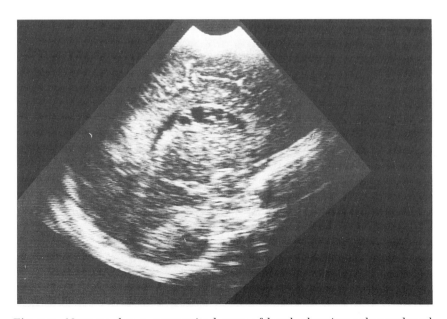

Fig. 6.6. Neonate day 1, parasagittal scan of head, showing subependymal cysts/intraventricular adhesions. Proven rubella.

2. Cardiomegaly (Fig. 6.7). Anaemia may cause high-output failure, and dilated cardiac chambers. Endocardial fibroelastosis has been described with coxsackie B3 infection, and perhaps mumps.

3. Poor cardiac contractility with myocarditis (coxsackie, parvovirus, syphilis, and toxoplasmosis).

4. Cardiac arrhythmias, for example supraventricular tachycardia (Fig. 6.8). A case of intermittent bradycardia with a transient pericardial effusion has been described with CMV.

5. Calcification anywhere.

6. Pulmonary hypoplasia can reflect oligohydramnios, fetal akinesia, or longstanding massive ascites.

7. Structural abnormalities (peripheral pulmonary artery stenosis, ventricular septal defect, atrial septal defect, pulmonary valvular stenosis) are features of the expanded congenital rubella syndrome (Carrington 1991); not all are recognizable antenatally.

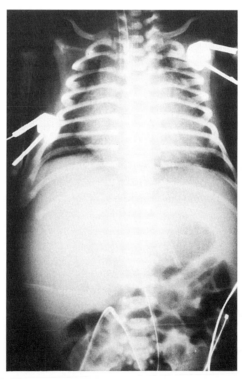

Fig. 6.7. Chest X-ray of neonate, showing cardiomegaly and hepatospleno-megaly. Metaphysitis is also present. Proven syphilis.

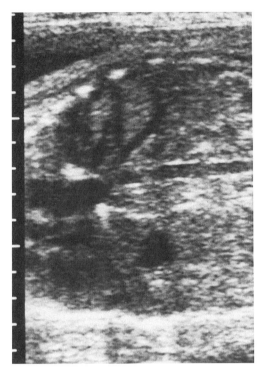

Fig. 6.8. 38 weeks, polyhdramnios. Coronal scan of fetal upper abdomen, left side down, caudad to the right. Dilated hepatic veins due to supraventricular tachycardia and heart failure. Proven Coxsackie B1 infection.

Abdomen

1. Ascites, oedema as features of generalized hydrops.

2. Hepatomegaly, splenomegaly (Fig. 6.9) are major markers for the common fetal infections (CMV, parvo, rubella, syphilis, toxoplasmosis), but can occur with any infection which causes fetal hepatitis, anaemia, or cardiac failure.

3. Non-visualization of the stomach (fetal akinesia), with polyhydramnios and other signs of infection.

4. Calcification anywhere. A single calcific focus in the liver as an isolated finding, however, is common and usually benign (Nyberg *et al.* 1990).

Limbs

1. Peripheral reduction defects (unilateral limb hypoplasia, rudimentary digits) can follow varicella–zoster.

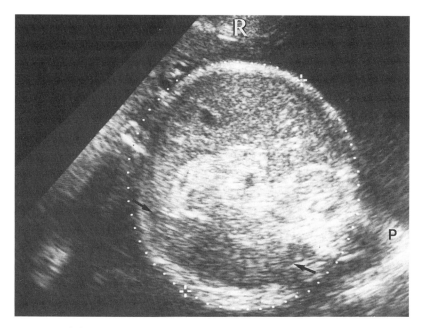

Fig. 6.9. Polyhydramnios. Transverse scan of fetal abdomen, R, right, P, posterior. Splenomegaly (arrows) and hepatomegaly. The stomach was not visualized. Proven toxoplasmosis (same case as Fig. 6.5).

2. Multiple joint deformities (Fig. 6.2) have been described with a number of infections which cause profound intracranial abnormality.

Amniotic fluid

Abnormalities of volume are non-specific findings. In one study (Drose *et al.* 1991), of ten proven cases of fetal CMV infection with other sonographic abnormalities six showed decreased amniotic fluid, and three had polyhydramnios.

Placenta

Fetal hydrops can be associated with placental oedema, so that it becomes bulky (Fig. 6.10) and less commonly, echogenic. Microscopy shows villous oedema, often with relative immaturity, hypercellularity, abnormal erythropoiesis, and/or inflammatory infiltrates.

Ultrasound-guided investigation and treatment

The ultrasonologist has two tasks related to fetal infection; to determine whether the fetus is infected and affected when there is proven maternal infection, and to

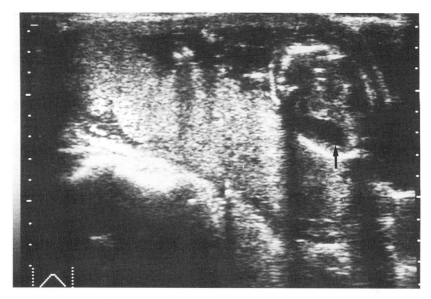

Fig. 6.10. 18 weeks, 'routine' scan. Longitudinal view of uterus, showing dilated fetal ventricles (arrow), oligohydramnios, and bulky placenta. Abdominal calcification and ascites were also evident. Proven CMV.

suggest appropriate investigations when abnormalities suspicious of infection are found unexpectedly on ultrasound scans. How aggressive the investigation should be depends on the stage of pregnancy at which infection occurred and the age at diagnosis, bearing in mind that most early infections or those that have caused sonographic abnormalities give a very poor prognosis. Depending on local laws and mores, a termination of pregnancy should be offered if a pre-viable infected fetus shows sonographic abnormality, parvovirus being an (arguable) exception.

Cordocentesis has had a major impact on the management of suspected fetal infection. It can be used to identify the organism by culture, immuno-electron microscopy, antigen detection with monoclonal antibodies, or hybridization studies with labelled DNA and RNA probes (Grose *et al.* 1989). Assays of specific IgM can be performed, although they are not reliable before 23 weeks, or in parvovirus infection (Carrington 1991). Non-specific signs of infection (haematological indices and liver enzyme assays) can be used to indicate whether the fetus is, at that time, affected as well as infected. Amniocentesis has a place in the culture of some organisms (CMV, toxoplasmosis), and body fluids (for example ascites) may also be a source of organisms. Chorionic villus sampling and early amniocentesis will be used increasingly in the future, and polymerase chain reaction (PCR) techniques may simplify investigation. Invasive studies should be restricted to situations where suspicion of an infection is strong.

Rubella

At present, termination of pregnancy should be offered to all women with a primary infection, or symptomatic reinfection, occurring before 17 weeks' gestation (Carrington 1991). This could be reduced if fetal infection could be excluded. Rubella antigen can be detected in amniotic fluid by an enzyme-linked immunoassay (ELISA), and rubella-specific IgM can be detected in cord blood after 19 weeks, but a single negative result is not conclusive with either test. Tissue obtained from chorionic villus biopsy at 12 weeks' gestation has been reported to show a characteristic cytopathic effect in appropriate cell lines, and a positive result with *in situ* hybridization using a DNA probe (Grose *et al.* 1989).

Cytomegalovirus

Since the infected fetus excretes the virus in urine, viral cultures of amniotic fluid can confirm infection in 1–3 days, (Grose and Weiner 1990). The sensitivity of this test is not known. Cordocentesis may have a place, either for further reassurance if amniotic fluid culture is negative, or to assess the current status of an infected fetus. Hohlfield *et al.* (1991*b*) have suggested that haematological abnormalities and elevated gamma-glutamyl transferase levels indicate an affected fetus, but it is not known whether negative results show that the fetus is one of the 90 per cent of infected infants who will be asymptomatic at birth. Some 5–15 per cent of such infants will later develop sensorineural hearing loss, chorioretinitis, developmental delay, or defects in dental enamel (Alford *et al.* 1990). Parents of a pre-viable infected fetus may find these odds unacceptable. If they elect to continue the pregnancy, the outcome should be documented.

Varicella–zoster

Infection has been confirmed by the demonstration of specific IgM in cord blood. Viral cultures of white cells may be diagnostic in the early phase; hybridization studies of DNA from white cells obtained by cordocentesis may provide a diagnosis if investigations are delayed (Grose and Itani 1989). The use of serial ultrasound scans has been suggested to identify limb reduction defects, intracranial abnormality, and microphthalmia. It may be possible to identify severe scarring. It is not known how many of those fetuses who were infected in the first or second trimester will be severely affected, but this seems to be rare (Wesselingh and Gordon, Chapter 6A, this volume).

Parvovirus

Maternal infection is associated with a 9 per cent pregnancy loss rate, from fetal anaemia and cardiac failure, with its greatest impact being in the second trimester (Public Health Laboratory Service Working Party on Fifth Disease 1990). Once hydrops develops, most untreated fetuses, but not all, succumb (Schwarz *et al.* 1988; Cameron *et al.* 1991). However, by treatment with transfusions, it is one of the few salvageable causes of infection-induced sonographic abnormality in the fetus.

Fetal infection can be proven by identifying viral inclusions in fetal red cells or ascitic fluid, with *in situ* DNA hybridization; fetal IgM is usually not contributory. However, cordocentesis carries the risk of causing prolonged bleeding in thrombocytopenic fetuses (Peters and Nicolaides 1990), and protocols have been suggested for non-invasive investigation following maternal infection. These consist of ultrasound scans every 1–2 weeks, with quantitation of maternal AFP levels, elevations of which can predate hydrops by several weeks (Carrington 1991; Holzgreve 1990). Surveillance should continue for 6–8 weeks after maternal exposure to parvovirus (Rodis *et al.* 1990) or longer if the AFP levels are abnormal. Fetal demise has occurred as late as 16 weeks after infection. Transfusion should be restricted to those fetuses with evidence of cardiac failure. The place of transfusion has been questioned, since it may depress natural compensatory erythropoiesis, and neither the natural history nor the teratogenic potential of parvovirus B19 infection is known (Morey *et al.* 1991; Public Health Laboratory Service Working Party on Fifth Disease 1990). Survivors should be monitored for evidence of long-term myocardial damage (Morey *et al.* 1991).

Toxoplasmosis

The pioneering work on the use of cordocentesis by Daffos, in Paris, is well known. Diagnosis of fetal infection may require a combination of studies; demonstration of the parasite in amniotic fluid and/or cord blood via cell culture and/or mouse inoculation, and assays of specific fetal IgM levels after 19 weeks (Hohlfield *et al.* 1989). Fetal toxoplasma infection has also been confirmed by amniocentesis and chorionic villus sampling in early second trimester (Foulon *et al.* 1990).

A normal ultrasound scan does not exclude profound cerebral injury. Termination of pregnancy before viability should, therefore, be offered if fetal infection occurred in the first trimester, or if there is any sonographic abnormality (Hohlfield *et al.* 1991*a*). Some workers would extend this to any infected pre-viable fetus. As was discussed in the previous chapter, in a continuing pregnancy proven maternal infection is treated immediately with spiramycin in an attempt to decrease the risk of transplacental transmission of infection (Hohlfield *et al.* 1989, 1991*a*), but its efficacy is not proven (Jeannel *et al.* 1990). Treatment with pyrimethamine, sulphadiazine, and folinic acid must be commenced if there is a sonographic abnormality, or when fetal infection is confirmed. Close monitoring for evidence of toxicity to the mother is necessary (Ho-Yen and Joss 1991).

Syphilis

In general, maternal syphilis does not warrant invasive fetal investigation, since serology on neonatal cord blood is not reliable, and all infants of infected untreated mothers require treatment (Wendel 1989). The maternal HIV status should be assessed, since HIV infection can make standard treatment for syphilis inadequate and genital ulcerative lesions, such as chancres, are thought to increase the efficiency of sexual transmission of HIV (Ikeda and Jenson 1990). Some 30–40 per cent of fetuses with antenatal syphilis are stillborn, making a strong argument for routine radiography of all stillbirths, since at least 95 per cent of cases of congenital syphilis show bony abnormalities (Wendel 1989).

Treatment of maternal syphilis which produces a Jarisch–Herxheimer reaction can cause transient fetal distress or premature labour; in the compromised fetus, it may precipitate fetal demise (Wendel 1989). If ultrasound shows fetal hydrops due to syphilis before 32 weeks, we suggest admitting the mother to hospital for the duration of treatment. Between 32 and 37 weeks, amniocentesis for lung maturity should be considered (avoiding the placenta in case there is concurrent maternal HIV infection). If the lungs are mature, or the pregnancy is more than 37 weeks, the hydropic fetus should be delivered before treatment is commenced. Syphilis is not a cause of hydrops before 20 weeks.

Investigations initiated on the basis of sonographic findings

The reader is referred to major textbooks (for example Romero *et al.* 1988; Nyberg *et al.* 1990) for differential diagnoses and protocols for the investigation of hydrops, ventricular dilatation, microcephaly, abdominal calcification, and arrythmias. Requests for serological tests should be directed to the most likely causes, rather than a blanket 'TORCH screen' (Best and Sutherland 1990).

The lists of causes of non-immune hydrops show a striking paucity of conditions with a good outcome. There is an argument, which may not be acceptable to the parents, for restricting antenatal investigation of second-trimester hydrops to the few salvageable causes, and offering termination of pregnancy if none is found.

Vigorous efforts should be made to arrive at a diagnosis after delivery, or to document the natural history of fetal infections in continuing pregnancies, within the limits of the finances and priorities of one's country. Further information is essential in order to assist the counselling of parents and the management of other cases.

Acknowledgments

We are grateful to Dr G. LeQuesne for permission to publish Figure 6.3, and to Dr J. Moore for Figure 6.8.

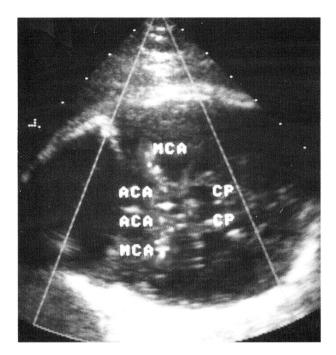

Plate 1 Transverse section of the fetal brain demonstrating the anterior communicating (ACA) and middle cerebral arteries (MCA) by colour flow imaging. The cerebral peduncles are indicated CP. (Reproduced with permission from the British Journal of Obstetrics and Gynaecology.)

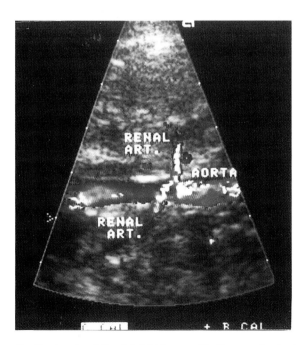

Plate 2 Longitudinal axis of the fetal kidney with the renal arteries and aorta demonstrated by colour flow imaging.

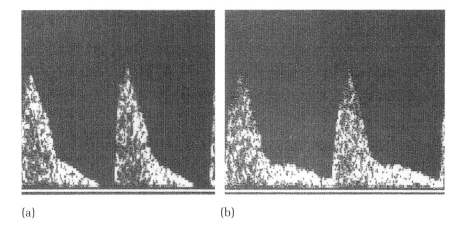

(a)   (b)

Plate 3 Flow velocity waveforms from the fetal renal artery at 26 (a) and 38 (b) weeks' gestation with absence of end-diastolic frequencies in the former and presence in the latter.

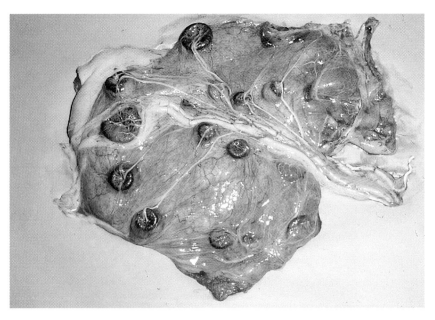

Plate 4 Photograph taken at post-mortem examination of the uterine wall showing placental cotyledons and bifurcations of the umbilical vessels. In sheep there are two umbilical veins and two umbilical arteries, in contrast to humans in which there are two umbilical arteries and a single umbilical vein.

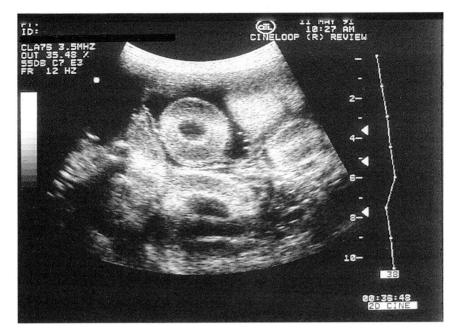

(a)

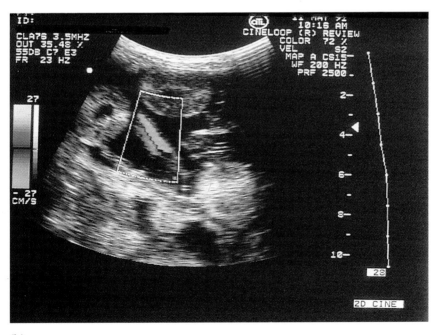

(b)

Plate 5 Ultrasound images at 80 days' gestation of placental cotyledons showing (a) their circular shape at this age and (b) flow through an umbilical artery and vein as displayed by colour flow Doppler examination.

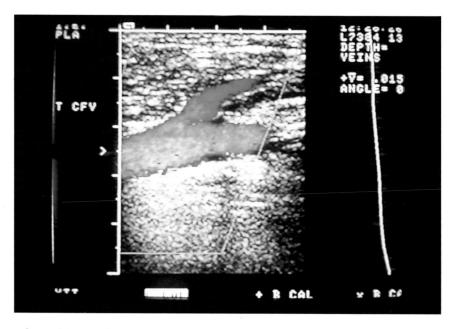

Plate 6(a) A colour Doppler image of a normal sapheno-femoral junction. Colour fills the entire lumen.

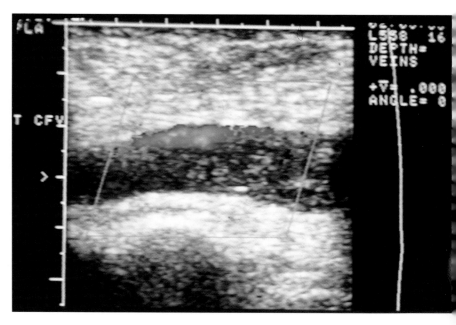

Plate 6(b) A colour Doppler image of a common femoral vein which is almost completely occluded by thrombus; a small residual lumen is seen superiorly with the flowing blood shown as blue.

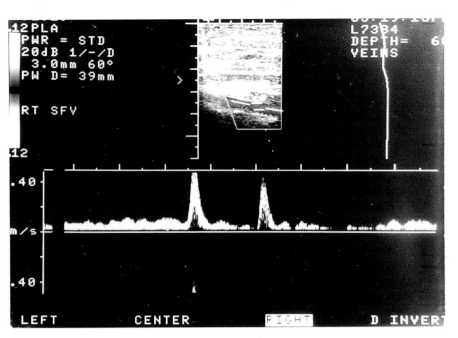

Plate 7(a) A normal augmentation response following two squeezes on the patient's calf.

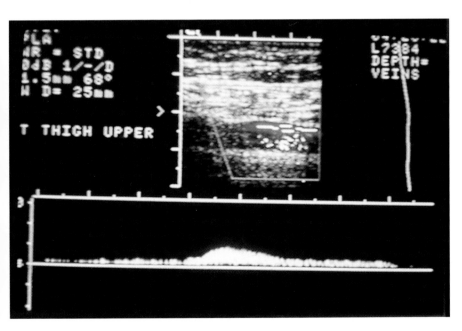

Plate 7(b) Abnormal, damped augmentation in a patient with deep vein thrombosis in the popliteal and lower superficial femoral veins.

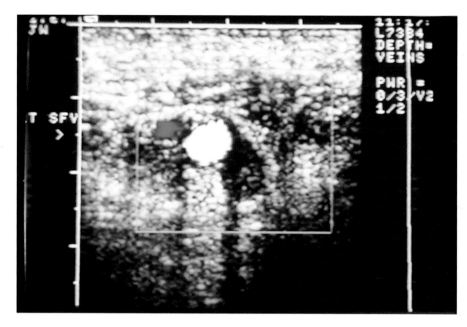

Plate 8 A patient with double superficial femoral veins on either side of the artery (pink). One vein is patent (blue) the other is occluded by thrombus.

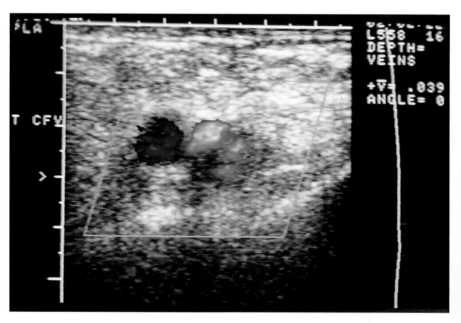

Plate 9 A transverse view of a common femoral vein which has a small thrombus attached to one side but most of the lumen is filled with flowing blood (blue).

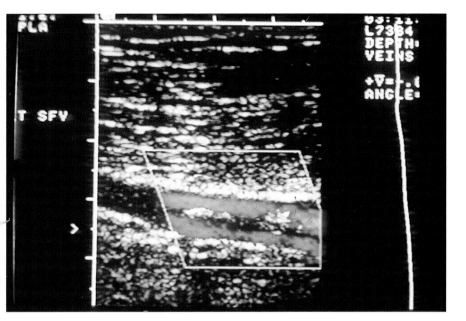

Plate 10 Recanalization after thrombosis. A ridge of echogenic old thrombus is seen projecting into the lumen of the vein with flowing blood (blue) on either side. The vein walls are also thicker and more echogenic than usual as a result of the previous thrombus.

References

Alford, C. A., Stagno, S., Pass, R. F., and Britt, W. J. (1990). Congenital and perinatal cytomegalovirus infection. *Reviews of Infectious Diseases*, **12**, 7, S745–53.

Alkalay, A. L., Pomerance, J. J., and Rimoin, D. L. (1987). Fetal varicella syndrome. *Journal of Pediatrics*, **111**, 3, 320–3.

Amstey, M. S., Miller, R. K., Menegus, M. A., and di Sant'Agnese, P. A. (1988). Enterovirus in pregnant women and the perfused placenta. *American Journal of Obstetrics and Gynecology*, **158**, 775–82.

Ben-Ami, T., Yousefzadeh, D., Backus, M., Reichman, B., Kessler, A., and Hammerman-Rozenberg, C. (1990). Lenticulostriate vasculopathy in infants with infections of the central nervous system and Doppler findings. *Pediatric Radiology*, **20**, 575–9.

Best, J. M. and Sutherland, S. (1990). Diagnosis and prevention of congenital and perinatal infections. *British Medical Journal*, **301**, 888–9.

Cameron, A. D., Ryan, G., Kingdom, J. C. P., Morrow, R. J., Murphy, K., Mackie, P., *et al.* (1991). Non-immune hydrops fetalis and parvovirus infection. *Ultrasound in Obstetrics and Gynaecology*, **1**, supplement 1, 89.

Carrington, D. (1991). Rubella and parvovirus in pregnancy. *Current Obstetrics and Gynaecology*, **1**, 72–7.

Dickinson, J. and Gonik, B. (1990). Teratogenic viral infections. *Clinical Obstetrics and Gynaecology*, **33**, 2, 242–52.

Drose, J. A., Dennis, M. A., and Thickman, D. (1991). Infection *in utero*: US findings in 19 cases. *Radiology*, **178**, 369–74.

Foulon, W., Naessens, A., de Catte, L., and Amy, J. J. (1990). Detection of congenital toxoplasmosis by chorionic villus sampling and early amniocentesis. *American Journal of Obstetrics and Gynecology*, **163**, 1511–13.

Grose, C. and Itani, O. (1989). Pathogenesis of congenital infection with three diverse viruses: varicella–zoster virus, human parvovirus, and human immunodeficiency virus. *Seminars in Perinatology*, **13**, 4, 278–93.

Grose, C. and Weiner, C. P. (1990). Prenatal diagnosis of congenital cytomegalovirus infection: two decades later. *American Journal of Obstetrics and Gynecology*, **163**, 2, 447–50.

Grose, C., Itani, O., and Weiner, C. P. (1989). Prenatal diagnosis of fetal infection: advances from amniocentesis to cordocentesis–congenital toxoplasmosis, rubella, cytomegalovirus, varicella virus, parvovirus and human immunodeficiency virus. *Pediatric Infectious Diseases Journal*, **8**, 459–68.

Hartwig, N. G., Vermeij-Keers, E., Van Elsacker-Niele, A. M. W., and Fleuren, G. J. (1989). Embryonic malformations in a case of intrauterine parvovirus B19 infection. *Teratology*, **39**, 295.

Hohlfield, P., Daffos, F., Thulliez, P., Aufrant, C., Couvreur, J., Macaleese, J., *et al.* (1989). Fetal toxoplasmosis: Outcome of pregnancy and infant followup after *in utero* treatment. *Journal of Paediatrics*, **115**, 5, 765–9.

Hohlfield, P., MacAleese, J., Capella-Pavlovski, M., Giovangrandi, Y., Thulliez, P., Forestier, F., and Daffos, F. (1991*a*). Fetal toxoplasmosis: ultra-sonographic signs. *Ultrasound in Obstetrics and Gynaecology*, **1**, 241–4.

Hohlfield, P., Vial, Y., Mailland, C., and Bossart, H. (1991*b*). CMV fetal infection: pre-natal diagnosis. *Ultrasound in Obstetrics and Gynaecology*, **1**, supplement 1, 87.

Holzgreve, P. D. W. (1990). Fetal anomalies. *Current Opinion in Obstetrics and Gynaecology*, **2**, 215–22.

Ho-Yen, D. O. and Joss, A. W. L. (1991). Toxoplasma and cytomegalovirus infections in pregnancy. *Current Obstetrics and Gynaecology*, **11**, 62–6.

Ikeda, M. K. and Jenson, H. B. (1990). Evaluation and treatment of congenital syphilis. *Journal of Pediatrics*, **117**, 6, 843–52.

Jeannel, D., Costagliola, D., Niel, G., Hubert, B., and Danis, M. (1990). What is known about the prevention of congenital toxoplasmosis? *Lancet*, **336**, 359–61.

Members of the joint study group on fetal abnormalities (1989). Recognition and management of fetal abnormalities. *Archives of Disease in Childhood*, **64**, 971–6.

Morey, A. L., Nicolini, U., Welch, C. R., Economides, D., Chamberlain, P. F., and Cohen, B. J. (1991). Parvovirus B19 infection and transient fetal hydrops. *Lancet*, **337**, 496.

Nyberg, D. A., Mahoney, B. S., and Pretorius, D. H. (ed.) (1990). *Diagnostic Ultrasound of Fetal Anomalies. Text and Atlas.* Mosby Year Book, St. Louis.

Peters, M. T. and Nicolaides, K. H. (1990). Cordocentesis for the diagnosis and treatment of human fetal parvovirus infection. *Obstetrics and Gynecology*, **75**, 501–4.

Public Health Laboratory Service Working Party on Fifth Disease. (1990). Prospective study of human parvovirus (B19) infection in pregnancy. *British Medical Journal*, **300**, 1166–70.

Rodis, J. F., Quinn, D. L., Gary, W., Anderson, L. J., Rosengren, S., Cartter, M. L., *et al.* (1990). Management and outcomes of pregnancies complicated by human B19 parvovirus infection: A prospective study. *American Journal of Obstetrics and Gynecology*, **163**, 1168–71.

Romero, R., Pilu, G., Jeanty, P., Ghidini, A., and Hobbins, J. C. (ed.) (1988). *Prenatal Diagnosis of Congenital Anomalies.* Appleton & Lange, Norwalk.

Schwarz, T. F., Roggerdorf, M., Hottentrager, B., Deinhardt, F., Enders, G., Gloning, K. P., *et al.* (1988). Human parvovirus B19 infection in pregnancy. *Lancet*, **ii**, 566–7.

Shapiro, I., Degani, S., and Sharf, M. (1991). Prenatal sonographic diagnosis of congenital cataract. *Ultrasound in Obstetrics and Gynaecology*, **1**, supplement 1, 52.

Wendel, G. D. (1989). Early and congenital syphilis. *Obstetrics and Gynecology Clinics of North America*, **16**, 479–94.

7
Biophysical profile scoring : a critical review
S. Walkinshaw

Introduction

The aims of antepartum fetal monitoring are two-fold: first to detect the compromised fetus at a stage where therapeutic intervention may avoid death or other major sequelae; and secondly to prevent unnecessary obstetric intervention in the uncompromised fetus.

In 1990 it was stated that fetal biophysical profile (BPP) scoring offered such a method of antepartum fetal surveillance which was sensitive in the recognition of both the normal and the compromised fetus, and that the method allowed grading of the degree of fetal compromise (Manning *et al.* 1990*b*). Yet others (Mohide and Keirse 1989) commented that well-conducted clinical trials were still required to determine the role of the fetal biophysical profile and its advantages over other forms of fetal monitoring.

With widespread use of the BPP in North America, and its increasing acceptance in the UK (Wheble *et al.* 1989), how is it possible to both determine when to use this test and what advantages it offers over other forms of antepartum fetal monitoring?

This review will examine the scientific basis behind fetal biophysical monitoring, the use of the BPP in general clinical practice and in specific high-risk groups, and the difficulties and limitations of such testing.

The development of the fetal biophysical profile

Fetal biophysical profile scoring using real-time ultrasound developed from concerns over the high false-positive rates for non-stress (cardiotocographic) testing (see Thacker and Berkelman 1986) and from early studies demonstrating that variables, such as fetal breathing activity, were as accurate as fetal heart rate monitoring in the detection of fetal compromise (Platt *et al.* 1978). Further work suggested that the combination of the non-stress test and fetal breathing might significantly reduce a false-positive prediction of fetal compromise (Manning *et al.* 1979). As other variables, such as fetal movement and amniotic fluid volume, were also known to have some predictive power (Pearson and Weaver 1976; Manning *et al.* 1981), it then appeared logical to assume that combinations of biophysical variables might be more predictive of both well-being and compromise in high-risk pregnancies. In particular, it was hoped that simultaneous examination of multiple real-time events might circumvent the problem of physiological cyclic variation and periodicity of biophysical variables, thus reducing the high false-positive rates seen in individual studies.

Two main scoring systems are in common use. The commonest system is based on the score developed by Manning and colleagues (Manning *et al.* 1980) as outlined in Table 7.1. This scoring system has subsequently been modified.

Table 7.1 Biophysical profile scoring system A

Biophysical variable	Normal (score = 2)	Abnormal (score = 0)
Fetal breathing movements	At least one episode of FBM of at least 30 s duration in 30 min observation	Absent FBM or no episode of > 30 s in 30 min
Gross body movement	At least three discrete body/limb movements in 30 min (episodes of active continuous movement considered as single movement)	Two or fewer episodes body/limb movements in 30 min
Fetal tone	At least one episode of active extension with return to flexion of fetal limb(s) or trunk. Opening and closing of hand considered normal tone	Either slow extension, with return to partial flexion, or movement of limb in full extension. Fetal movement absent
Reactive FHR	At least two episodes of FHR acceleration of > 15 beats/min and of at least 15 s duration associated with fetal movement in 30 min	Less than two episodes of acceleration of FHR or acceleration of > 15 beats/min in 30 min
Qualitative AFV	At least one pocket of AF that measures at least 1 cm in two perpendicular planes	Either no AF pockets or a pocket < 1 cm in two perpendicular planes

From Manning *et al.* (1980)

Many regard a pool depth of 1 cm as too strict a definition of reduced liquor, and 2 cm pool depths are commonly used (Basket 1989; Manning 1990). In most recent studies an amniotic fluid score of zero is regarded as an abnormal score, irrespective of the presence of other variables (Manning 1990). It has also been suggested that the non-stress test (NST) can be excluded if all dynamic ultrasound variables are normal (Manning *et al.* 1987*a*).

The other scoring system used is that proposed by Vintzileos and colleagues (Vintzileos *et al.* 1983) and which is outlined in Table 7.2. It largely differs from that of Manning *et al.* in the addition of placental grading, felt to be an additional predictor, and in grading the scoring 0, 1, and 2.

Basis for fetal biophysical assessment

To utilize and interpret biophysical parameters visualized by real-time ultrasound, there must be an understanding of the response of those variables to hypoxaemia and acidaemia. The dynamic biophysical variables of fetal heart rate reactivity, fetal breathing activity, gross body movement, and fetal tone are controlled by extensive integrated systems within the central nervous system (CNS). If an activity is normal, then it is assumed that the CNS control mechanism and that part of the brain controlling that mechanism are functionally intact. The essential premise is that hypoxaemia results in depression of these central nervous system regulated biophysical activities. Experimental evidence clearly demonstrates a reduction or cessation of fetal breathing activity and fetal movements (Boddy *et al.* 1974) with hypoxaemia and a reduction in fetal heart rate reactivity is seen in hypoxaemic human fetuses (Visser *et al.* 1990). Human observations have confirmed that severe hypoxaemia is associated with loss of fetal tone.

The relationships between these biophysical variables are complex. It has been suggested that the response to hypoxaemia varies, with some variables being more sensitive to lesser degrees of hypoxaemia, related to the onset of neurodevelopmental function of the differing control areas (Vintzileos *et al.* 1983). Thus the non-stress test and fetal breathing activity are the first variables to be altered by hypoxaemia, and fetal tone the last variable. There is human evidence to support such a concept. In the study by Vintzileos *et al.* (1987*b*), the mean umbilical arterial pH was 7.28 where fetal breathing activity and the non-stress test were normal, 7.20 where only these variables were abnormal, and 7.16 where these variables and either movement or tone was absent. More direct data from antenatal percutaneous umbilical blood sampling in severely growth retarded fetuses shows that fetal breathing activity and the non-stress test are frequently abnormal in the presence of mild to moderate fetal hypoxaemia, whilst fetal activity and tone remain normal (Ribbert *et al.* 1990).

Table 7.2 Biophysical scoring system B

Test	Score	Criteria
Non-stress test	2 (NST 2)	5 or more FHR accelerations of at least 15 b.p.m in amplitude and at least 15 s duration associated with fetal movements in a 20 min period
	1 (NST 1)	2–4 accelerations of at least 15 b.p.m in amplitude and at least 15 s duration associated with fetal movements in a 20 min period
	0 (NST 0)	1 or fewer accelerations in a 20 min period
Fetal movements	2 (FM 2)	at least 3 gross (trunk and limbs) episodes of fetal movements with 30 min; simultaneous limb and trunk movements were counted as a single movement
	1 (FM 1)	1 or 2 fetal movements within 30 min
	0 (FM 0)	absence of fetal movements within 30 min
Fetal breathing movements	2 (FBM 2)	at least 1 episode of fetal breathing of at least 60 s duration within a 30 min observation period
	1 (FBM 1)	at least 1 episode of fetal breathing lasting 30–60 s within 30 min
	0 (FBM 0)	absence of fetal breathing or breathing lasting less than 30 s within 30 min
Fetal tone	2 (FT2)	at least 1 episode of extension of extremities with return to position of flexion, and also 1 episode of extension of spine with return to position of flexion
	1 (FT 1)	at least 1 episode of extension of extremities with return to position of flexion, or 1 episode of extension of spine with return to position of flexion
	0 (FT 0)	extremities in extension; fetal movements not followed by return to flexion; open hand
Amniotic fluid volume	2 (AF 2)	fluid evident throughout the uterine cavity; a pocket that measures 2 cm or more in vertical diameter
	1 (AF 2)	a pocket that measures less than 2 cm but more than 1 cm in vertical diameter
	0 (AF 0)	crowding of fetal small parts; largest pocket less than 1 cm in vertical diameter
Placental grading	2 (PL 2)	placental grading 0, 1, or 2
	1 (PL 1)	placental posterior difficult to evaluate
	0 (PL 0)	placental grading 3

From Vintzileos *et al.* (1983)

The final variable to consider is that of amniotic fluid volume. This is regarded as a more chronic response to asphyxial stress. The main sources of amniotic fluid in the latter half of pregnancy are the fetal lungs and kidneys (Seeds 1980). Experimental studies demonstrated that aortic body chemoreceptor stimulation by hypoxaemia results in redistribution of cardiac output, with particular reduction in renal and pulmonary perfusion (Cohn *et al.* 1974). More recent studies on the human fetus using pulsed and colour flow Doppler ultrasound appear to confirm this redistribution of output and reduction in renal perfusion in the presence of hypoxaemia (Wladimiroff *et al.* 1987; Vyas *et al.* 1989). These observations and previously described observations of adverse outcome in pregnancies with oligohydramnios (Chamberlain *et al.* 1984), support its use as a marker of chronic compromise.

Clinical studies with the BPP

Prospective blind studies

Both of the initial studies describing the BPP were of this nature (Manning *et al.* 1980; Platt *et al.* 1983) as was the initial description of the alternative scoring system (Vintzileos *et al.* 1983). Two other studies could be considered, that of Schifrin *et al.* (1981) using a variant of the Manning score where, although ultrasound findings were available to clinicians, management was based on a NST/contraction stress test protocol, and that of Vintzileos *et al.* (1987*b*) where profile scoring was performed immediately before elective Caesarean section.

All studies used heterogeneous groups of high-risk pregnancies, with data presented for the whole study group. All claim to demonstrate a better prediction of abnormal outcome with increasing numbers of abnormal variables. The results, analysed to show sensitivity, specificity, and predictive values are shown in Table 7.3.

The numbers are insufficient to allow comment on mortality in all studies, the highest number of non-malformed deaths being seven. Nevertheless, the false-positive rates are close to 90 per cent, with negative predictive values no different from the NST alone. Fetal distress is difficult to define and data are for cardiotocographic evidence of distress, except for that of Schifrin *et al.* (1981) where Apgar scores at 5 minutes are used. The positive predictive values do appear better for the BPP than for the NST, although false-positive rates remain over 50 per cent. Negative prediction is not altered by the addition of dynamic biophysical variables. Looking at more objective measures of outcome — birth asphyxia leading to asphyxial death or neurological sequelae, or umbilical arterial pH — Vintzileos and colleagues (Vintzileos *et al.* 1983, 1987*b*) demonstrate improved performance of the profile. However, it is not significantly better than the non-stress test. Examining acidosis alone, the BPP outperforms the NST, but

Table 7.3 Predictive value of the BPP in prospective blind study

	Sensitivity (%)	Specificity (%)	Predictive value positive (%)	Predictive value negative (%)
Perinatal mortality				
Manning *et al.* 1980 BPP (NST)	71 (71)	80 (77)	11 (9)	99 (99)
Platt *et al.* 1983 BPP (NST)	50 (50)	95 (91)	12 (7)	99 (99)
Fetal distress (FHR defined)				
Manning *et al.* 1980	71 (48)	86 (77)	44 (23)	95 (91)
Platt *et al.* 1983	36 (57)	96 (93)	29 (30)	97 (98)
Schifrin *et al.* 1981	100 (57)	98 (79)	86 (11)	100 (98)
Vintzileos *et al.* 1983	39 (50)	84 (73)	44 (39)	81 (81)
Asphyxia/acidosis				
Vintzileos *et al.* 1983	90 (100)	96 (76)	82 (44)	98 (100)
Vintzileos *et al.* 1987*b*	100 (100)	83 (93)	32 (52)	100 (100)

Figures in brackets denote values using NST alone

$$\text{Sensitivity} = \frac{\text{true-positives}}{\text{true-positives} + \text{false-negatives}}$$

$$\text{Specificity} = \frac{\text{true-negatives}}{\text{true-negatives} + \text{false-positives}}$$

$$\text{Predictive value positive} = \frac{\text{true-positives}}{\text{true-positives} + \text{false-positives}}$$

$$\text{Predictive value negative} = \frac{\text{true-negatives}}{\text{true-negatives} + \text{false-negatives}}$$

a combination of the NST and fetal breathing activity has the same predictive value as the full BPP. Only in the initial study of Manning *et al.* (1980) is it possible to similarly compare full BPP scoring with other combinations of dynamic variables. Using fetal breathing and the NST alone, positive and negative predictive values of 0.38 and 0.93 are obtained for fetal distress, with a sensitivity of 60 per cent. This is not significantly different from full BPP scoring.

The conclusion from these studies is that assessment of dynamic ultrasound parameters is at least as good as the non-stress test in the prediction of mortality and morbidity. The positive predictive value, and hence the false-positive rate, may be better, though no study is large enough to achieve a statistically significant result, with the exception of that of Vintzileos *et al.* (1983). There appears little evidence from these studies of an advantage to examining multiple variables if one or two are normal. The question of comparisons between the full BPP and combinations of two or more variables has rarely been addressed. Where such analysis has been undertaken, full BPP monitoring has shown no advantage, both for negative and for positive predictive values.

Randomized controlled studies

Only two such studies have been carried out (Manning *et al.* 1984; Platt *et al.* 1985), and both compared the full BPP with the non-stress test only. They contain almost 1400 pregnancies and address the problem of perinatal morbidity only. In neither is randomization satisfactory (Mohide and Keirse 1989), using coin flip or sequential numbers. The study of Manning *et al.* (1984) excludes suspected growth-retarded pregnancies.

The results are summarized in Table 7.4. Although there are differences in sensitivity in most cases, these do not achieve statistical significance. As in the prospective studies, there are no differences in the negative predictive values, confirming that there appears little advantage in multiple parameter testing if

Table 7.4 Results from randomized trials

		Sensitivity (%)	Specificity (%)	Positive prediction (%)	Negative prediction (%)
Low Apgar at 5 minutes					
Manning 1984	BPP	77	97	57[*]	99
	NST	57	85	13	98
Platt 1985	BPP	25	97	25	97
	NST	33	96	20	98
Fetal distress in labour					
Platt 1985	BPP	31	98	50	96
	NST	13	95	13	95
Overall abnormal outcome					
Manning 1984	BPP	76	97	56[*]	99
	NST	58	85	18	97
Platt 1985	BPP	32	99	88[*]	93
	NST	14	96	33	88

[*]Statistically significant results

the non-stress test is normal. There are, however, differences in the positive predictive value using the morbidity markers of low Apgar scores and cardio-tocographic fetal distress in combination with corrected perinatal loss, and these are significant. These data support those from the prospective studies, and support a possible role for the BPP in reducing false-positive results from non-stress testing. However, there are no randomized studies comparing the BPP with other dynamic variables, either singly, or in groups of two or three. The question of how extensive should biophysical testing be remains unanswered.

Open interventional studies

The widespread use of the biophysical profile is based on large longitudinal clinical studies (Baskett *et al.* 1984, 1987; Manning *et al.* 1985, 1987*c*, 1990*a–c*; Vintzileos *et al.* 1987*a*). In these studies, the score, in conjunction with other clinical variables, was used to guide clinical management (see Table 7.5). Comparisons were made with historical controls or with contemporary un-monitored pregnancies. Comparisons between different parameters were made using outcome variables following intervention based on those variables. Given the equivocal results from both blinded and randomized studies, interpretation of open studies must be cautious, especially when claims of superior prediction over less extensive monitoring are discussed.

The corrected intrauterine death rate within a week of a normal BPP is 0.7 per 1000 (Manning *et al.* 1985, 1987*c*; Baskett *et al.* 1987), a false-negative rate superior to that of any single parameter. However, the problems with high false-positive rates have not been completely resolved. Manning and colleagues (Manning *et al.* 1990*b*) demonstrated a clear relationship between decreasing score and corrected perinatal mortality, but the sensitivity for the prediction of intrauterine death is less than 50 per cent. In the large studies of Manning *et al.* (1985) and Baskett *et al.* (1987) the false-positive rates for prediction of death *in utero* are 99 per cent and 94 per cent, respectively. Even a score of 0 has a false-positive prediction of death of over 50 per cent (Manning *et al.* 1990*a*), although many of the survivors may have sequelae of severe asphyxia.

For perinatal morbidity, Baskett *et al.* (1984) showed little difference in both sensitivity and negative predictive values for fetal distress or low Apgar scores between the BPP and individual biophysical variables. False-positive rates were reduced using multiple parameters (see Table 7.6). The more detailed analysis of abnormal scores and morbidity carried out by Manning and colleagues (Manning *et al.* 1990*b*) demonstrates a significant inverse trend in increasing rates of fetal distress, low Apgar scores, and umbilical vein acidosis with decreasing BPP scores. This supports the data of Vintzileos (Vintzileos *et al.* 1987*b*) describing the gradual hypoxia concept, giving further credence to the concept of sequential loss of acute biophysical activities with increasing compromise.

Table 7.5 Clinical management based on the BPP score

Test score result		Interpretation	Management
10/10		Risk of fetal asphyxia extremely rare	Intervention only for obstetrical and maternal factors. No indication for intervention of fetal disease
8/10	(normal fluid)		
8/8	(NST not done)		
8/10	(abnormal fluid)	Probable chronic fetal compromise	Determine that there is functioning renal tissue and intact membranes — if so deliver for fetal indications
6/10	(normal fluid)	Equivocal test, possible fetal asphyxia	If the fetus is mature — deliver. In the immature fetus, repeat test within 24 h — if < 6/10, deliver
6/10	(abnormal fluid)	Probable fetal asphyxia	Deliver for fetal indications
4/10		High probability fetal asphyxia	Deliver for fetal indications
2/10		Fetal asphyxia almost certain	Deliver for fetal indications
0/10		Fetal asphyxia certain	Deliver for fetal indications

From Manning 1987c

However, no comparable data on single variables or other combinations less than the full score are presented for comparison. The false-positive rates for an abnormal score remain high (see Table 7.6), even when considering objective measures of distress such as acidosis at delivery. Therefore, despite the wealth of data, it still remains unproven whether full scoring is necessary in all cases.

Use of biophysical profile scoring in specific high-risk groups

Diabetes mellitus

Sudden unexpected death remains a feared complication of pregnancy in the diabetic mother. Although the precise mode of death remains unclear, there is some evidence that it may be hypoxaemic in nature (Bradley *et al.* 1988). A number of studies have examined the use of the BPP in diabetic pregnancies (Golde *et al.* 1984; Dicker *et al.* 1988; Johnson *et al.* 1988), with 255 established

Table 7.6 Perinatal morbidity in prospective open studies

Predictive	Sensitivity (%)	Specificity (%)	Predictive value positive (%)	value negative (%)
Fetal distress				
Baskett *et al.* 1984				
BPP	13.4	97.8	33	94
NST	22.5	90.5	15	94
Manning *et al.* 1990*b*				
BPP	30.3	91.6	41	87
Low Apgar score				
Baskett *et al.* 1984				
BPP	27.2	97.5	16	99
NST	33.0	89.5	05	99
Manning *et al.* 1990*b*				
BPP	38.8	89.5	17	96
Low cord pH				
Manning *et al.* 1990*b*				
BPP	87.5	64.8	23	98

insulin-dependent diabetics and 188 gestational diabetics being examined. All were managed by BPP monitoring, available to their obstetricians.

There were three stillbirths, all in the study of Golde *et al.* (1984); two being lethal malformations and one occurring in a woman with diabetic ketoacidosis. Prediction of morbidity is poorly addressed in these studies, the positive predictive value for various indices of distress being 5–11 per cent in the study of Dicker *et al.* (1988) and all babies having low 5 minute Apgar scores in the study of Johnson *et al.* (1988) having normal BPP scores. Nevertheless, all claim an important role for the BPP in the management of the diabetic pregnancy.

In the absence of unexplained deaths it is difficult to be certain that the BPP is as reassuring as is claimed. All three stillbirths in diabetic pregnancies in the original analysis of Manning *et al.* (1985) occured within one week of a normal profile. In a prospective blind study of the use of BPP monitoring in insulin-dependent diabetes, we have observed two such unexplained deaths 3 and 5 days following a normal score (Walkinshaw *et al.* unpublished data).

No comparative trials of the predictive value of the BPP against less extensive monitoring have been performed, and the advantage of the BPP over other forms of monitoring in diabetic pregnancies is unsubstantiated.

In physiological terms, such testing may not be appropriate. Diabetic pregnancies are associated with excess liquor; the conventional definition of a 2 cm pool may be less sensitive for these pregnancies. Fetal breathing activity is affected by maternal glucose levels (Natale *et al.* 1978). In over 200 BPP examinations in over 30 insulin diabetic pregnancies, I have yet to note absent fetal breathing. Thus fetal breathing may be a less sensitive parameter in diabetic pregnancies. By contrast, the absence of breathing activity or the presence of reduced liquor in the diabetic pregnancy may be more indicative of compromise in these pregnancies than expected. Such physiological considerations reinforce the views of Vintzileos (Vintzileos *et al.* 1987*a*) that individual interpretation of profile components in conjunction with clinical information is likely to lead to better management than adherence to a score.

Allo-immunization

Allo-immunized pregnancies make up a small proportion of tested pregnancies in most studies. It has been suggested that BPP assessment may be of value in the recognition of fetal deterioration due to anaemia (Manning *et al.* 1987*b*). Very few data are available and are anecdotal. Our own experience suggests that biophysical profile assessment adds little to the assessment or management of the severely affected fetus (Walkinshaw and Barron, unpublished data), profiles being normal in severely anaemic hydropic fetuses prior to transfusion. The management of severe allo-immunization will continue to depend on careful assessment of the maternal history, antibody levels, amniotic fluid optical density, ultrasound assessment of early hydrops, and fetal blood sampling, rather than fetal biophysical assessment.

Twin pregnancies

Lodeiro *et al.* (1986) examined 49 twin pairs using the scoring system from Table 7.2. All fetuses subsequently having fetal distress (either low 5 minute Apgar score or cord pH less than 7.20) had an abnormal score, in four cases this being accurately predicted in only one of the twins. Baskett (1989) described experience with 141 twin pregnancies using the scoring system in Table 7.1. Two deaths were noted in severely growth-retarded fetuses with abnormal scores. No such potentially 'asphyxial' deaths were noted in those with normal scores.

Although the numbers are small and there are no comparative data provided on individual variables, BPP monitoring may have potential in twin pregnancies. Maternal variables and external stimuli which may affect biophysical activities are controlled as they are identical for each fetus, thus differences in scores may be highly significant. Unfortunately there are few data on the synchronicity or otherwise of cyclical fetal biophysical behaviour in twin pairs, and, therefore, there will remain the uncertainty over sleep or asphyxia even if only one score is abnormal.

Premature rupture of the membranes (PROM)

Much of the assessment of biophysical assessment in PROM has used the profile described in Table 7.2. PROM itself does not appear to affect the total biophysical score, although the incidence of reactive non-stress test appears higher and the incidence of absent fetal breathing lower than in intact membranes (Vintzileos *et al.* 1986*a*).

In a small prospective study, a normal BPP was associated with a neonatal sepsis rate of 2.7 per cent, whereas an abnormal score was associated with a sepsis rate of 93.7 per cent (Vintzileos *et al.* 1985). The most sensitive indices appear to be the non-stress test and fetal breathing. Others have confirmed the value of fetal breathing activity in the prediction of fetal infection (Goldstein *et al.* 1988). The presence of fetal breathing appears to be the best predictor of the absence of fetal infection (Vintzileos *et al.* 1986*b*) although this negative prediction lasts only 24 hours compared with the 7 day negative prediction for most other risk states. The BPP may indeed be superior to Gram staining of amniotic fluid in the prediction of fetal infection (Vintzileos *et al.* 1986*c*). The prospective use of daily BPP examination with prompt intervention in this group appears to reduce the incidence of neonatal sepsis from 23.2 per cent noted in two historical control groups to 6.7 per cent (Vintzileos *et al.* 1987*c*).

It may well be that BPP assessment can distinguish the infected fetus from cases where there is colonization or maternal evidence of clinical amnionitis only. As such it may be an important test in the management of this group of high-risk pregnancies. Whether full scoring is necessary, or whether less frequent liquor assessment with a daily NST and fetal breathing assessment would suffice remains to be evaluated. Whether prompt antibiotic therapy in cases with normal profiles and evidence of maternal infection or colonization only would prolong pregnancy and improve outcome is a potential therapeutic use of profile assessment which also requires study.

Suspected growth retardation

The pathophysiology of the growth-retarded fetus appears well suited to surveillance by biophysical parameters, and as such this group has made up a substantial proportion of all pregnancies studied.

Scores of 6 or less occur in only 3.4 per cent of patients tested (Manning 1990) but in pregnancies complicated by proven intrauterine growth retardation (IUGR), the rate of abnormal testing is much higher, 16.3 per cent in the studies of Baskett and colleagues (Baskett 1989). In the Winnepeg studies, suspected

IUGR accounts for 22.8 per cent of tested pregnancies (Manning *et al.* 1987*c*), but almost 40 per cent of fetuses with a score of 4 or less were growth retarded. All intrauterine deaths, excluding anomaly and allo-immunization, where the score was zero, occurred in growth-retarded fetuses, and over 80 per cent of liveborn infants with scores of zero were growth retarded (Manning *et al.* 1990*a*). Even in tested pregnancies, the perinatal mortality for proven IUGR remains higher than for other tested groups (Manning *et al.* 1987*b*; Manning 1990).

Despite its obvious application, as an individual group such pregnancies have been poorly studied. Suspected IUGR fetuses were excluded from one of the two randomized studies (Manning *et al.* 1984). Retrospective analysis of a large number of proven IUGR infants managed by the BPP showed a mortality of only 12.5 per 1000, compared with historical controls and with expected rates (Manning 1990). Comparative data with other testing strategies have not been presented.

In our own studies (Walkinshaw *et al.* 1992 and unpublished studies) we have evaluated a group of 143 fetuses selected on fetal weight estimates as suspected IUGR. Serial BPP assessments were carried out, the results not being available for clinical management and BPP assessment not being available outside the study. An abnormal outcome was described as any one of the following:

(1) delivery for fetal distress based on cardiotocographic evidence and/or fetal scalp blood acidosis

(2) umbilical venous pH less than 7.20

(3) neonatal intubation and positive pressure ventilation for asphyxia

(4) unexplained intrauterine death.

Twenty-seven per cent of these fetuses had a score of 6 or less. The predictive values of an abnormal score were: sensitivity 51.5 per cent, specificity 82.7 per cent, positive predictive value 47.2 per cent, negative predictive value 85 per cent. As the study was non-interventional and blind, we were able to assess the relative predictive performances of other combinations, less than the full BPP (see Table 7.7). We concluded that, as yet, there is no clear advantage to be gained in using full BPP assessment in this group of pregnancies. This is especially so if variables are normal. It would appear that first line assessment using the non-stress test and amniotic fluid volume provides equal reassurance to the full BPP. Addition of fetal breathing should one of the original parameters be abnormal improves the false-positive rate. This is very much in agreement with the strategies proposed by Vintzileos *et al.* (1987*a*) and by Mills *et al.* (1990).

Further work, and preferably randomized trials, are required before the full BPP becomes a 'routine' first line assessment in suspected IUGR.

Table 7.7 Prediction of outcome where EFW below the 5th centile

	Sensitivity (%)	Specificity (%)	Predictive value negative (%)	Predictive value positive (%)
NST	28.0	91.8	79	54
AFV	40.0	83.6	80	45
FM	36.0	78.1	78	36
FBM	32.0	70.0	75	27
FT	16.0	97.3	77	67
NST+AFV*	48.0	80.8	82	46
NST+FM	52.0	74.0	82	41
NST+FBM	48.0	65.7	79	32
AFV+FM	64.0	72.0	85	44
AFV+FBM	60.0	60.3	81	34
FM+FBM	44.0	57.5	75	26
NST+AFV+FM**	36.0	85	79	45
NST+AFV+FBM	36.0	89.0	80	53
AFV+FM+FBM	32.0	82.6	78	40
NST+FM+FBM	24.0	87.7	77	40
BPP	56.0	82.2	85	52

* One or both abnormal
** Two or three abnormal

Prolonged pregnancy

Johnson *et al.* (1986) reviewed experience with 307 pregnancies beyond 42 weeks using the BPP as the primary method of monitoring. Women with abnormal scores were delivered, an abnormal score being 6 or less, or a score of 8 if amniotic fluid volume was the abnormal variable. Women with a normal score but a favourable cervix were also delivered. Given the structure of the study it is virtually impossible to determine the true predictive abilities of the score. Those with normal scores who were allowed to labour spontaneously had low perinatal morbidity. In the abnormal score group, despite intervention, rates for morbidity and operative delivery for distress were high. Similar intervention rates were noted by Baskett (1989). However, most of this morbidity was evident in the subgroup classified as abnormal due to reduced amniotic fluid. It is not clear whether amniotic fluid volume assessment alone would have performed equally well. The studies of Crowley *et al.* (1984) and Phelan *et al.* (1985) suggest that amniotic fluid alone can achieve comparable results.

Shine *et al.* (1984) used weekly biophysical profiles, slightly modified from the score of Manning *et al.* (1980), to study 129 prolonged pregnancies. The score was a highly sensitive predictor of post-term dysmature infants, as defined postnatally, and who were significantly more acidotic than those with normal scores and term controls. However, once again, a combination of non-stress test and amniotic fluid volume alone would have had similar predictive ability.

In an attempt to resolve the relative predictive abilities of the profile and conventional assessment with the NST and amniotic fluid volume measurement, we examined 117 women at a mean gestation of 293 days, just prior to induction of labour (Walkinshaw *et al.* in preparation). Biophysical monitoring was performed as in Table 7.2 but using a 2 cm liquor pool cut-off. Results of testing were not available to staff conducting the labour. An abnormal outcome was defined as for our suspected IUGR study. The results are summarized in Table 7.8. The second half of this table shows the results of Hann *et al.* (1987) and Majeed (1989), using the scoring system in Table 7.2, excluding placental morphology in the case of Majeed (1989). Hann *et al.* (1987) studied 131 pregnancies beyond 41 weeks and used neonatal morbidity markers as outcome measures. Majeed (1989) studied 205 pregnancies beyond 290 days. Although not blinded, induction policies were fixed prior to recruitment, depending on consultant preference. An abnormal perinatal outcome was defined as one of perinatal death, fetal distress in labour, meconium aspiration syndrome, low 5 minute Apgar score, or signs of dysmaturity.

Table 7.8 Predictive value in prolonged pregnancy

	Sensitivity (%)	Specificity (%)	Predictive value positive (%)	Predictive value negative (%)
Walkinshaw *et al.* (in preparation)				
NST	15.8	93.9	33	85
AFV	36.8	91.8	47	88
NST + AFV	47.3	86.7	41	89
BPP	42.1	85.7	36	88
Majeed (1989)				
NST	22.2	98	80	78
AFV	79.6	74	52	91
BPP	55.6	97	88	86
Hann *et al.* (1987)				
NST	12.5	95	14	94
AFV	25.0	92	17	95
BPP	12.5	95	14	94

Our own studies suggest little advantage in using full BPP scoring. A combination of the non-stress test and amniotic fluid volume assessment performs just as well. Looking at acidosis alone as an outcome measure, results were similar. Hann *et al.* (1987) could not demonstrate any difference between biophysical profile scoring and either the NST or amniotic fluid assessment alone. Majeed (1989) does suggest that the profile has advantages in terms of sensitivity and positive predictive value over individual parameter testing, but if individual parameters are normal, no advantage accrues from examining other variables. Her data do not examine the combination of non-stress test and amniotic fluid, so it is uncertain if the high sensitivity of amniotic fluid would combine with the high predictive value of the non-stress test.

From all these studies, it would appear that if conservative management of prolonged pregnancy is felt desirable, monitoring using liquor volume and the non-stress test can suffice.

Limitations and possible modifications of fetal biophysical profile scoring

The two major problems in the interpretation of fetal BPP scoring are the normal physiological variability of individual parameters and the question of the weighting of each parameter.

Physiological variability

The acute biophysical variables of breathing, movement, and heart rate variability must be interpreted within the confines of fetal physiology. All exhibit cyclical patterns and these alter with gestational age (Patrick *et al.* 1980, 1982; Natale *et al.* 1984; Gagnon *et al.* 1987; Natale and Nasello–Paterson 1988). By late pregnancy biophysical activity is highly dependent on behavioural state. The maximum durations of fetal apnoea and inactivity increase with gestation (Patrick *et al.* 1980, 1982). Fetal heart rate variability and the extent of movement associated acceleration are also gestation dependent (Natale *et al.* 1984; Gagnon *et al.* 1987). There may be interrelationships between variables which could affect the overall score. Recent work has suggested that oligohydramnios affects the amplitude and speed of fetal movement (Sival *et al.* 1990).

The decision, therefore, to limit ultrasound assessment to 30 minutes and to use fixed definitions for profile scoring is arbitrary, and simply reflects clinical practicalities. Inherent in such a decision must be an acceptance of a high false-positive rate, the asleep or preterm rather than the asphyxiated fetus.

In practical terms, mean durations of fetal apnoea and inactivity are shorter in the preterm and thus 30 minutes may be sufficient observation time to define an at-risk fetus. However, observation later in pregnancy, particularly of the post-term fetus, may require extended testing. The reduced variability and reduced acceleration amplitude observed in the normal preterm fetus (Gagnon *et al.* 1987) should lead to alterations in the definition of a reactive non-stress test to include gestation, and this is our current practice.

The criterion for liquor volume is based on perceived risk at varying cut-off points (Chamberlain *et al.* 1984). There remains a dispute whether 1, 2, or 3 cm maximum liquor pools should be used. Amniotic fluid volume alters with gestation (Brace and Wolf 1989) and it may be more appropriate to define the score for amniotic fluid volume based on gestational norms rather than on fixed value. Some consideration must be taken of whether maximum pool depth is the most appropriate assessment of oligohydramnios. Four quadrant amniotic fluid index (AFI) (Moore and Cayle 1990) may be an alternative.

Weighting of variables

The decision to score 0 or 2 (Manning *et al.* 1980) was arbitary, and chosen to mimic the Apgar scoring system. With increasing experience, weighting has been subtly introduced. The non-stress test has been devalued, not being used if ultrasound variables are normal (Manning *et al.* 1987*a*). This implies that less weight is placed on this variable. The allocation of an abnormal score where only liquor volume is abnormal implies higher weight to that variable (Manning *et al.* 1987*b*). The recent analysis of Manning *et al.* (1990*c*) looked at the problem of predictive accuracy by score composition. They concluded that the positive predictive accuracy of some of the morbidity end points was better with some test combinations than with others. In particular abnormal scores (less than or equal to 4) where the non-stress test and liquor volume were normal were much less predictive of an abnormal outcome than expected. These analyses imply that the weighting of some biophysical variables should not be equal, and confirms the arguments of Vintzileos (Vintzileos *et al.* 1987*a*) that interpretation must be within the clinical situation.

As discussed under the individual risk groups, for certain pathological groups certain variables may be more or less important. Thus absent fetal breathing activity in the fetus of a diabetic mother with high blood glucose concentrations or with preterm ruptured membranes may be more sinister than a similar finding in a normal pregnancy at 42 weeks' gestation. Very little work is available on the differing weighting of individual components for different pathological groups.

Conclusions

Major questions over the role and place of fetal biophysical profile scoring remain, in part because adequate and appropriate comparative studies have yet to be performed.

There is little doubt that biophysical activities are influenced by hypoxaemia acidaemia in the human fetus. The recent detailed studies from Vintzileos *et al.* (1991) confirm the sequential loss of biophysical activities with increasing fetal hypoxaemia and acidaemia. As such, observation of these variables undoubtedly has a role in fetal surveillance. What remains to be demonstrated is whether full five or six component testing is of any greater benefit than less extensive fetal monitoring, and in which high-risk pregnancies the BPP has a central role.

There appears little doubt that if the non-stress test and fetal breathing are normal, little is to be gained by more extensive testing. Biophysical profile scoring may be of benefit if one or other of these is abnormal, though this remains to be assessed in an appropriate randomized trial.

In individual high-risk groups, randomized trials have not been undertaken, and evidence is scanty to support the use of the BPP as the front line test in most groups. There may be a role for the BPP in twin pregnancies and in preterm premature rupture of the membrane but this needs further evaluation.

Definitions for a normal BPP score were produced over 10 years ago and it is now appropriate to re-examine these. The definitions of abnormal amniotic fluid, of fetal heart reactivity, and the duration of the test at different gestations require urgent reappraisal to better reflect fetal physiology.

In conclusion, interpretation of the variables used in the score requires detailed knowledge of fetal physiology in different risk groups, the changes in that physiology with gestation, and an inherent understanding of the limitations of such assessments. Although these criteria will be met within centres who have developed the profile, in the UK at least, it is likely that most testing will be performed by non-obstetric staff and a total score reported. At present, too few obstetricians are sufficiently aware of the problems of interpretations within the score, and it seems likely that its use will be devalued. The comments by Mohide and Keirse (1989) are unfortunately still relevant.

Reference

Baskett, T. F. (1989). Fetal biophysical profile. In *Progress in obstetrics and Gynaecology, Vol 7* (ed. J. Studd), pp. 145–60. Churchill Livingstone.

Baskett, T. F., Gray, J. H., Prewitt, S. J., Young, L. M., and Allen, A. C. (1984). Antepartum fetal assessment using a fetal biophysical profile score. *Am. J. Obstet. Gynecol.*, **148**, 630–3.

Baskett, T. F., Allen, A. C., Gray, J. H., Young, D. C., and Young, L. M. (1987). Fetal biophysical profile and perinatal death. *Obstet. Gynecol.*, **70**, 357–9.

Boddy, K., Dawes, G. S., Fisher, R., *et al.* (1974). Fetal respiratory movements, electrocortical and cardiovascular responses to hypoxaemia and hypercapnia in sleep. *J. Physiol.*, **243**, 599.

Brace, R. A. and Wolf, E. J. (1989). Normal amniotic fluid volume changes throughout pregnancy. *Am. J. Obstet. Gynecol.*, **161**, 382–8.

Bradley, R. J., Nicolaides, K. H., Brudenell, J. M., and Campbell, S. (1988). Early diagnosis of chronic fetal hypoxaemia in diabetic pregnancy. *Br. Med. J.*, **296**, 94–6.

Chamberlain, P. F., Manning, F. A., Morrison, I., *et al.* (1984). Ultrasound evaluation of amniotic fluid volume. I. The relationship of marginal and decreased amniotic fluid volumes to perinatal outcome. *Am. J. Obstet. Gynecol.*, **150**, 245–9.

Cohn, N. E., Sacks, E. T., Heyman, M. A., *et al.* (1974). Cardiovascular responses to hypoxemia and acidemia in fetal lambs. *Am. J. Obstet. Gynecol.*, **120**, 817–21.

Crowley, P., O'Herlihy, C., and Boylan, P. (1984). The value of ultrasound measurement of amniotic fluid volume in the management of prolonged pregnancies. *Br. J. Obstet. Gynaecol.*, **91**, 444–8.

Dicker, D., Feldberg, D., Yeshaya, A., Peleg, D., Karp, M., and Goldman, J. A. (1988). Fetal surveillance in insulin-dependent diabetic pregnancy: Predictive value of the biophysical profile. *Am. J. Obstet. Gynecol.*, **159**, 800–4.

Gagnon, R., Campbell, K., Hunse, C., and Patrick, J. (1987). Patterns of human fetal heart rate accelerations from 26 weeks to term. *Am. J. Obstet. Gynecol.*, **157**, 743–8.

Golde, S. H., Montoro, M., Good-Anderson, B., *et al.* (1984). The role of nonstress tests, fetal biophysical profile and contraction stress tests in the outpatient management of insulin-requiring diabetic pregnancies. *Am. J. Obstet. Gynecol.*, **148**, 269–73.

Goldstein, I., Romero, R., Merrill, S., Wan, M., O'Connor, T. Z., Mazor, M., *et al.* (1988). Fetal body and breathing movements as predictors of intraamniotic infection in preterm premature rupture of membranes. *Am. J. Obstet. Gynecol.*, **159**, 363–8.

Hann, L., McArdle, C., and Sachs, B. (1987). Sonographic biophysical profile in the postdate pregnancy. *J. Ultrasound Med.*, **6**, 191–5.

Johnson, J. M., Harman, C. R., Lange, I. R., and Manning, F. A. (1986). Biophysical profile scoring in the management of the postterm pregnancy: An analysis of 307 patients. *Am. J. Obstet. Gynecol.*, **154**, 269–73.

Johnson, J. M., Lange, I. R., Harman, C. R., Torchia, M. G., and Manning, F. A. (1988). Biophysical profile scoring in the management of the diabetic pregnancy. *Obstet. Gynecol.*, **72**, 841–6.

Lodeiro, J. G., Vintzileos, A. M., Feinstein, S. J., Campbell, W. A., and Nochimson, D. J. (1986). Fetal biophysical profile in twin gestations. *Obstet. Gynecol.*, **67**, 824–7.

Majeed, R. (1989). Fetal biophysical profile: Its role in antepartum surveillance in prolonged pregnancy. M. Obstet. Gynaecol. Thesis, University of Liverpool.

Manning, F. A. (1990). The fetal biophysical profile score: current status. *Obstetrics and Gynecology Clinics of North America*, **17**, 147–62.

Manning, F. A., Platt, L. D., Sipos, L., and Keegan, K. A. (1979). Fetal breathing movements and the nonstress test in high-risk pregnancies. *Am. J. Obstet. Gynecol.*, **135**, 511–15.

Manning, F. A., Platt, L. D., and Sipos, L. (1980). Antepartum fetal evaluation: Development of a fetal biophysical profile. *Am. J. Obstet. Gynecol.*, **136**, 787–95.

Manning, F. A., Hill, L. M., and Platt, L. D. (1981). Quantitative amniotic fluid volume determination by ultrasound: Antepartum detection of intrauterine growth retardation. *Am. J. Obstet. Gynecol.*, **139**, 254.

Manning, F. A., Lange, I. R., Morrison, I., and Harman, C. R. (1984). Fetal biophysical profile score and the nonstress test: A comparative trial. *Obstet. Gynecol.*, **64**, 326–31.

Manning, F. A., Morrison, I., Lange, I. R., Harman, C. R., and Chamberlain, P. F. (1985). Fetal assessment based on fetal biophysical profile scoring: Experience in 12 620 referred high risk pregnancies. I. Perinatal mortality by frequency and etiology. *Am. J. Obstet. Gynecol.*, **151**, 343–50.

Manning, F. A., Morrison, I., Lange, I. R., Harman, C. R., and Chamberlain, P. F. (1987*a*), Fetal biophysical profile scoring: Selective use of the nonstress test. *Am. J. Obstet. Gynecol.*, **156**, 709–12.

Manning, F. A., Menticoglou, S. M., Harman, C. R., Morrison, I., and Lange, I. R. (1987*b*) Antepartum fetal risk assessment: the role of the fetal biophysical profile score. In *Ballière's clinical obstetrics and gynaecology*, Volume 1 (ed. M. J. Whittle), pp. 55–72, publisher Ballière Tindall.

Manning, F. A., Morrison, I., Harman, C. R., Lange, I. R., and Menticoglou, S. (1987*c*). Fetal assessment based on fetal biophysical profile scoring: Experience in 19 221 referred high risk pregnancies. II. An analysis of false negative fetal deaths. *Am. J. Obstet. Gynecol.*, **157**, 880–4.

Manning, F. A., Harman, C. R., Morrison, I. R., and Menticoglou, S. M. (1990*a*). Fetal assessment based on fetal biophysical profile scoring III. Positive predictive accuracy of the very abnormal test (biophysical profile score = 0). *Am. J. Obstet. Gynecol.*, **162**, 398–402.

Manning, F. A., Harman, C. R., Morrison, I., Menticoglou, S. M., Lange, I. R., and Johnson, J. M. (1990*b*). Fetal assessment based on fetal biophysical profile scoring IV. An analysis of perinatal mortality and morbidity. *Am. J. Obstet. Gynecol.*, **162**, 703–9.

Manning, F. A., Morrison, I. R., Harman, C. R., and Menticoglou, S. M. (1990*c*). The abnormal fetal biophysical profile score V. Predictive accuracy according to score composition. *Am. J. Obstet. Gynecol.*, **162**, 918–27.

Mills, M. S., James, D. K., and Slade, S. (1990). Two-tier approach to biophysical assessment of the fetus. *Am. J. Obstet. Gynecol.*, **163**, 12–16.

Mohide, P. and Keirse, M. (1989). In *Effective care in pregnancy and childbirth*. Volume 1. *Pregnancy* (ed. I. Chalmers, M. Enkin and M. J. N. C. Keirse), pp. 477–92. Oxford University Press, Oxford.

Moore, T. R. and Cayle, J. E. (1990). The amniotic fluid index in normal human pregnancy. *Am. J. Obstet. Gynecol.*, **162**, 1168–73.

Natale, R. and Nasello-Paterson, C. (1988). Patterns of fetal breathing activity in the human fetus at 24 to 28 weeks' gestation. *Am. J. Obstet. Gynecol.*, **158**, 317–21.

Natale, R., Patrick, J., and Richardson, B. (1978). Effects of maternal venous plasma glucose concentrations on fetal breathing movements. *Am. J. Obstet. Gynecol.*, **132**, 36–41.

Natale, R., Nasello, C., and Turliuk, R. (1984). The relationship between movements and accelerations in fetal heart rate at twenty-four to thirty-two weeks' gestation. *Am. J. Obstet. Gynecol.*, **148**, 591–5.

Patrick, J., Campbell, K., Carmichael, L., *et al.* (1980). A definition of human fetal apnoea and the distribution of fetal apnoeic intervals in the last ten weeks of pregnancy. *Am. J. Obstet. Gynecol.*, **136**, 471–7.

Patrick, J., Campbell, K., Carmichael, L., *et al.* (1982). Patterns of gross fetal body movements over 24-hour observation intervals in the last ten weeks of pregnancy. *Am. J. Obstet. Gynecol.*, **142**, 363–71.

Pearson, J. F. and Weaver, J. B. (1976). Fetal activity and fetal well-being; an evaluation. *Br. Med. J.*, **1**, 1305–7.

Phelan, J. O., Platt, L. D., Yeh, S-Y., Broussard, P., and Paul, R. H. (1985). The role of ultrasound assessment of amniotic fluid volume in the management of the postdate pregnancy. *Am. J. Obstet. Gynecol.*, **151**, 304–8.

Platt, L. D., Manning, F. A., LeMay, M., and Sipos, L. (1978). Human fetal breathing: Relationships to fetal condition. *Am. J. Obstet. Gynecol.*, **132**, 514–18.

Platt, L. D., Eglinton, G. S., Sipos, L., Broussard, P. M., and Paul, R. H. (1983). Further experience with the fetal biophysical profile. *Obstet. Gynecol.*, **61**, 480–5.

Platt, L. D., Walla, C., Paul, R. H., Trujillo, M. D., Loesser, C. V., Jacobs, N. D., *et al.* (1985). A prospective trial of the fetal biophysical profile versus the nonstress test in the management of high-risk pregnancies. *Am. J. Obstet. Gynecol.*, **153**, 624–33.

Ribbert, L. S. M., Snijders, R. J. M., Nicolaides, K. H., and Visser, G. H. A. (1990). Relationship of fetal biophysical profile and blood gas values at cordocentesis in severely growth-retarded fetuses. *Am. J. Obstet. Gynecol.*, **163**, 569–71.

Schifrin, B. S., Guntes, V., Gergely, R. C., Eden, R., Roll, K., and Jacobs, J. (1981). The role of real time scanning in antenatal fetal surveillance. *Am. J. Obstet. Gynecol.*, **140**, 525–30.

Seeds, A. E., (1980). Current concepts of amniotic fluid dynamics. *Am. J. Obstet. Gynecol.*, **138**, 575–86.

Shime, J., Gare, D. J., Andrews, J., Betrand, M., Salgado, J., and Whillans, G. (1984). Prolonged pregnancy: Surveillance of the fetus and the neonate and the course of labor and delivery. *Am. J. Obstet. Gynecol.*, **148**, 547–51.

Sival, D. A., Visser, G. H., and Prechtl, H. F. R. (1990). Does reduction in amniotic fluid affect fetal movements? *Early Hum. Devel.*, **23**, 233–46.

Thacker, S. B. and Berkelman, R. L. (1986). Assessing the diagnostic accuracy and efficacy of selected antepartum fetal surveillance techniques. *Obstet. Gynecol. Survey*, **41**, 121–41.

Vintzileos, A. M., Campbell, W. A., Ingardia, C. J., and Nochimson, D. J. (1983). The fetal biophysical profile and its predictive value. *Obstet. Gynecol.*, **62**, 271–8.

Vintzileos, A. M., Campbell, W. A., Nochimson, D. J., *et al.* (1985). The fetal biophysical profile in patients with premature rupture of the membranes. An early indicator of fetal infection. *Am. J. Obstet. Gynecol.*, **152**, 510.

Vintzileos, A. M., Feinstein, S. J., Lodeiro, J. G., Campbell, W. A., Weinbaum, P. J., and Nochimson, D. J. (1986*a*). Fetal biophysical profile and the effect of premature rupture of the membranes. *Obstet. Gynecol.,* **67**, 818–23.

Vintzileos, A. M., Campbell, W. A., Nochimson, D. J., and Weinbaum, P. J. (1986*b*). Fetal breathing as a predictor of infection in premature rupture of the membranes. *Obstet. Gynecol.*, **67**, 813–17.

Vintzileos, A. M., Campbell, W. A., Nochimson, D. J., and Weinbaum, P. J. (1986*c*). Fetal biophysical profile versus amniocentesis in predicting infection in preterm premature rupture of the membranes. *Obstet. Gynecol.*, **68**, 488.

Vintzileos, A. M., Campbell, W. A., Nochimson, D. J., and Weinbaum, P. J. (1987*a*). The use and misuse of the fetal biophysical profile. *Am. J. Obstet. Gynecol.*, **156**, 527–33.

Vintzileos A. M., Gaffney S. E., Salinger L. M., Kontopoulos V. G., Campbell W. A., and Nochimson D. J. (1987*b*). The relationships among the fetal biophysical profile, umbilical cord pH, and Apgar scores. *Am. J. Obstet. Gynecol.*, **157**, 627–31.

Vintzileos, A. M., Bors-Koefoed, R., Pelegano, J. F., *et al.* (1987*c*). The use of the fetal biophysical profile improves pregnancy outcome in premature rupture of the membranes. *Am. J. Obstet. Gynecol.*, **157**, 236.

Vintzileos, A. M., Fleming. A. D., Scorza, W. E., Wolf, E. J., Balducci, J., Campbell, W. A., and Rodis J. F. (1991). Relationship between fetal biophysical activities and umbilical cord blood gas values. *Am J. Obstet. Gynecol.*, **165**, 707–13.

Visser, G. A., Sadovsky, G., and Nicolaides, K. H. (1990). Antepartum heart rate patterns in small-for-gestational-age third trimester fetuses: correlations with blood gas values obtained at cordocentesis. *Am. J. Obstet. Gynecol.*, **162**, 698–703.

Vyas, S., Nicolaides, K. H., and Campbell, S. (1989). Renal artery flow-velocity waveforms in normal and hypoxaemic fetuses. *Am. J. Obstet. Gynecol.*, **161**, 168–72.

Walkinshaw, S. A., Cameron, H., McPhail, S., and Robson S. 1992 The prediction of fetal compromise and acidosis by biophysical profile scoring in the small for gestational age fetus. *J. Perinatal Med.* **20**, 227–32

Wheble, A. M., Gillmer, M. D. G., Spencer, J. A. D., and Sykes, G. S. (1989). Changes in fetal monitoring practice in the UK *Br. J. Obstet. Gynaecol.*, **96**, 1140–5.

Wladimiroff, J. W., Winjgaard, J. A. G. W., Degani, S., Noordam, J., van Eyck, J., and Tonge, H. M. (1987). Cerebral and umbilical arterial flow velocity waveforms in normal and growth retarded pregnancies. *Obstet. Gynecol.*, **69**, 705–9.

8

Human fetal responses to chronic hypoxaemia: Doppler studies of the cerebral and renal circulation
S. Vyas

Introduction

Invasive animal experiments have helped to elucidate the fetal cardiovascular adjustments that occur in response to hypoxaemia. Peeters *et al.* (1979) reduced the percentage of oxygen in the gas mixture inhaled by ewes to examine the effect of a reduction in fetal arterial oxygen content on the distribution of blood flow in sheep fetuses at term. Radioactively labelled microspheres were injected during maternal hypo-oxygenation and fetal organ perfusion was determined from the amount of radioactivity measured at post-mortem. The perfusion of fetal organs at different degrees of hypoxaemia was measured, and the responses fell into four groups:

Group 1. Blood flow increased in inverse relation to arterial oxygen content. This response was found in the heart, brain, and adrenal glands.

Group 2. Blood flow decreased progressively with a reduction in arterial oxygen content. This response was found only in the lungs.

Group 3. Blood flow was maximal at a certain arterial oxygen content. The gut, carcass, and kidneys had steady blood flow until the arterial oxygen content was reduced to 3 mM/l, thereafter it fell.

Group 4. Blood flow was unrelated to arterial oxygen content. The thyroid, thymus, and most importantly, the placenta did not show any alteration in blood flow.

These data provide evidence of a redistribution of cardiac output that selectively increases the perfusion of Group 1 organs, at the expense of those in Group 2 and 3 in response to hypoxaemia. The effect would be to overcome the reduction in blood oxygen content per unit volume by increasing the amount of blood delivered to selected organs per unit time.

These complex circulatory adjustments are usually summarized by the term 'brain sparing effect'. Evidence of this effect can be seen in the human fetus during the antenatal period from ultrasound biometric measurements, which show an alteration in the head to abdomen circumference ratio in favour of head growth in some small for gestational age (SGA) fetuses (Campbell and Thoms 1975).

Two relatively new techniques, cordocentesis and Doppler ultrasound, have made the study of the fetal response to hypoxaemia in humans possible. Cordocentesis provides access to the fetal circulation, and has made possible precise measurements of the fetal blood gas, acid–base, and metabolic status (Soothill *et al.* 1986, Nicolaides *et al.* 1989). These measurements thus represent a 'Gold Standard' against which different techniques of assessing fetal well being can be evaluated. This chapter summarizes the changes in the fetal cerebral and renal circulations in small for gestational age (SGA) fetuses determined by Doppler ultrasound, and correlates these changes with fetal blood gas and acid–base status in samples obtained by cordocentesis.

Human Doppler studies

Doppler ultrasound provides a non-invasive and safe technique for the assessment of the fetus. The combination of ultrasound imaging and pulsed Doppler ultrasound in a Duplex system (Eik-Nes *et al.* 1982) enables the study of blood flow characteristics in specific fetal circulations.

Currently, analyses of the flow velocity waveform (FVW) involve the calculation of blood velocity and indices which are thought to represent downstream impedance to blood flow. Although volume flow measurements are theoretically possible, inaccuracies in the measurement of the vessel diameter have limited their extrapolation to normal physiology. The three commonly used indices of impedance are:

A/B ratio $= A/B$ (Stuart *et al.* 1980)
Resistance Index, $RI = A - B/A$ (Pourcelot 1974)
Pulsatility Index, $PI = A - B/$mean (Gosling and King 1975)

where A is the maximum systolic Doppler shift and B is the end-diastolic Doppler shift. For the pulsatility index the denominator (mean) is the mean of the maximum frequency envelope over the complete cardiac cycle.

The A/B ratio and RI are related:

$$A/B = 1/(1 - RI).$$

As the flow velocity waveform (FVW) becomes more pulsatile all three indices increase. However, when end-diastolic frequencies (EDF) are absent ($B = 0$), RI and A/B become unity and infinity, respectively, and cease to be useful. In contrast, the denominator in the calculation of the PI will continue to be influenced by the shape of the FVW, and is therefore the only index of value in quantifying FVWs which have absent EDF.

Doppler studies of the umbilical artery provide information on perfusion of the fetoplacental circulation, abnormalities of which may limit placental exchange and lead to fetal hypoxaemia, hypercapnia, and acidaemia. Doppler studies of selected fetal organs are valuable in detecting the haemodynamic rearrangements that occur in response to hypoxaemia.

Fetal cerebral circulation in appropriate for gestational age fetuses

Studies of the fetal cerebral circulation have included examination of the common carotid artery, the intracranial portion of the internal carotid artery, and branches of the circle of Willis, notably the middle cerebral artery.

To obtain FVWs from the common carotid artery, a longitudinal section of the fetal neck is first obtained. The common carotid artery is a relatively straight vessel, and the range gate is placed on its proximal portion before it branches into the internal and external carotid arteries.

Bilardo *et al.* (1988) obtained common carotid artery FVWs from 70 fetuses of appropriate size for gestation (AGA). The coefficient of variation for the measurement of mean blood velocity was 12.5 per cent and 7.9 per cent for the measurement of *PI*. End-diastolic frequencies were usually absent until 32 weeks' gestation, but increased progressively thereafter. Common carotid artery mean blood velocity increased linearly with advancing gestation, and the *PI* remained constant until 32 weeks, when it fell steeply. Bilardo *et al.* (1988) combined the findings from the study of the common carotid artery and aorta and expressed them as ratios of the *PI* and mean blood velocity. There was a linear increase in the common carotid velocity/aortic velocity ratio, whilst the common carotid *PI*/aortic *PI* ratio remained constant to 32 weeks' gestation when it fell steeply. Thus, both curves were principally influenced by the large changes with advancing gestation that occur in common carotid artery *PI* and velocity. The authors speculated that a progressively increasing fraction of cardiac output was directed to the fetal brain, and postulated that this redistribution was in response to falling PO_2 (Soothill *et al.* 1986; Nicolaides *et al.* 1989).

Van den Wijngaard *et al.* (1989) used Duplex pulsed Doppler ultrasound to obtain FVWs from the fetal intracranial circulation of 55 AGA fetuses at 25–41 weeks' gestation. To obtain FVWs from the internal carotid artery, a transverse section of the fetal brain is first obtained at the level of the biparietal diameter. The transducer is then moved towards the base of the skull to the level of the cerebral peduncles. The pulsations of the internal carotid artery are seen just anterior to the cerebral peduncles, and the range gate is placed on these pulsations to obtain FVWs (Wladimiroff *et al.* 1986). Pulsations running laterally from those of the internal carotid artery are thought to represent the middle cerebral artery, whilst FVWs from the posterior cerebral artery are obtained by placing the range gate lateral to the cerbral peduncles. FVWs from the anterior cerebral artery are obtained by placing the range gate further anterior to the cerebral peduncles.

Van den Wijngaard *et al.* (1989) reported successful examinations of these vessels as follows:

Internal carotid artery	89%
Middle cerebral artery	91%
Posterior cerebral artery	58%
Anterior cerebral artery	64%

End-diastolic frequencies were present in all vessels examined, suggesting that the brain is served by a low impedance vascular bed. The *PI* in all the vessels remained constant until 34 weeks, when it fell.

Kirkinen *et al.* (1987) used a similar methodology to examine 83 AGA fetuses at 25–42 weeks' gestation and also described a reduction in impedance to flow with gestation in 'intracranial arteries'. The authors were unsure of the exact origin of the Doppler shifted signals, but argued that they were most likely to originate from the short intracranial portion of the internal carotid artery, the middle cerebral artery, or, a mixture of both. Woo *et al.* (1987) used similar methodology in their longitudinal study of 15 normal pregnancies. They noted a reduction in a modified A/B ratio with advancing gestation, greatest after 30 weeks. In this study EDF were absent at 24–26 weeks' gestation in an unspecified number of cases.

Although FVWs can be obtained from the fetal intracranial vasculature from 25 weeks onwards, there is uncertainty as to the origin of these signals (Kirkinen *et al.* 1987). As a result of this uncertainty there are discrepancies in the results. Thus, EDF were found in all fetuses in the studies of Van den Wijngaard *et al.* (1989) and Kirkinen *et al.* (1987) but not in that of Woo *et al.* (1987).

The problem of accurate identification of the intracranial vasculature has been overcome by the introduction of colour flow imaging. This relatively new technique produces a real-time image in which the velocity and direction of movement in the scan plane are colour coded. The identification of small vessels is, therefore, dependent on the demonstration of red blood cell movement rather than the imaging of vessel walls, the diameter of which may be beyond the resolution of B-mode imaging.

To obtain FVWs from the middle cerebral artery using colour flow imaging, a transverse view of the fetal brain is obtained at the level of the biparietal diameter. The transducer is then moved towards the base of the skull to the level of the lesser wing of the sphenoid bone. The middle cerebral artery can be seen as a major lateral branch of the circle of Willis, running anterolaterally towards the lateral edge of the orbit (Plate 1). The range gate is then placed on the proximal portion of this vessel to obtain FVWs.

In their cross-sectional study of 172 AGA fetuses between 18 and 43 weeks' gestation Vyas *et al.* (1990*b*) used colour flow imaging to identify the middle cerebral artery for subsequent pulsed Doppler studies. FVWs of satisfactory quality were obtained in 154 cases (90 per cent). Failure to obtain FVWs was always due to deep engagement of the fetal head in the maternal pelvis or a per-sistent occipito-anterior or posterior position, rather than ambiguity about the intracranial vascular anatomy. The intraobserver coefficient of variation for the measurement of fetal middle cerebral artery *PI* was 5.3 per cent. End-diastolic frequencies were present in 32 of 41 fetuses (78 per cent) at 18–25 weeks' gestation, 36 of 47 (77 per cent) at 26–33 weeks and all 66 fetuses after 34 weeks (Fig. 8.1). The relationship of fetal middle cerebral artery *PI* with gestation was best described by a quadratic equation.

The middle cerebral artery mean blood velocity was also measured in 106 of the 154 fetuses. The intraobserver coefficient of variation for this measurement was 11.1 per cent. The relationship with gestation was best described by a linear equation following $\log_{10}$ transformation. In the 106 fetuses in which both Doppler parameters were measured there was an inverse relationship between middle cerebral artery mean blood velocity and *PI*.

The similarity in the pattern of reduction in impedance to flow in the cerebral vasculature with gestation in these studies suggests that the fall in common carotid artery *PI* during normal of pregnancy is due predominantly to a reduc-tion in impedance to flow in the cerebral vasculature. Furthermore, the increase in middle cerebral artery mean blood velocity is significantly associated with the decrease in impedance to flow.

Mean blood velocity in the intracranial vasculature has not been previously reported, possibly due to difficulties in vessel imaging by B-mode ultrasound and, therefore, accurate measurement of the angle of insonation.

Fetal cerebral circulation in small for gestational age fetuses

Marsal *et al.* (1984) first reported an increase in EDF from the common carotid artery in SGA fetuses, whilst Wladimiroff *et al.* (1986) described similar altera-tions in FVWs from the intracranial circulation. This morphological change is associated with a fall in the *PI* of the FVWs. Wladimiroff *et al.* (1986) expressed the internal carotid artery and umbilical artery *PI* as a ratio, and improved the predictive value of poor perinatal outcome over the individual measurements.

More recently Van den Wijngaard *et al.* (1989) investigated the middle cerebral, anterior and posterior communicating, and internal carotid arteries in 14 SGA fetuses. They confirmed the characteristic finding of increased EDF and a reduced *PI*, indicating a fall in impedance to flow. This effect was most prominent in the fetal middle cerebral artery.

Bilardo *et al.* (1990) examined the mean blood velocity and *PI* of FVWs from the fetal aorta and common carotid artery in 41 SGA and 10 appropriate for gestational age (AGA) fetuses. All fetuses also had fetal blood sampling per-formed by cordocentesis after the Doppler examination. Since the fetal Doppler and blood gas parameters alter with gestation, the observed values were expressed as the number of standard deviations by which they differed from the

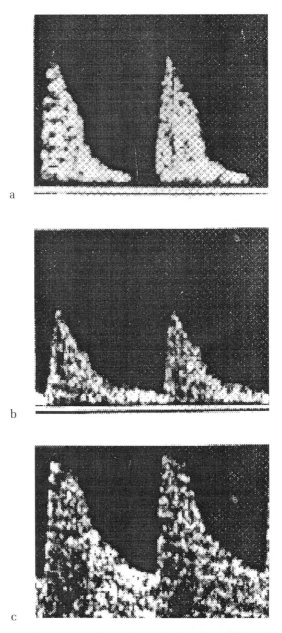

a

b

c

Fig. 8.1. Flow velocity waveforms from the fetal middle cerebral artery: (A) at 22 weeks' gestation with end-diastolic frequencies absent; (B) at 37 weeks' gestation with end-diastolic frequencies present, and (C) in a hypoxaemic fetus at 28 weeks, gestation where end-diastolic frequencies were increased. (Reproduced with permission from the *British Journal of Obstetrics and Gynaecology.*)

expected normal mean for gestation. This procedure corrects for the effect of gestational age on observed values, which are then expressed as delta (Δ) values. There were significant correlations between the reduction of the *PI* of FVWs from the common carotid artery (ΔPI) and ΔPO_2 and ΔpH. Furthermore, common carotid artery mean blood velocity was increased in the SGA fetuses, and there was a significant association between the magnitude of this increase and ΔPO_2 and ΔpH. Blood gases and pH were correlated individually, and, as an 'asphyxia index' to the Doppler measurements. The asphyxia index was derived by principal component analysis, and defined by the equation:

$$\text{Asphyxia} = -\Delta PO_2 + 1.43\,(\Delta PCO_2) - 180.2\,(\Delta pH).$$

Although there were significant correlations between the blood gas results and both the *PI* and mean blood velocity in the individual vessels, better correlations were found with the ratio of common carotid artery and descending thoracic aorta mean blood velocity and *PI*. The best predictor of asphyxia (as judged by the lowest residual standard deviation and highest correlation coefficient) was an index comprising the aortic mean blood velocity and the *PI* of FVWs from the common carotid artery. This index was also derived by principle component analysis, and defined by the equation:

$$\text{Aortic–carotid index} = \Delta AoVm + 4.2\,(\Delta CCPI).$$

When the aortic–carotid index was abnormal, all fetuses had an asphyxia index above the mean, 89 per cent of the fetuses had an asphyxia index one standard deviation above the mean and 60 per cent greater than two standard deviations above the mean. A normal index was always associated with normal blood gases.

Taken as a whole, these results provide strong evidence of the brain-sparing effect in human SGA fetuses, as a reduction in impedance to blood flow would facilitate an increase in cerebral perfusion. Bilardo *et al.* (1990) suggested that the decrease in aortic mean blood velocity and increase in *PI* represented the cumulative vasoconstrictor influence of the visceral organs and carcass.

However, the studies of Van den Wijngaard *et al.* (1989) did not include data on fetal blood gases, whilst Bilardo *et al.* (1990) measured fetal blood gases, but examined the common carotid artery. This vessel supplies the tissues of the face and neck in addition to the brain. Thus, during fetal hypoxaemia the common carotid artery would reflect the opposing vasoconstrictive effects of the tissues of the head and neck and the vasodilatory effects of the cerebral circulation.

In an effort to elucidate the fetal cerebral vascular response to hypoxaemia, Vyas *et al.* (1990*b*) related umbilical cord blood gases with Doppler indices of velocity and impedence to flow in the fetal middle cerebral artery.

The *PI* of FVWs from the fetal middle cerebral artery of 81 SGA fetuses was significantly lower than the reference range (Fig. 8.2). There was a significant quadratic relation between ΔPI and ΔPO_2 (Fig. 8.3). Similarly, there was a significant quadratic relation between ΔPI and ΔpH. The middle cerebral artery

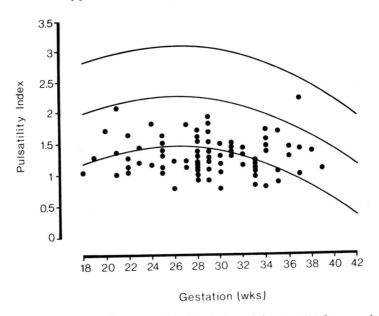

Fig. 8.2. Middle cerebral artery pulsatility index of the 81 SGA fetuses plotted on the reference range for gestation (mean and individual 90 percent CI). (Reproduced with permission from the *British Journal of Obstetrics and Gynaecology.*)

mean blood velocity (Vm) was measured in 58 cases, and was significantly higher than the reference range (Fig. 8.4). There was a significant correlation between ΔVm and ΔPO_2 (Fig. 8.5). The relation of ΔVm to ΔpH was best described by a quadratic equation and there was a significant correlation between ΔPI and ΔVm in the 58 SGA fetuses in which both measurements were performed. There were no significant associations between ΔPCO_2 and ΔPI or ΔVm.

These data provide evidence of vasodilatation in the cerebral vasculature during mild to moderate hypoxaemia. With severe degrees of hypoxaemia (2–4 standard deviations below the normal mean for gestation), usually associated with acidaemia, the reduction in *PI* reached a maximum which probably represents maximum vessel dilatation. In extreme hypoxaemia (a PO_2 value greater than four standard deviations below the normal mean for gestation) the reduction in *PI* was proportionally less (Fig. 8.3). Vyas *et al.* (1990*a*) had previously demonstrated that fetal head compression by the ultrasound transducer is associated with an increase in the *PI* of FVWs from the middle cerebral and internal carotid arteries. This increase in impedance to blood flow is presumably due to an increase in intracranial pressure. It could be hypothesized that a similar mechanism may operate in the severely hypoxaemic and acidaemic SGA fetus, where the vasodilatation mediated decrease in *PI* is blunted by increased

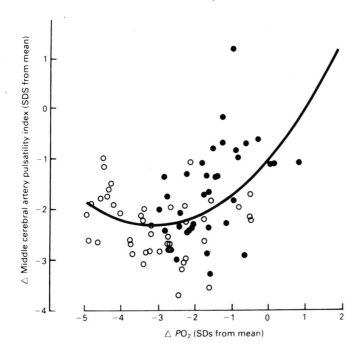

Fig. 8.3. The relationship between fetal hypoxemia (ΔPO_2) and fetal middle cerebral artery pulsatility index, both expressed as the number of standard deviations by which the observed values differed from the respective normal mean for gestation. The open circles indicate acidaemic fetuses and the closed circles represent non-acidaemic fetuses. (Reproduced with permission from the *British Journal of Obstetrics and Gynaecology*.)

intracranial pressure, possibly due to cerebral oedema. This phenomenon has been described in hypoxaemic monkey fetuses (Myers *et al.* 1984).

The middle cerebral artery mean blood velocity was higher in the SGA group, and there are significant correlations between the increased mean blood velocity and fetal hypoxaemia and acidaemia. However, the relationship between the increase in mean blood velocity and the decrease in *PI* was weaker in SGA than AGA fetuses ($r = -0.366$ and $r = -0.667$, respectively). These findings suggest that, in SGA fetuses the reduction in downstream impedance to blood flow is a smaller contributer to the increase in mean blood velocity than in AGA fetuses; other factors such as cardiac contractility, vessel compliance and blood viscosity may play a more significant role. This independence of blood velocity and *PI*, however, works in favour of middle cerebral artery velocity measurements in predicting severe fetal acidaemia. Thus, the sensitivity of middle cerebral artery mean blood velocity for the

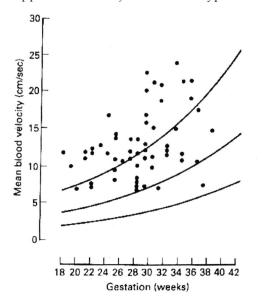

Fig. 8.4. Middle cerebral artery mean blood velocity of the 58 SGA fetuses (●) plotted on the reference range for gestation (mean and individual 90 per cent CI). (Reproduced with permission from the *British Journal of Obstetrics and Gynaecology.*)

prediction of acidaemia is 70 per cent, with a specificity of 77 per cent, which is superior to that of the middle cerebral artery *PI*.

Fetal renal circulation in appropriate for gestational age fetuses

Studies of the human fetal visceral circulation are of considerable interest as animal studies have demonstrated that in fetal hypoxaemia there is a redistribution of blood flow. Hitherto, studies of the fetal visceral circulation were not possible since the arterial supply could not be imaged for accurate pulsed Doppler studies. This problem has been overcome with the introduction of colour flow imaging, and the fetal renal artery was the first visceral vessel to be investigated using this method (Vyas *et al.* 1989).

To obtain FVWs from the fetal renal artery, first a longitudinal view of the fetal kidneys and aorta is obtained by real-time ultrasonography. Using colour flow imaging, the renal artery can be seen running directly towards the transducer, from its origin as a lateral branch of the abdominal aorta to the hilum of the kidney (Plate 2). In this orientation the beam-vessel angle for the renal artery is close to 0°, whilst that for the abdominal aorta is close to 90°. This ensures that the signals from the renal artery are optimized, with no contamination from the aorta. The Doppler range gate is placed over the renal artery, rather than one of its branches. In practice, the length of the vessel

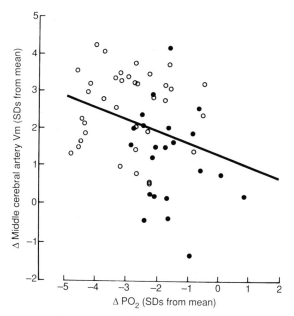

Fig. 8.5. The relationship between fetal hypoxaemia (ΔPO_2) and fetal middle cerebral artery mean blood velocity, both expressed as the number of standard deviations by which the observed values differed from the respective normal mean for gestation. The open circles indicate acidaemic fetuses and the closed circles represent non-acidaemic fetuses. (Reproduced with permission from the *British Journal of Obstetrics and Gynaecology*.)

imaged is insufficient for an accurate measurement of the angle of insonation, so mean blood velocity has not been reported.

To date 212 AGA fetuses have been examined and FVWs of satisfactory quality were obtained in 192 cases (91 per cent). The intra-observer coefficient of variation for the measurement of fetal renal artery *PI* was 5.4 per cent. The FVWs are highly pulsatile and the presence of EDF becomes more common with gestation. Thus, EDF were present in 6 of 46 cases (13 per cent) at 18–25 weeks' gestation, 13 of 67 cases (20 per cent) at 26–34 weeks, and 70 of 79 cases (89 per cent) at 35–43 weeks (Plate 3). This morphological alteration in the FVW with gestation was also reflected in the fall in *PI* which remained constant until 32 weeks' gestation, falling steeply thereafter. The relationship of *PI* with gestation was best described by a quadratic equation.

During renal angiogenesis there is lengthening of the developing nephrons and branching of the arterioles. This process begins in the early second trimester and is completed by the late third trimester (Hudlicka and Tyler 1986). Thus, the observed reduction in impedance to flow in the renal artery with gestation is likely to be the result of a maturational process representing an increase in the total arteriolar cross-sectional area.

Assuming that fetal arterial blood pressure does not change with gestation, then fetal renal perfusion increases. This may offer an explanation for the increase in fetal urine production rate with gestation (Rabinowitz *et al.* 1989). This is in agreement with studies on chronically catheterized fetal lambs, where total renal blood flow (ml/min) and filtration fraction are significantly higher near term when compared to earlier in the third trimester (Robillard *et al.* 1981).

Pearce *et al.* (1988) reported that there is a slight but significant increase in the *PI* of FVWs from the fetal aorta with gestation, whilst Bilardo *et al.* (1988) demonstrated that it remains constant. Since approximately 40 per cent of the cardiac output is distributed to the umbilical circulation (Rudolph and Heymann 1967), where the *PI* falls with gestation, Pearce *et al.* (1988) suggested that impedance to flow in the other major branches of the aorta must increase to produce a minimal net effect on impedance to flow in the aorta. The findings of Vyas *et al.* (1989) demonstrate that this is not the case. Furthermore, the fetal kidneys receive only 3 per cent of the cardiac output (Rudolph and Heymann 1967) and the net effect of changes in impedance to flow in the renal circulation on impedance to flow in the aorta would be expected to be minimal.

Bilardo *et al.* (1988) and Van Den Wijngaard *et al.* (1989) suggested that the decrease in impedance to flow in the cerebral circulation during normal pregnancy represents a physiological increase in cerebral perfusion in response to falling PO_2 (Soothill *et al.* 1986; Nicolaides *et al.* 1989). Were this the case, consideration of the hypoxaemic sheep fetus model (Cohn *et al.* 1974; Peeters *et al.* 1979) would lead one to expect the *PI* of FVWs from the fetal renal artery to increase with advancing gestation. This is not the case. The steepest fall in *PI*, in both the fetal renal and cerebral circulations, in normal pregnancy occurs at the time of fastest arteriolar proliferation (Hudlicka and Tyler 1986). This suggests that reduction of impedance to flow in both these circulations during normal pregnancy represents arteriolar proliferation rather than a redistribution of blood flow in response to progressive hypoxaemia.

Fetal renal circulation in small for gestational age fetuses

The animal model suggests that the increase in cerebral perfusion occurs at the expense of perfusion of the viscera. In order to investigate this hypothesis in the human fetus, Vyas *et al.* (1989) related the degree of fetal hypoxaemia measured in umbilical cord blood samples to the *PI* of FVWs from the fetal renal artery. Although the initial report was based on a small number of fetuses, the current analyses are based on the investigation of 48 SGA fetuses (Vyas 1990). As a group the renal artery *PI* of the SGA fetuses were significantly higher than the normal mean for gestation (Fig. 8.6). For the whole group, there was no significant association between ΔPI and ΔPO_2. However, for fetuses at greater than 24 weeks' gestation there was a significant association between ΔPI and

ΔPO_2 (Fig. 8.7; n = 39). For the subgroup of fetuses at or below 24 weeks' gestation six of the nine fetuses had renal artery *PI* values within the 90 per cent confidence intervals of the reference range for gestation; ΔPI was not significantly related to ΔPO_2 (n = 9, r = 0.004). These findings suggest a gestation-related 'maturation' in renal vascular responsiveness to hypoxaemia.

A sonographic diagnosis of oligohydramnios was made when the vertical diameter of the largest pool of amniotic fluid was less than 1 cm (Manning *et al.* 1980). There was no significant difference in mean ΔPI between the oligo-hydramnios and non-oligohydramnios sub-groups. In SGA pregnancies beyond 24 weeks' gestation, the renal artery *PI* was above the 95th centile of the reference range in 15 of 16 cases (94 per cent) in which an ultrasound diagnosis of oligohydramnios was made. This suggests that increased impedance to flow in the renal vasculature may result in a reduction in fetal urine production, and therefore, a concomitant reduction in amniotic fluid volume. However, in the same group oligohydramnios was present in only 15 of the 28 cases (54 per cent) in which the renal artery *PI* was above the 95th centile of the reference range. Since the amniotic fluid volume reflects the chronic state, and renal artery *PI* the acute state, it is possible that oligohydramnios will develop in the remaining 13 cases (46 per cent) in later pregnancy if the renal artery *PI* remains elevated due to chronic hypoxaemia. This hypothesis needs further evaluation.

Previous studies using pulsed Doppler ultrasound have alluded to alterations in the organ perfusion of SGA human fetuses. Hackett *et al.* (1987) found that when there was absence of EDF in the fetal descending thoracic aorta, there was an increased incidence of neonatal nercrotizing enterocolitis and

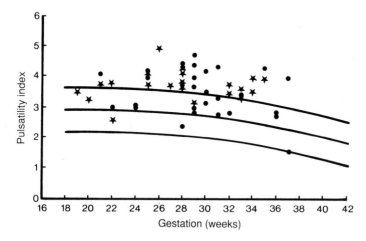

Fig. 8.6. The renal artery pulsatility index of the 48 SGA fetuses (●) plotted on the reference range for gestation (mean and individual 95 per cent CI). In 21 cases there was oligohydramnios (*).

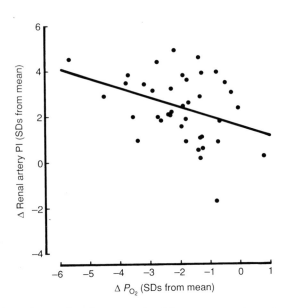

Fig. 8.7. The relationship between fetal hypoxaemia (ΔPO_2) and fetal renal artery pulsatility index, both expressed as the number of standard deviations by which the observed values differed from the respective normal mean for gestation, for fetuses > 24 weeks' gestation.

haemorrhage. The authors speculated that these neonatal complications were the result of hypoperfusion of the fetal gut and liver, respectively. However, exact information was not obtained as the arterial supply of individual organs could not be identified. The use of colour flow imaging has facilitated the investigation of the renal artery, and we presume that the finding are representative of visceral vasoconstriction in chronically hypoxaemic SGA fetuses.

The mechanism underlying this increase in impedance to flow has been investigated by Robillard *et al.* (1986) in chronically catheterized hypoxaemic fetal lambs. Changes in renal blood flow were measured by indwelling pulsed Doppler probes, and changes in renal vascular resistance were calculated after taking account of the perfusion pressure (mean aortic pressure – mean inferior vena cava pressure). In each fetus, the left kidney was denervated by severing and stripping the renal nerves around and along the renal artery and vein, followed by the application of 10 per cent phenol in absolute alcohol; the renal pedicle on the right was explored, but only 0.9 per cent saline was applied. Renal vascular resistance was increased and renal blood flow fell in both kidneys in response to fetal hypoxaemia. However, the changes in renal blood flow were always smaller in the denervated than in the intact kidney. The conclusion was that renal vasoconstriction in response to fetal hypoxaemia is modulated by other factors in addition to neuronal stimulation.

Conclusions

The studies described in this chapter have demonstrated that hypoxaemia is associated with alterations in human fetal blood flow that mirror the brain-sparing effect previously demonstrated in animal studies. This effect is presumably modulated by chemoreceptors in the aorta and carotid body, and it appears to be triggered by even moderate reductions of PO_2.

Prolonged intrauterine hypoxaemia could have permanent effects on fetal neurological development, especially if sustained from an early and more vulnerable stage of brain development. In practice, the Doppler abnormalities are seen days or even weeks before alterations in the fetal heart rate patterns or the biophysical profile, which appear to require more severe, or possibly prolonged degrees of hypoxaemia and/or acidaemia to trigger a measurable change. It is too early to say whether Doppler studies of the fetal circulation will be better than other fetal assessment techniques in optimizing the time of delivery to ensure survival of the infant without long-term handicap.

References

Bilardo, C. M., Campbell, S., and Nicolaides, K. H. (1988). Mean blood velocity and flow impedence in the fetal descending thoracic aorta and common carotid artery in normal pregnancy. *Early Hum. Dev.*, 18, 213.

Bilardo, C. M., Nicolaides, K. H., and Campbell, S. (1990). Doppler measurement of fetal and uteroplacental circulations: relationship with umbilical venous blood gases measured at cordocentesis. *Am. J. Obstet. Gynecol.*, 162, 115.

Campbell, S. and Thoms, A. (1975). Ultrasound measurement of the fetal head to abdomen circumference ratio in the assessment of growth retardation. *Br. J. Obstet. Gynaecol.*, 84, 165.

Cohn, H. E., Sacks, E. J., Heyman, M. A., and Rudolph, A. M. (1974). Cardiovascular responses to hypoxaemia and acidaemia in fetal lambs. *Am. J. Obstet. Gynecol.*, 120, 817.

Eik-Nes, S. H., Marsal, K., Brubakk, A. O., Kristofferson, K., and Ulstrin, M. (1982). Ultrasonic measurement of human fetal blood flow. *J. Biomed Eng.*, Jan, 4(1) 28–36.

Gosling, R. G. and King, D. H. (1975). Ultrasonic angiology. In *Arteries and veins* (ed. A. W. Harcus and L. Adamson p. 61 Chruchill Livingstone, Edinburgh.

Hackett, G. A. S., Campbell, S., Gamsu, H., Cohen-Overbeek, T., and Pearce, J. M. F. (1987). Doppler studies in the growth retarded fetus and prediction of neonatal necrotising enterocolitis, haemorrhage, and neonatal morbidity. *Br. Med. J.*, 294, 13.

Hudlicka, O. and Tyler, K. R. (1986). *Angiogenesis*, p. 76. Academic Press, London.

Kirkinen, P., Muller, R., Huch, R., and Huch, A. (1987). Blood flow velocity waveforms in human fetal intra-cranial arteries. *Obstet. Gynecol.*, 70, 617.

Manning, F., Platt, L., and Sipos, L. (1980). Antepartum fetal evaluation: Development of a fetal biophysical profile. *Am. J. Obstet. Gynecol.*, 136, 787.

Marsal, K., Lingman, G., and Giles, W. (1984). Evaluation of the carotid, aortic and umbilical blood velocity waveforms in the human fetus. In *Proceedings XI Annual Conference of the Society of Fetal Physiology*, C33 Oxford.

188   *Doppler studies in fetal chronic hypoxaemia*

Myers, R. E., de Courtney-Myers, G. M., and Wagner, K. R. (1984). Effects of hypoxia on fetal brain. In *Fetal physiology and Medicine*, (ed. R. W. Beard and P. W. Nathanielsz, p. 419. Butterworth, London.

Nicolaides, K. H., Economides, D. L., and Soothill, P. W. (1989). Blood gases, pH and lactate in appropriate and small for gestational age fetuses. *Am. J. Obstet. Gynecol.*, 161, 996.

Pearce, J. M., Campbell, S., Cohen-Overbeek, T., Hackett, G., Hernandez, J., and Royston, P. (1988). Reference ranges and sources of variation for indices of pulsed Doppler flow velocity waveforms from the uteroplacental and fetal circulation. *Br. J. Obstet. Gynaecol.*, 95, 248.

Peeters, L. L. H., Sheldon, R. E., Jones, M. D., Makowski, E. L., and Meschia, G. (1979). Blood flow to fetal organs as a function of arterial oxygen content. *Am. J. Obstet. Gynecol.*, 135, 637.

Pourcelot, L. (1974). Applications clinique de l'examen Doppler transcutanie. In *Velocimetric ultrasonor Doppler* (ed. P. Peronneau), INSERM Vol. 34, pp. 213.

Rabinowitz, R, Peters, M. T., Vyas, S., Campbell, S., and Nicolaides, K. H. (1989). Measurement of fetal urine production in normal pregnancy by real-time ultrasonography. *Am. J. Obstet. Gynecol.*, 161, 1264.

Robillard, J. E., Weitzman, R. E., Burmeister, L., and Smith, F. G. (1981). Developmental aspects of the renal response to hypoxemia in the lamb fetus. *Circ. Res.*, 48, 128.

Robillard, J. E., Nakamura, K. T., and Dibona, G. F. (1986). Effect of renal denervation on renal responses to hypoxaemia in fetal lambs. *Am. J. Physiol.*, 19, F294.

Rudolph, A. M. and Heymann, M. A. (1967). The circulation of the fetus *in utero*. Methods for studying distribution of blood flow, cardiac output and organ blood flow. *Circ. Res.*, 21, 163.

Soothill, P. W., Nicolaides, K. H., Rodeck, C. H., and Campbell, S. (1986). Effect of gestational age on fetal and intervillous blood gas and acid–base values in human pregnancy. *Fetal Therapy*, 1, 168.

Stuart, B., Drumm, J., Fitzgerald, D. E., and Duignan, N. M. (1980). Fetal blood velocity waveforms in normal pregnancy. *Br. J. Obstet. Gynaecol.*, 87, 780.

Van den Wijngaard, J. A. G. W., Groenenberg, I. A. L., Wladimiroff, J. W., and Hop, W. C. J. (1989). Cerebral Doppler ultrasound in the human fetus. *Br. J. Obstet. Gynaecol.*, 96, 845.

Vyas, S. (1990). Investigation of placental and fetal renal and cerebral circulations by colour Doppler ultrasound. Unpublished MD thesis. University of London.

Vyas, S., Nicolaides, K. H., and Campbell, S. (1989). Renal artery flow velocity waveforms in normal and hypoxaemic fetuses. *Am. J. Obstet. Gynecol.*, 161, 168.

Vyas, S., Campbell, S., Bower, S., and Nicolaides, K. H. (1990a). Maternal abdominal pressure alters fetal cerebral blood flow. *Br. J. Obstet. Gynaecol.*, 97, 740.

Vyas, S., Nicolaides, K. H., Bower, S., and Campbell, S. (1990b). Middle cerebral artery flow velocity waveforms in fetal hypoxaemia. *Br. J. Obstet. Gynaecol.*, 97, 797.

Wladimiroff, J. W., Tonge, H. M., and Stewart, P. A. (1986). Doppler ultrasound assessment of cerebral blood flow in the human fetus. *Br. J. Obstet. Gynaecol.*, 93, 471.

Woo, J. S., Liang, S. T., Lo, R. L. S., and Chan, F. Y. (1987). Middle cerebral artery Doppler flow velocity waveforms. *Obstet. Gynecol.*, 70, 613.

9
Ultrasound in the developing world: appropriate technology?
S. P. Munjanja

Introduction

Obstetric ultrasound has become an indispensable tool in maternity care in developed countries. Its value in the management of several pregnancy complications has been well documented, although there is little evidence that its routine use produces a clear benefit (Neilson and Grant 1989). Rigorous scientific assessment of obstetric ultrasound has arrived late in the day, when the technique has become established in maternity practice and both providers and consumers demand its use. Most women in the developed world will, therefore, undergo ultrasound scanning as a routine investigation at least once during a pregnancy.

In the developing world the situation is quite different. Obstetric ultrasound is not available to the majority of pregnant mothers. However, the same combination of desire for technology and commercial interest that spurred the use of obstetric ultrasound in the developed world has now arrived in the developing world. History risks repeating itself, with probably a far less favourite outcome than has been attained in the developed world.

This is, therefore, an appropriate moment to ponder whether obstetric ultrasound is a useful technology in the developing world.

In assessing the value of this technology several factors will be taken into account. First, there will be a discussion on factors surrounding the provision and maintenance of obstetric ultrasound services. Secondly, factors in the delivery of the maternity services which have a bearing on obstetric ultrasound will be discussed. Finally, the relevance of the technique with regard to the obstetric pathology present in the population will be discussed.

It is striking how little evaluative research has been done or published on obstetric ultrasound in the developing world. Therefore, in approaching the subject of this chapter, one has to rely on published work in the developed countries, and apply this to the situations in the developing world.

Procurement of ultrasound equipment

In most developing countries decisions on buying ultrasound equipment (or any other expensive equipment) are made centrally by the senior staff of departments or ministries of health. Within such a centralized system clinicians are often at the periphery of the decision-making process, and their opinions have little impact on the type and quality of equipment which is eventually purchased.

Many developing countries have no formula for health resource allocation. The tendency to base allocation on historical need means that urban health centres and tertiary centres will get more resources to the detriment of other areas of the health service. Formulae for determining health resource allocation have been developed (Department of Health and Social Security 1976; Bourne *et al.* 1990), but their derivation requires epidemiological information which is difficult to obtain in developing countries. The final decision on what equipment is bought, and who gets it, is the result of a complex balancing act between competing national demands, and between competing medical disciplines. In countries composed of several ethnic, religious, or language groups, political factors may play a significant role in determining the regional allocation of expensive equipment. Radiology and obstetric departments may have to share one machine, a situation which leaves neither department satisfied. When ultrasound equipment is bought, it is often the case that cheaper, but outdated, equipment is ordered.

Another method of acquiring ultrasound equipment is through aid donated by agencies or countries. When this happens, the donor country or agency makes a short list of models of ultrasound equipment which are available within the terms of the aid package, effectively restricting the choice of the recipients. The choice is usually restricted to the country of origin of the aid, and to a few manufacturers within that country. A country which concludes several aid agreements with different donor countries will find itself with several different models. This equipment will usually be outdated and no longer in demand on the home market. Good quality up-to-date equipment is rarely brought into developing countries through aid agreements.

A third way in which ultrasound equipment is purchased is by individuals for use in the private health sector. The equipment is bought to fulfil individual practice needs and such individuals have no interest in a grand national health strategy. Although it would make sense for such health professionals to team up in order to obtain favourable purchase agreements from suppliers, in practice this does not happen. As a result one may find that even in the small private sector in developing countries, there will be several different models of ultrasound equipment. Where one supplier has managed to sell several machines to such a small market, this will usually be the result of aggressive marketing on their part, rather than co-operation from the buyers.

To overcome some of these problems, the World Health Organization has made recommendations for ultrasound equipment which they consider appropriate for developing countries (WHO 1985*a*). This information should be made more widely available.

Maintenance of obstetric ultrasound equipment

It is usual in developed countries for the purchaser to conclude a maintenance agreement with the supplier for the guarantee period. In theory, this is also the case in developing countries, but in practice this means nothing at all if the maintenance service is not present in the country. Sometimes, the equipment is supplied by an importer who has no maintenance or repair service whatsoever. Equipment brought in through intergovernmental aid agreements is not supported by a maintenance service since it is deemed to be a donation.

If such equipment breaks down completely and cannot be repaired, it may not be replaced, resulting in a permanent break of service. The institution or health centre involved will have qualified for an 'aid' machine because its yearly funding cannot support the purchase of such equipment. Even if the equipment is eventually replaced, the usual delay is at least one year because such expensive items have to be applied for through the yearly health budget allocation.

The main problem regarding maintenance and repair is that not enough machines are bought from each manufacturer to justify the setting up of facilities in each country. Present-day equipment suffers few breakdowns and most of these occur well after the guarantee period is over. A manufacturer who has supplied three or four machines would, therefore, find it quite expensive to provide the skilled manpower and equipment required for maintenance and repair as this would be underutilized.

In developing countries, the departments or ministries of health do have electrical engineers looking after medical equipment. However, it is rare for them to have someone who is familiar enough with ultrasound equipment to attend to breakdowns. In any case there would not be enough equipment to keep such personnel busy. Initially, equipment breakdown will usually be attended to by the hospital electrical engineer, before being disassembled for posting back to the manufacturer. This causes long breaks in the service. In Zimbabwe we have experienced breaks of service of 3–6 months whenever we have sent equipment abroad to the manufacturer for repairs.

For a quicker service, the manufacturer will offer to send a technician to do the repairs on the spot but this option is too expensive for the users, who would of course have to pay the air fares and accommodation for this person.

The problems with procurement and maintenance of obstetric ultrasound equipment in the developing countries undermine the possible contribution this equipment could make to obstetric management. The obstetric ultrasound service in many developing countries is characterized by poor quality equipment bought without sufficient maintenance support.

Organization of maternity services in relation to obstetric ultrasound

The appropriateness of any item of medical technology depends on the health care delivery system of which it is a part. It is difficult for any technology, no matter how good, to make an impact if it does not fit in well with the rest of the health care delivery system. Similarly, some of the claims made regarding the contribution of ultrasound to obstetrics in developed countries may have less to do with the technique itself than with the system of which it is a part.

The maternity referral system

Certain features exist in the maternity services of developing countries which diminish the importance of the technique to obstetric management. The first of these is the pyramidal hierarchy which exists within the maternity services (Fig. 9.1). These features in African countries have been described by Philpott (1980) and Nylander and Adenkule (1990).

Within such a system, due to insufficient resources, sophisticated facilities and skills are restricted to a few centres in the country. Between this level and

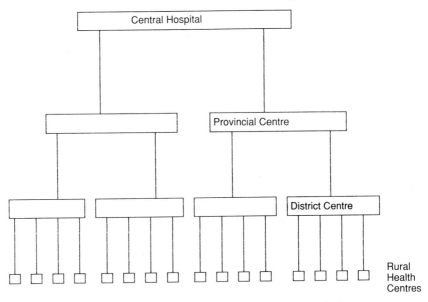

Fig. 9.1. Organization of health services in Zimbabwe.

the most basic rural health centre exist two other levels, the district health centre and the provincial health centre. Similar forms of differentiation are present even in the developed countries; the highly sophisticated units are called 'centres of excellence'. What distinguishes the hierarchy in the developing countries is the very wide gap in skills and technology between the levels. Indeed, in most of Africa, only 29–36 per cent of births are attended by trained personnel, according to the World Health Organization (WHO 1985*b*). This is a further indication of the skills gap between the highest and lowest forms of care.

Fig. 9.1, illustrates the organization of health services in Zimbabwe, which is typical of Sub-Saharan African Countries. Ultrasound equipment is only available at the central hospitals and in some provincial hospitals. Since referrals only occur to the next level within the system, a pregnant women requiring a scan at a rural health centre may have to visit two other centres before the investigation is done. This presents the staff and patients with substantial transport and communication problems. First, it may take a week or two before the patient reaches the ultrasound department, by which time the obstetric condition may have changed (for example a malpresentation has corrected itself). The value of ultrasound in giving immediate information for prognostic purposes is lost. Secondly, there is no direct communication between the person requesting the investigation and the ultrasonographer. Extra information cannot be obtained at short notice and there is no direct feedback to the staff of the rural health centre. They may never know if their diagnoses are confirmed or rejected if the patient delivers at the central hospital. This reduces the educational value of the technique in contributing towards obstetric management. Thirdly, due to transport problems, patients may wait up to a week at a district or provincial health centre before the examination is done. The woman and/or her fetus may come to harm because the staff are 'waiting for a scan'. Specialists from central hospitals visiting provincial centres have been told during medical rounds that so-and-so is 'waiting for a scan', as if that were a form of management. Monitoring and/or treatment of the patient is suspended because ultrasound is deemed to be the investigation that will determine the main course of action.

An added problem is that patients have to pay for transport and in some countries, such as Zimbabwe, pay for the examination itself. The costs are often beyond the means of rural families. This would be less unacceptable if all of the referrals were appropriate. Due to excessive reliance on ultrasound, acquired during their years of training as students and junior doctors, the provincial medical staff frequently make inappropriate requests for the investigation. Common examples in Zimbabwe are 'poor' fetal movements between 20–24 weeks, or malpresentation between 30–36 weeks. What justification can there be for a woman to travel up to 200 kilometres for these indications?

Training

Most obstetricians and midwives learn how to perform ultrasound examination by apprenticeship, whereas radiologists and radiographers undergo formal training leading to a recognized certificate. In developing countries, this latter type of training is not readily available due to a shortage of facilities and personnel. Apart from a few radiologists and radiographers who will go to developed countries for training, most health personnel performing ultrasound examinations undergo apprenticeship training, or are self-taught.

Informal training has the major advantages that it is cheaper and can be done within the country. However, it is difficult to ensure that satisfactory standards are established and maintained because of the wide variety of skills of the tutors. Ultrasound equipment is now much easier to use and the operating instructions are soon learnt. However, interpretation of anthropometric data is a skill which is obtained much more slowly. Especially where people have taught themselves, it is quite common to see women whose dates have been altered by one week following a third trimester scan, or to see unnecessary concern raised about cerebral ventricular size in early pregnancy in a normal fetus.

Zimbabwe has introduced formal training for radiographers leading to a diploma in ultrasonography. The experience gained from involvement with this course leads one to believe that regional co-operation in such training is necessary. Not only will the turnover of candidates be increased, but it may be easier to obtain adequate facilities if resources are combined from several countries. The course is modelled on the British Diploma in Ultrasonography, but certain aspects of this syllabus are difficult to fulfil in Zimbabwe.

Obstetric ultrasonography scanning in practice

The experience in Harare, Zimbabwe, will be used to discuss the applicability and relevance of ultrasonography in obstetrics in the developing world.

Harare Maternity Hospital is one of two tertiary level obstetric units in the country. It serves as a referral unit not only for Harare, but for four provinces adjoining the city. The unit is run jointly by government and university specialists who also teach midwives, undergraduate, and postgraduate students. About 18 000 women are delivered every year, all of them high risk. The perinatal mortality of the unit ranges between 50–60 per thousand and has shown no change over the past few years.

The Harare Maternity Hospital ultrasound unit is run by radiographers in consultation with obstetricians who have experience in scanning. No routine scanning is available, even to the high-risk patients booked at Harare Maternity Hospital. The service is only available to those who are deemed to need it. Because of the numbers involved the indications are highly selective. The unit scans an average of 35 patients a day on one machine, the daily workload ranging from 20 to 60. These high-risk patients demand skilled ultrasonography. Yet due to the workload, it is difficult to differentiate levels of scanning. Thus the quality of scanning which they get is that normally associated with a routine scan.

Table 9.1 illustrates the characteristics of the population served by the Harare Maternity Hospital Ultrasound unit.

In 1990 the unit performed 9109 ultrasound examinations, of which over 7000 were for obstetrical indications. The information from the first consecutive 7000 examinations confirms that the majority of these patients presented very late and this data is shown in Table 9.2.

The indications for requesting ultrasound examination are summarized in Table 9.3.

To determine the potential usefulness of ultrasonography in obstetric management, we should examine the indications for scanning in more detail with regard to the population served.

Estimation of gestational age

The assessment of various fetal anthropometric parameters to determine gestational age is a major component of obstetric scanning. The accuracy with which this can be done is greatest in early pregnancy (Robinson and Fleming 1975; Campbell *et al.* 1985) but decreases with advancing gestation. It is least

Table 9.1 Characteristics of population served by Harare Central Hospital ultrasound unit (1990)

Median gestation at antenatal booking	28.4 weeks
Median gestation at first scan	31.1 weeks
Proportion of non-Harare patients	16 per cent

Table 9.2 Number of patients presenting for the first scan by trimester

Period (weeks)	Number	Percentage
0–13	594	8.5
14–26	2245	32.1
27–40	4161	59.4
Total	7000	100

Table 9.3 Main indications for obstetric ultrasound examination at Harare Central Hospital in 1990

Indication	Percentage
Estimation of gestational age	34.7
Suspicion of multiple pregnancy	14.8
Concern for fetal viability	13.1
Abnormal presentation/lie	10.0
Placental localization	10.0
Suspected abnormal fetal growth	7.7
Types of abortion	5.1
Exclusion of fetal abnormality	2.5
Suspected trophoblastic disease	0.6
Suspected ectopic pregnancy	0.6
Others	0.9
Total	100

accurate in the third trimester. Even so, routine early pregnancy scanning for dating has not been shown to have beneficial effects on perinatal outcome, and so far the only significant impact demonstrated has been on the rate of inductions for 'post-term' pregnancy (Eik-Nes *et al.* 1984; Neilson and Grant 1989).

Estimation of gestational age was the commonest indication for obstetric scanning in Harare, but nearly 60 per cent of the women presented in the third trimester (Table 9.2), when the value of this estimation is minimal. For various reasons, antenatal booking occurs very late, so that the median gestation at the first visit is 28 weeks. The three-week gap between booking (28 weeks) and presenting for the first scan (31 weeks) reflects the period between the patient being seen at the peripheral health centre and being referred to Harare Maternity Hospital. So ingrained is the late booking behaviour that the overwhelming majority of those women who are scanned in the first trimester have complications in pregnancy, such as threatened abortion, which make them seek medical attention.

The time, money, and effort spent on scanning this large number of late bookers cannot be justified by the scientific evidence. About 16 per cent of these patients come from outside Harare and will have had to be transported for distances ranging from 50–200 kilometres, usually at their own expense. Efforts have been made to stop this practice, but medical staff wanting to obtain an estimate of the gestational age simply used another reason for referring the patients, knowing that fetal measurements would still be done. An initiative has started to encourage early antenatal booking but the initial response is slow (Munjanja, unpublished observations). It is obvious that we will have to wait for many years before the median booking gestation falls below 20 weeks. Until then, one of the major reasons for recommending early ultrasonography in pregnancy will be of little relevance to the Zimbabwean population.

Diagnosis of multiple pregnancy

Because of late booking, few twin pregnancies are identified before the third trimester. The opportunity for serial ultrasonography for fetal growth monitoring is limited by this, and also by the fact that delivery occurs early in multiple pregnancy. In the Harare population, the mean gestation at delivery of a twin pregnancy is 35.9 weeks (Neilson *et al.* 1988). Ultrasonography in multiple pregnancy, therefore, tends to be limited to making the diagnosis, and ruling out placenta praevia.

Fetal viability

Ultrasound for early pregnancy bleeding and for fetal viability in the last two trimesters accounts for 18.4 per cent of the examinations at Harare Maternity Hospital. The pattern of referrals here is different, there being an even spread throughout pregnancy. This is because the women will book whenever the problem arises.

The practice of referring patients from outlying health centres with suspected intrauterine death has practical implications for both the woman and the specialist institution. If the diagnosis is confirmed, the woman will be induced at the referral hospital, since the smaller centres have inadequate facilities for labour induction. At this distressing time, she will not be near the midwives she has known during the pregnancy or her relatives. Thus the hospital performing ultrasound becomes congested with inductions for confirmed intrauterine death. The fear of disseminated intravascular coagulation is still great, even though the risk is now known to be small.

Intrauterine growth retardation

The diagnosis of intrauterine growth retardation is bedevilled by the problems of definition of the phenomenon and the interpretation of the anthropometric data (Keirse 1984). Two requirements must be met before ultrasonography can be used to detect a small for dates fetus. Firstly, the dates must be accurately known. This means gestational age will have been confirmed or assigned by an early pregnancy scan. Secondly, growth charts appropriate for the population should be available for various anthropometric parameters, both for the fetus and the neonate.

The late booking creates a fundamental problem for later monitoring of fetal growth by ultrasonography, so that its contribution to the management of this problem is diminished.

Until recently the growth charts used with obstetric ultrasonography in developing countries were obtained from developed countries. This situation is now changing and nomograms have been published for African populations (Okupe *et al.* 1984; Munjanja *et al.* 1988). The use of local nomograms is particularly important in the third trimester since this is when interpopulation variation is at its greatest (Munjanja 1988).

Fetal malformations

The actual value of ultrasonography in the diagnosis of fetal malformations depends on several conditions:

1. The degree to which malformations contribute to perinatal mortality and morbidity should be accurately known.
2. The woman should present early enough in pregnancy to allow termination of pregnancy, if necessary.
3. The woman and her culture should be agreeable to termination of pregnancy.
4. Ancillary laboratory services should be available to improve the diagnostic capability of the services as a whole.
5. Facilities for termination of pregnancy or for neonatal surgery should be available.

This is a tall order for most developing countries.

The contribution of fetal malformations to perinatal mortality and morbidity is not known with any degree of accuracy, so it cannot be determined whether ultrasonography is worthwhile or not. In Zimbabwe, congenital malformations account for 4–6 per cent of perinatal deaths every year, but this is likely to be an underestimate due to the poor investigation of the large group of 'macerated, cause unknown' stillbirths.

Because the women present late for antenatal booking, termination of pregnancy cannot be performed for serious malformations when these are detected. Occasionally the woman simply refuses to believe the diagnosis of a major malformation; this is a strange paradox in a community normally characterized by excessive faith in the powers of technology. The strength of this denial may be such that the woman happily proceeds to term whilst everyone else around her is worried about it. African cultures on the whole do not believe in termination of pregnancy, and would rather leave the outcome to nature or to fate. The mortality rate for infants with malformations or handicap is quite high, so families do not have to support these children for a long time as would be the case in developed countries. If the woman wishes to terminate her pregnancy, the decision may pit her against her immediate family. Most developing countries allow termination of pregnancy on the grounds of fetal malformation, but have created bureaucratic regulations to prevent this facility being abused. A lot of paperwork may be required to obtain permission to terminate a pregnancy. The diagnosis of a major fetal malformation, especially in the third trimester, may, therefore, pose more problems that it solves.

Ancillary laboratory facilities are required for ultrasonography to reach its fullest potential in the diagnosis of fetal malformations. A wide range of laboratory procedures are now possible with tissue obtained from chorionic villus sampling (Loeffler 1985), amniocentesis (Crane 1983), and fetal blood sampling (Nicolaides and Rodeck 1987). These sophisticated laboratory facilities are usually lacking in developing countries. For example, in Zimbabwe no facilities exist for performing any investigations on amniotic fluid, fetal blood, or chorionic villi, and there is the same situation in the neighbouring countries apart from the Republic of South Africa. Amniotic fluid from Zimbabwe and Malawi can be sent to the Republic of South Africa, although the average time between doing an amniocentesis and getting the result is 4 weeks. Most terminations are, therefore, performed between 19–22 weeks, which would be an unacceptable situation were it not the lesser of two evils.

Some malformations detected by ultrasonography are amenable to surgery performed in the neonatal or infant period. Where laboratory facilities are lacking, little additional information is available before the baby is born. It may not be known before birth, for example, if a fetus with duodenal atresia or stenosis has an associated chromosomal malformation. The planning for neonatal surgery is, therefore, affected.

Placentography

Ultrasonography has brought a change to the management of antepartum haemorrhage at Harare Maternity Hospital. Previously, all mothers were hospitalized until term, awaiting an examination in theatre. The use of ultrasonography has freed the beds by allowing those who do not have a low-lying placenta to be discharged. Even those women from outlying centres with placenta praevia can be sent back as facilities for Caesarean section exist in district and provincial units. The repeat examinations necessitated by the discovery of a low-lying placenta in early pregnancy are not a problem when the women book so late.

Research in obstetric ultrasound

The little work that has been published in developing countries refers mostly to the establishment of growth standards (Okupe *et al.* 1984; Ayagande and

Okonofua 1986; Munjanja *et al.* 1988). No randomized controlled trials have been published from Sub-Saharan African countries. As already discussed, due to the structure of the health services, ultrasound equipment is placed in referral units which, by their nature, serve high-risk populations. They drain large geographical areas, and hence are physically far from the majority of the normal population that would be required say for a randomized controlled trial on routine ultrasonography.

Moreover, with a weak information infrastructure, research is hampered by the difficulties of following up patients for results. The major obstacle to any meaningful research will remain the late antenatal booking pattern in these countries.

This situation is unfortunate because a randomized controlled trial, in which denial of ultrasonography is one arm of the study, could be mounted in developing countries for reasons given above and hence without ethical difficulties, which might not be the case in developed countries.

Conclusions

At this stage, ultrasonography is clearly not an appropriate technology in most developing countries, except in tertiary referral centres, although the situation may change. The equipment is bought in a haphazard manner and is usually outdated. There are little or no maintenance facilities in most countries, resulting in long or permanent breaks of service. The quality of training in the technique is very variable. The structure of the health service severely limits the wide applicability of the technique, until each district and provincial centre has its own equipment.

Most importantly, the late booking behaviour of the obstetric population drastically reduces the value of the examination, with the exception of placentography.

The high perinatal mortality rates found in developing countries will not respond to expensive technology placed in a few isolated centres (TambyRaja 1982). Rather, attention must be placed on low cost but widely applicable technologies to improve nutrition, sanitation, and health education (Harrison 1980; TambyRaja 1982).

It is accepted, however, that in appropriate clinical situations, ultrasonography is very useful in high-risk centres in developing countries. In addition, the trend towards the acquisition of technology will not be easily reversed.

For these reasons, the following suggestions are being made:

1. Before ultrasound equipment is bought, a critical assessment of its likely potential in any population should be made. Epidemiological data is necessary for this assessment.

2. Ultrasound equipment should be bought through the budget of the ministries of health so that recurrent costs (maintenance, repair, replacement) are included at the beginning. The equipment should not be brought in as part of an aid project.

3. Obstetricians, radiologists, and radiographers who will perform the examinations should be fully consulted before purchase.

4. Local and regional co-operation is necessary in the purchase of equipment in order to get favourable terms from manufacturers. Regional co-operation will ensure that maintenance facilities are set up for each area.

5. Regional collaboration is necessary in the training of doctors, radiographers, and midwives. It is not viable at this stage for every country to set up its own diploma course.

6. There will be no need to set up sophisticated laboratory facilities in support of ultrasonography until the population is ready to take advantage of it.

Acknowledgements

During the preparation of this chapter I received the assistance of two people to whom I am grateful, Miss Violet Charangwa typed the manuscript and Dr J. P. Neilson helped me with some useful suggestions.

References

Ayagande, S. O., and Okonofua, F. E. (1986). Normal growth of fetal biparietal diameter in an African population. *Int. J. Gynecol. Obstet.*, **24**, 35–42.

Bourne, D. E., Pick, W. M., Taylor, S. P., McIntyre, D. E., and Klopper, J. M. L. (1990). A methodology for resource allocation for health care in South Africa. Part III. A South African Health Resource Allocation Formula. *S. Afr. Med. J.*, **77**, 456–9.

Campbell, S., Warsof, S. L., Little, D., and Cooper, D. J. (1985). Routine ultrasound screening for the prediction of gestational age. *Obstet. Gynaecol.*, **65**, 613–20.

Crane, J. P. (1983). Genetic amniocentesis. In *Progress in obstetrics and gynaecology* (ed. J. Studd) pp. 34–46, Churchill Livingstone, Edinburgh.

Department of Health and Social Security (1976). *Report of the resource allocation working party*. HMSO, London.

Eik-Nes, S. H., Okland, O., Aure, J. C., and Ulmstein, M. (1984). Ultrasound screening in pregnancy: a randomized controlled trial. *Lancet*, **i**, 1347.

Harrison, K. A. (1980). Approaches to reducing perinatal and maternal mortality in Africa. In *Maternity services in the developing world. What the community needs*, (ed. R. H. Philpott) pp. 52–95, Royal College of Obstetricians and Gynaecologists, London.

Keirse, M. J. N. C. (1984). Epidemiology and aetiology of the growth retarded baby. *Clin. Obstet. Gynaecol.*, **11**, 415–36.

Loeffler, F. E. (1985). Chorionic villus biopsy. In *Progress in obstetrics and gynaecology* Vol. 5 (ed J. Studd). pp. 22–35 Churchill Livingstone, Edinburgh.

Munjanja, S. P. (1988). Intrauterine growth: A Zimbabwean study. MD Thesis. University of Birmingham.

Munjanja, S. P., Masona, D., and Masvikeni, S. (1988). Fetal bi-parietal diameter and head circumference measurement: results of a longitudinal study in Zimbabwe. *Int. J. Gynecol. Obstet.*, **26**, 223–8.

Neilson, J. and Grant, A. (1989). Ultrasound in pregnancy. In *Effective care in pregnancy and childbirth* Vol. 1 (ed. I. Chalmers M. Enkin, and M. J. N. C. Keirse), pp. 419–39. Oxford University Press.

Neilson, J. P., Verkuyl, D. A. A., Crowther, C., and Bannerman, C. (1988). Preterm labour in twin pregnancies: prediction by cervical assessment. *Obstet. Gynecol*, **72**, 719–23.

Nicolaides, K. H. and Rodeck, C. H. (1987). Fetal blood sampling. *Clin. Obstet. Gynaecol.*, **1**, 623–48.

Nylander, P. P. S. and Adekunle, A. O. (1990). Antenatal care in developing countries. *Clin. Obstet. Gynaecol.*, **4**, 169–86.

Okupe, R. F., Cocker, O. O., and Gbajumo, S. A. (1984). Assessment of fetal biparietal diameter during normal pregnancy by ultrasound in Nigerian women. *Br. J. Obstet. Gynaecol.*, **91**, 629–32.

Philpott, R. H. (1980). The organization of services in Africa. In *Maternity services in the developing world: What the community needs* (ed. R. H. Philpott), pp. 131–42. Royal College of Obstetricians and Gynaecologists, London.

Robinson, H. P. and Fleming, J. E. E. (1975). A critical evaluation of crown–rump length measurements. *Br. J. Obstet. Gynaecol.*, **82**, 702–10.

TambyRaja, R. L. (1982). Trends in perinatal mortality in the developing world. In *Recent advances in obstetrics and gynaecology* (ed. J. Bonnar), pp. 201–14 Churchill Livingstone, Edinburgh.

WHO (1985a). Diagnostic imaging for developing countries. *WHO Chron.* **39**, 143–8.

WHO (1985b). *Coverage of maternity care.* World Health Organization, Division of Family Health, Geneva.

10
Ultrasound for research with fetal sheep
John P. Newnham and Robert W. Kelly

Introduction

Research with experimental animals has made a major contribution to our understanding of fetal growth and development. Of all the species available for research the fetal sheep has been one of the most extensively studied (Hecker 1983), due to the many similarities which exist between fetal humans and fetal sheep. Placental size, fetal growth patterns, and birth-weight in sheep are similar to humans. Additionally, in most countries, sheep are easy to obtain and maintain; their docile nature makes them ideally suited to life in the laboratory; and manipulation and incision of the pregnant uterus for the purpose of fetal surgery will seldom result in preterm labour (Alexander 1974).

There are also important differences between human and ovine biology, an understanding of which is vital when extrapolating findings from sheep studies to human medicine. In sheep the gestation period (150 days) is approximately half that of the human, and preterm birth does not occur in the absence of infection. Placental weight in sheep increases to a maximum at about 70–90 days' gestation and then declines (Mellor 1980; Kelly *et al.* 1987), whereas in humans placental weight increases until 34–36 weeks but thereafter does not usually decrease. Fetal growth in sheep is more rapid than in humans and is sensitive to a variety of influences which include maternal nutrition, breed, maternal age, parental size, and number of fetuses. In the field, the perinatal mortality rates of sheep are high with an average loss of 15–20 per cent resulting in part from the low fat content of the newborn lamb, the thermal disadvantage of the neonate from the high surface area to weight ratio, and the close relationship between maternal nutrition and lamb survival (Alexander 1974; Kelly and Newnham 1990).

The use of sheep by medical researchers has spanned many centuries. In 1667 transfusion of blood from a sheep into a man led to the first medical description of transfusion incompatibility (Mollison 1983). Dr Guillotin in 1790 perfected, using sheep, the 'philanthropic decapitating machine' that was used during the French revolution (quoted in Hecker 1983). Modern research with fetal sheep was initiated by Barcroft and colleagues during the 1930s, in a series of experiments aimed at determining the mechanisms whereby the fetus can tolerate an environment of low oxygen tension (Barcroft and Kennedy 1939). In 1965 Meschia and colleagues (1965) introduced the technique of chronic catheterization using indwelling plastic catheters, thus allowing continuous access to body fluids over periods of weeks or even months. However, surgical manipulation and chronic catheterization of the fetus are not without complications; the techniques are not simple, are costly, frequently result in loss of the fetus, and the presence of indwelling catheters may interfere with normal fetal growth and development (Mellor 1980; Newnham *et al.* 1986). Small sample sizes reduce statistical power and present an important source of error for measurements which have high variances.

Ultrasound in its various forms offers a unique opportunity to gain access to the pregnant uterus and fetus without the need for surgery. The techniques developed so far have widespread application not only for medical research, but also for veterinary studies and the agricultural industry.

Diagnosis of pregnancy and number of fetuses

Large animals industries, including sheep farming, have a major interest in the diagnosis of pregnancy and determination of the number of fetuses present. Nutritional requirements of non-pregnant, single bearing, and twin bearing ewes are different, so that knowledge of pregnancy status allows more efficient and cost effective management of feed supply and assistance at lambing. Until the introduction of ultrasound techniques, the diagnosis of pregnancy and number of fetuses was based on a variety of techniques, including rectal–abdominal palpation, X-rays, and measurement of hormone levels. The first ultrasonic techniques employed either A-mode, static B-mode, or Doppler. Transrectal Doppler achieved some popularity for the diagnosis of pregnancy (Deas 1977), but its use was limited by reports that 50 per cent of ewes so examined suffered some form of rectal damage (Tyrrell and Plant 1979).

Real-time ultrasound scanning of pregnant sheep was pioneered in Australia and reported in 1980 by Fowler and Wilkins. The same authors (1984) later reported a trial of 5530 scans with an accuracy for pregnancy diagnosis of 99.4 per cent; for non-pregnancy diagnosis of 99.8 per cent; for confirmation of a single fetus of 98.7 per cent; for detection of two fetuses of 93.8 per cent; and for triplet detection of 52.3 per cent. The major source of error was in underestimating litter sizes by failing to examine the entire uterine contents.

With ultrasound imaging, confirmation of pregnancy can be made with confidence by 30 days after conception (Fowler and Wilkins 1984; White *et al.* 1984; Kelly *et al.* 1989). One operator with several assistants can scan 80–120 ewes per hour, and can thus evaluate up to about 1000 sheep each working day. It has been estimated that in the United Kingdom the number of ewes scanned increased from 1000 in 1983 to 2 million in 1986; this represented scanning of 13 per cent of the national flock by 60 commercial operators (Russel 1985).

Technique

The position in which ultrasound scanning of sheep is most simple is shown in Fig. 10.1. In a reclined sitting attitude, sheep are docile and not distressed. For greatest ease, the ewe is held by the forelimbs from behind by a seated assistant. The ultrasound operator is seated in a legless chair facing the ultrasound machine and the hindlimbs of the ewe may be held in a restraining plate.

A satisfactory image requires the absence of air between the transducer and the skin. This can be achieved either by close shearing of the anterior abdominal wall and the liberal use of gel or vegetable oil, or by placing the transducer on the skin in the bare inguinal region adjacent to the udder. With the ewe in a sitting position, the latter technique makes use of the loose bare skin by carrying it upwards over the uterus and often obviates the need to clip wool from the abdominal wall. In ewes which have access to roughage such as hay, silage, or straw, intestinal gas may need to be reduced by witholding food for 8–12 hours before the examination.

Fetal imaging

The uterus consists of a central short corpus from which arise two horns. Most of the fetus will be found in one or other of the two horns. In twin pregnancies, it is most common for the two fetuses to each occupy one of the horns.

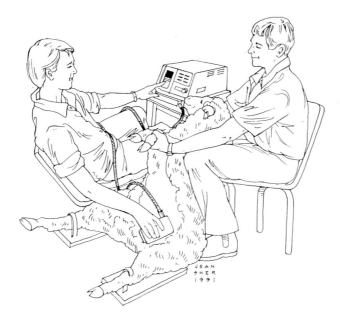

Fig. 10.1. Illustration demonstrating positions of the sheep, ultrasound operator, and assistant for ultrasound examination of the pregnant ewe.

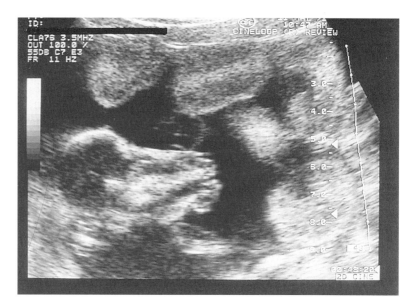

(a)

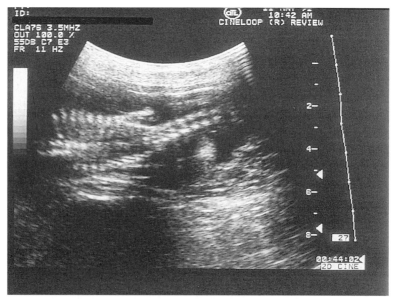

(b)

Fig. 10.2. Ultrasound images of a fetal sheep at 80 days' gestation demonstrating (a) the fetal head, (b) thorax and neck.

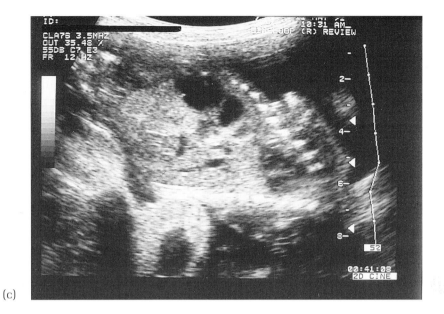

(c)

(d)

Fig. 10.2. Ultrasound images of a fetal sheep at 80 days' gestation demonstrating (c) chest wall and abdomen, and (d) rumen.

Many of the differences in anatomy between fetal humans and fetal sheep are self-evident (Fig. 10.2(a)–(d)). Fetal sheep have long and prominent limbs and a relatively narrow thorax. In the upper abdomen of the fetus one can usually see two fluid-filled pouches of the rumen, while in humans there is a single stomach.

Demonstration of fetal breathing movements by A-scan was first reported in 1971 (Boddy and Robinson), and by real-time ultrasound observation in 1981 (Wittmann *et al.*). Wittmann and co-workers demonstrated a close correlation between fetal breathing movements and tracheal pressure traces obtained from catheters implanted in the fetus. Since that time advances in ultrasound imaging systems have improved the quality of the image that can be obtained.

Measurement of fetal head size and determination of gestational age

The fetal head can be imaged and measured without difficulty from about 40 days' gestation onwards (Kelly and Newnham 1989). After 100 days' gestation measurement of the fetal head becomes increasingly difficult because of its relatively large size and shadowing as calcification of the bones increases. In early pregnancy growth of the fetal head occurs at a greater rate than that of the body (Joubert 1956). The biparietal diameter (BPD), which largely reflects growth of the fetal brain, is of similar appearance to that of the human. However, growth of the lower jaw occurs at an even greater rate than that of the skull, and measurement of the occipito–snout length (OSL) can be made without difficulty. A description of these measurements is shown in Fig. 10.3. Figure 10.4 displays the 95 per cent confidence intervals for BPD and OSL measurements plotted against gestational age in pregnancies with a single fetus. These data were obtained by serial measurement at 2 week intervals of 40 3–6-year-old multiparous Merino ewes fed at a maintenance level throughout pregnancy (Kelly and Newnham 1989). The oestrous cycles had previously been synchronized using protestagen-impregnated intravaginal sponges and flock mated with rams fitted with sire–sire harnesses and crayons (to mark mated ewes). Laparoscopy was performed at day 10 of pregnancy to determine ovulation rates; in sheep a single corpus luteum is strong evidence that only a single fetus has been conceived because identical twins are rare. Twenty of these animals were sacrificed at 90 days' gestation to allow comparison between ultrasound and post-mortem measurements.

As shown in Fig. 10.4, the growth rate of the OSL exceeds that of the BPD. However, after 80 days' gestation the error values for prediction of gestational age by OSL measurements were greater than those of BPD measurements, probably because of the difficulty in imaging the full length of the fetal head and jaws as their length increased. The most accurate time to determine gestational age using head measurements was found to be between 40 and 80 days' gesta-

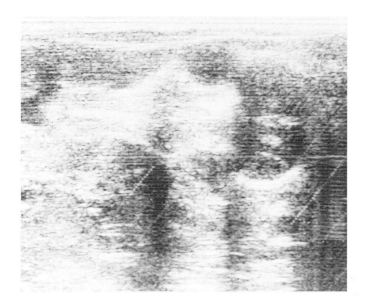

(a)

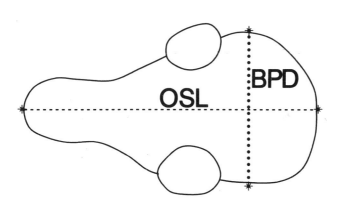

(b)

Fig. 10.3. (a) Ultrasound image and (b) illustration of the fetal head showing measurements of the biparietal diameter (BPD) and occipito–snout length (OSL). (Reproduced with permission from Kelly and Newnham 1989.)

tion. Of the two measurements, OSL provides the greatest precision. Predictive formulae to estimate gestational age were developed using regression coefficients and their standard errors. These data are displayed in Table 10.1 and indicate that measurement of OSL at 40–80 days' gestation has 95 per cent confidence limits of about ± 5 days for the estimation of gestational age.

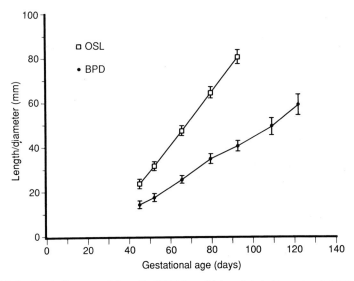

Fig. 10.4. Occipito–snout length (OSL) and biparietal diameter (BPD) plotted against gestational age. Data are mean and 95 per cent confidence intervals.

The effects of twin gestation on fetal head growth were investigated by serial measurement of 67 4–5-year-old Merino ewes each carrying two fetuses and in which laparoscopy at 10 days' gestation had demonstrated two corpora luteum (Kelly and Newnham 1989). OSL and BPD measurements between 40 and 80 days' gestation were not significantly different in twins when compared with singles. Averaging the head measurements of the twins resulted in a reduction in error of 22–28 per cent for OSL and 30–40 per cent for BPD.

Growth rates of fetal sheep in late pregnancy are sensitive to the level of maternal nutrition. However, in this study we were, in general, unable to demonstrate an effect of differential feeding of the ewe on ultrasound measurements of fetal head growth when measured prior to 80 days' gestation.

Post-mortem measurement of the fetal head by calipers indicated no biases in the ultrasound measurements which had been made the day before slaughter. However, comparison of these measurements with data from post-mortem examination of British bred sheep reported by Joubert (1956) indicates that head growth of fetal sheep may differ between breeds. Such differences must be considered if our data for prediction of gestational age for Australian Merinos are to be applied to other populations.

Assessment of amniotic fluid volume

Fluid surrounding the fetus can be readily identified because of its lack of echogenicity. A proportion of this fluid in sheep is allantoic rather than amniotic,

Table 10.1. Prediction of gestational age in single fetuses by measurement of the biparietal diameter and occipito–snout length

Measurement (mm)	Gestational age (days)	
	Biparietal diameter	Occipito– snout length
10	37.2 (4.9)	—
12	41.1 (4.9)	—
14	44.9 (4.8)	—
16	48.7 (4.7)	—
18	52.5 (4.7)	—
20	56.2 (4.6)	40.7 (1.8)
22	59.9 (4.6)	43.1 (1.8)
24	63.6 (4.5)	45.3 (1.9)
26	67.3 (4.5)	47.5 (1.9)
28	70.9 (4.4)	49.5 (2.0)
30	74.4 (4.4)	51.5 (2.0)
32	78.0 (4.4)	53.3 (2.1)
34	81.5 (4.3)	55.2 (2.2)
36	84.9 (4.3)	56.9 (2.2)
38	88.4 (4.3)	58.7 (2.3)
40	91.8 (4.2)	60.3 (2.4)
42	95.2 (4.2)	62.0 (2.4)
44	98.6 (4.2)	63.6 (2.5)
46	101.9 (4.1)	65.2 (2.6)
48	105.2 (4.1)	66.8 (2.7)
50	108.5 (4.1)	68.4 (2.8)
52	—	70.0 (2.9)
54	—	71.6 (3.0)
56	—	73.1 (3.1)
58	—	74.7 (3.2)
60	—	76.3 (3.4)
62	—	77.9 (3.5)
64	—	79.5 (3.7)
66	—	81.2 (3.9)
68	—	82.8 (4.1)
70	—	84.6 (4.3)
72	—	86.3 (4.6)

Data are mean (± SE)
Adapted from Kelly and Newnham (1989)

but it is difficult on ultrasound examination to discriminate between the two compartments. In humans the allantois is rudimentary.

Assessment of amniotic fluid volume is an important component of the ultrasound examination of human pregnancy. This assessment may be subjective or, alternatively, can be based on measurement of pocket sizes. Summation of the vertical pocket depths in each of the four uterine quadrants produces the amniotic fluid index score (Moore 1990). Moore and Brace (1989) have determined, in sheep, the relationship between true amniotic volume and the amniotic fluid index. Near-term pregnant ewes were sacrificed and a catheter placed in the amniotic cavity after all amniotic and allantoic fluid had been drained. Amniotic fluid index measurements were made at periodic intervals while the amniotic fluid volume was restored. Over the volume ranges of 0–2000 ml, a close linear relationship was observed between amniotic fluid index and the actual amniotic fluid volume. In pregnant ewes at term the amniotic fluid volume of 600–1200 ml is much greater than the 150–250 ml in humans; however, the amniotic fluid index values in these two species are similar because of the differences in size and shape of the uterus and fetus.

Placental growth

In humans, accurate assessment of placental size by ultrasound imaging is not feasible. However, in sheep the placenta consists of discrete cotyledons (Plate 4) which can be imaged and their dimensions measured (Kelly *et al.* 1987). These cotyledons are attached to 60–150 endometrial thickenings called caruncles (Alexander 1974). Attachment of chorionic tissue to these sites is evident 30 days after fertilization. Each cotyledon consists of fetal tissue surrounded by maternal tissues. Usually about 70 per cent of the caruncles will be occupied by cotyledons, but this percentage declines with increasing age and parity of the ewe, and is 10 per cent greater when the fetus is male. As the number of fetuses per pregnancy increases there is a greater proportion of caruncles which are occupied, and individual cotyledons increase in size to compensate for the reduced number of cotyledons per fetus.

On ultrasound examination the cotyledons appear round or oval in shape (Plate 5(a)). In late pregnancy the cotyledons frequently change in shape as the ratio of fetal to maternal tissue increases. We have determined the 'average maximum dimension' by measuring the maximum diameter of a representative sample of up to 20 cotyledons. For each examination scanning commences at the caudal right side of the abdomen and advances progressively to the left to ensure that no single cotyledon is measured on more than one occasion. To investigate the accuracy of this method, 40 pregnant ewes carrying a single fetus were examined at frequent intervals commencing at 45 days' gestation (Kelly *et al.* 1987). Half the ewes were sacrificed on day 94 and the remainder on day 141. At post-mortem examination each cotyledon was dissected from the uterus and the maximum diameter and weight recorded. Close correlations were observed between the cotyledon diameters observed by ultrasound examination and the post-mortem measurement, and between ultrasound measurement of cotyledon size and placental weight when the number of cotyledons was included in the analysis. The relationship between cotyledon diameter and placental weight was better at day 94 than at day 141, due in part to the irregular shape of many cotyledons in late pregnancy and the difficulty in scanning cotyledons adjacent to the main fetal mass. The mean cotyledon diameter plotted against gestational age for weekly measurement of 15 ewes bearing a single fetus in another experiment is shown in Fig. 10.5. Cotyledon diameters increased between 40 and 80 days' gestation, after which there was a plateau in values. However, between about 90–140 days' gestation there is usually a modest reduction in total placental weight (Kelly and Newnham 1990). This disparity between change in cotyledon diameter and placental weight in the last one-third of pregnancy indicates that changes in ultrasound measurements over this time need to be interpreted with caution. However, for evaluation of cotyledon growth in the first 70–90 days of pregnancy, and as a measurement system to compare the effects of interventions at any one gestational age, ultrasonic measurement of cotyledon diameters provides a non-invasive method of assessment of placental size in sheep.

Assessment of blood flow by Doppler ultrasound

Application of the Doppler principle allows an estimation of volume blood flow (Gill 1979) and vascular resistance (Fitzgerald and Drumm 1977). The use of quantitative blood flow has been limited by potential errors inherent in the

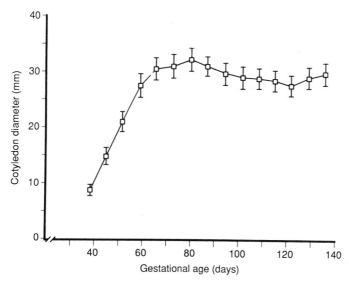

Fig. 10.5. Cotyledon diameter plotted against gestational age in 15 pregnant ewes examined serially between 40–140 days' gestation. Data are means and 95 per cent confidence intervals.

measurement systems which are estimated to be up to 35 per cent for fetal descending aorta volume flow and up to 50 per cent for umbilical venous flow (Erskine and Ritchie 1985). These errors arise from inaccuracies in assessment of the angle of insonation, the diameter of the vessel, the mean and maximum blood velocities, and the estimated fetal weight. Description of the flow velocity waveform rather than volume flow will circumvent these sources of error. This method displays, by audio-frequency analysis of the Doppler signal, a spectrum of frequencies which are porportional to red blood cell velocity plotted against time. Use of ratios removes the need to measure the angle of insonation. The waveforms may be obtained by pulsed wave Duplex systems in which the vessel of origin is imaged, or by stand-alone, continuous-wave Doppler systems in which the vessel is not imaged but the origin is identified by its characteristic arterial signature. Most of the information contained within the arterial wave-form is described by the maximum frequency envelope (Thompson *et al.* 1986). Several indices have been developed to describe the velocity waveform, of which the most frequently used are the systolic/diastolic (or A/B) ratio (maximum systolic frequency divided by the minimum diastolic frequency), the resistance index (maximum systolic frequency minus least diastolic frequency divided by the maximum systolic frequency), and the pulsatility index (maximum systolic frequency minus minimum diastolic frequency divided by the mean frequency over the cardiac cycle). All three indices appear to measure the same phenomenon and correlate highly with each other (Thompson *et al.* 1986; Irion and Clark 1990).

Umbilical artery waveforms

Experiments with chronically catheterized fetal sheep have indicated that arterial waveforms and systolic/diastolic ratios obtained by external Doppler systems correlate highly with those obtained by electromagnetic flow probes placed directly on the artery (Nimrod *et al.* 1989; Irion and Clark 1990). Identification of the origin of the waveform by pulsed Duplex scanning has confirmed that umbilical arterial signatures in sheep are similar to those observed in human pregnancy (Newnham *et al.* 1987). While continuous wave Doppler systems are entirely satisfactory for obtaining umbilical arterial waveforms, concurrent use of ultrasound imaging is of assistance in determining the site of the umbilical cord. In sheep, the umbilical vessels branch to the many cotyledons and the umbilical cord is short. Multiple observations may be required to ensure the signal has been obtained from the umbilical cord and not from smaller cotyledonary vessels.

Elevated systolic/diastolic ratios are believed to reflect increased downstream resistance to flow. In humans, examination of the placenta from cases in which systolic/diastolic ratios were elevated has shown obliteration of the arteries in the tertiary stem villi (Giles *et al.* 1985). This relationship between abnormal

Doppler waveform studies and placental vascular disease has been confirmed by experiments with sheep in which the umbilical circulation has been compromised by embolization. Repetitive injection of microspheres into the umbilical arteries is followed by increases in both calculated umbilical–placental resistance and umbilical artery systolic/diastolic ratios (Trudinger *et al.* 1987; Morrow *et al.* 1989).

Changes observed in umbilical artery waveforms with advancing gestation are consistent with the alterations in placental vascular resistance which are known to occur in normal sheep pregnancy. Arterial waveforms can be obtained with continuous wave Doppler systems from 66 days' gestation onwards (Newnham *et al.* 1987). Thereafter, umbilical artery systolic/diastolic ratios decrease significantly with advancing gestation, the greatest reduction occurring between 66–109 days' gestation (Fig. 10.6). A similar effect of gestational age on placental vascular resistance had previously been demonstrated by Dawes (1962) who measured the pressure gradient between the fetal femoral artery and umbilical vein and then calculated the umbilical blood flow. He determined a fall in resistance within the umbilical circulation between 90–115 days with no significant alteration between 115–140 days' gestation. There was an increase in blood flow after 115 days' gestation which resulted from increased systemic arterial pressure. Thus results from Doppler

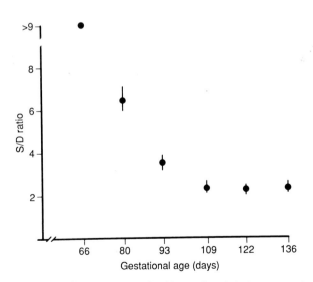

Fig. 10.6. Umbilical artery systolic/diastolic (S/D) ratios plotted against gestational age. Data are means and 95 per cent confidence intervals. (Reproduced with permission from Newnham *et al.* 1987.)

flow studies are consistent with those from previous experimentation and their availability has enabled measurements to be made at early stages in pregnancy.

However, the exact relationships between actual placental vascular resistance and Doppler waveforms are far from simple. Resistance represents the non-pulsatile component of the arterial input impedance, while the Doppler waveforms is also influenced by proximal compliance, cardiac function, and distribution of blood flow. Trudinger and co-workers (1987) observed increases in systolic/diastolic ratios after four days of embolization of the umbilical arterial circulation, while calculated umbilical vascular resistance did not increase until nine days of embolization. Adamson and co-workers (1990) also observed changes in umbilical artery waveform shape after embolization of the small vessels in the cotyledons, but it was necessary to increase this cotyledonary resistance six-fold to produce the abnormalities in waveforms which are seen in some growth-retarded human fetuses. Moreover, constriction of the umbilical arteries by angiotensin II infusion did not alter the shape of the arterial waveform, even when the constriction was severe enough to markedly decrease placental perfusion and to increase resistance in the umbilical arteries 13-fold. Thus, Doppler waveform studies must not be misinterpreted to be a measure of flow; major changes in placental blood flow can occur without concomitant alterations in the Doppler-derived arterial waveform.

Recently, Doppler ultrasound systems have been applied to laboratory studies in which sheep experiments are used to address problems of relevance to the medical management of human pregnancy. In exteriorized fetal sheep, occlusion of the umbilical veins has been used to produce the abnormal umbilical arterial waveform shape seen in humans. This intervention results in a redistribution of blood flow within the fetus which can be assessed by Doppler ultrasound examination (Fouron *et al.* 1991). The increased resistance to placental flow, combined with vasodilation of cerebral vasculature secondary to hypoxaemia, has been shown to predispose the fetus to diversion of poorly oxygenated blood towards the brain.

In chronically instrumented fetal sheep, van Huisseling *et al.* (1989) have induced fetal hypoxaemia by occlusion of the maternal common internal iliac artery. The resultant fetal heart rate decelerations were associated with increased Doppler-derived pulsatility indices. The alterations in heart rates and pulsatility indices were negated by the administration of atropine, indicating that any changes in Doppler indices during late decelerations are mediated by changes in heart rate (Mires *et al.* 1987) and are not the consequences of changes in placental vascular resistance.

Continuous wave Doppler systems have also allowed the non-invasive study of placental perfusion after surgical induction of intrauterine growth retardation. Giles *et al.* (1989) restricted fetal growth by pre-pregnancy carunclectomy, thus reducing the number of placental implantations sites. Eight of the fourteen pregnant ewes delivered small for gestational age fetuses, of which all but one had unaltered umbilical artery Doppler waveform studies before birth. It was concluded that this method of growth restriction in sheep does not equate to the disease of placental insufficiency seen in humans.

Uteroplacental artery waveforms

Ulteroplacental waveforms may be obtained by insonation of the maternal arteries leading into cotyledons. The effects of gestational age on systolic/diastolic ratios of waveforms from these vessels in sheep are shown in Fig. 10.7 (Newnham *et al.* 1987). In this study of 40 pregnant ewes, a small reduction in systolic/diastolic ratios was observed between 66–80 days' gestation, after which a plateau in values was seen. Concomitant imaging by Duplex scanning has confirmed the origin of these low resistance waveforms, but the technique is limited by our inability to identify the site of sampling in the arterial tree. It is likely that arteries close to cotyledons have a much greater diastolic flow than do arteries which are more proximal and in which there is a greater proportion of downstream bifurcations to high resistance non-placental tissue.

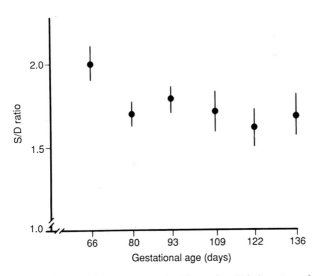

Fig. 10.7. Uteroplacental artery systolic/diastolic (S/D) ratios plotted against gestational age. Data are means and 95 per cent confidence intervals. (Reproduced with permission from Newnham *et al.* 1987.)

Ultrasound guided fetal blood sampling

Since the introduction of chronic catheterization of fetal blood vessels in 1965 (Meschia *et al.* 1965), a large proportion of research with fetal sheep has been reliant on our ability to sample blood through indwelling catheters. However, the cost and complexity of these preparations limit the number of animals which can be studied, and the effects of surgery and catherization on fetal well being remain incompletely understood (Mellor 1980). Ultrasound guidance provides the opportunity to introduce needles into vessels or organs, and has achieved widespread acceptance in human medicine for the aspiration of fetal blood from the umbilical cord (Daffos *et al.* 1985). The optimum site for sampling is usually the umbilical vein at the point where it is fixed at its placental insertion. In sheep, the umbilical cord is short and divides into numerous vessels which supply the cotyledons. Aspiration of blood from one of the two umbilical veins is possible, but the procedure is difficult, time-consuming, and success is dependent on fetal position. However, sampling from a cardiac ventricle is simple and the technique can be applied to large numbers of animals. We have previously reported 76 attempts at blood sampling from a cardiac ventricle in 32 fetal sheep between 101–136 days' gestation (Newnham *et al.* 1989) (Fig. 10.8). The ewes were held in a sitting position as shown in Fig. 10.1. Most procedures were performed with a linear array transducer and a small portable imaging system. A 'free hand' technique was usually employed. Four of the first nine fetuses died as a result of the procedure. However, of the next 67 procedures only three fetuses died, two in the hours immediately following the aspiration and one during labour several weeks later. Post-mortem examination revealed a pericardial haematoma in only one of the seven lambs which died following the procedure. The improved survival appeared to result from increasing operator experience and possibly from a policy of restricting the needle to the inferior aspect of the heart, well clear of the cardiac conduction system. Five samples were taken from four fetuses over a 90-minute-period to investigate the effects of repeated sampling. There were no complications in these four pregnancies, and arterial blood gas values remained constant throughout the sampling period.

Ultrasound guided fetal blood sampling from a cardiac ventricle is a straight-forward procedure which one operator and an assistant can comfortably perform on 30 sheep during a working day. It is anticipated that this technique will be of use in veterinary and agricultural studies in which fetal blood samples are required. In laboratory settings, the procedure cannot entirely replace the use of indwelling vascular catheters because it is not possible to be certain which ventricle has been the site of sampling. Nevertheless, for studies involving measurements which are not affected by the site of aspiration, ultrasound guided blood sampling from a cardiac ventricle may be considered

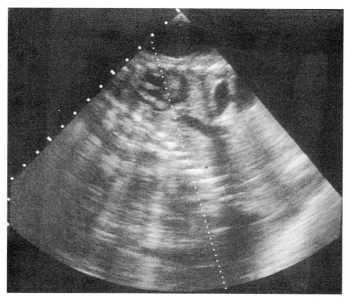

(a)

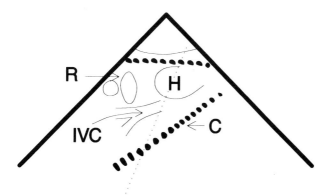

(b)

Fig. 10.8. (a) Ultrasound image and (b) illustration at 108 days' gestation displaying the fetal chest at the time of a fetal blood sampling procedure. Shown are the rumen, R; inferior vena cava, IVC; heart, H; and chest wall and ribs, C. The dotted line depicts the direction the needle will follow if introduced through a purpose built biopsy guide. (Reproduced with permission from Newnham *et al.* 1989.)

as a feasible alternative. The application of technologies with greater imaging resolution and biopsy guides will facilitate sampling from other vessels and organs. Studies need to be performed to investigate the degree of fetal stress induced by this intervention.

Conclusion

Research with fetal sheep has provided much of the information we have on the biology of reproduction. The application of ultrasound techniques to this research enhances our ability to determine the number of fetuses present, the gestational age, and to confirm fetal well being. Measurements of cotyledon size and Doppler waveform analysis provide information on placental growth and development. In laboratory settings these measurement systems present an alternative to some of the invasive techniques currently in use. The ability of ultrasound based systems to be applied to large numbers of animals offers new opportunities in veterinary and agricultural research. In the future, increasing resolution and accuracy of imaging and Doppler systems can be expected to provide exciting new avenues for probing the secrets of intrauterine growth and development.

References

Adamson, S. L., Morrow, R. J., Langille, B. L., Bull, S. B., and Ritchie, J. W. K. (1990). Site-dependent effects of increases in placental vascular resistance on the umbilical arterial velocity waveform in fetal sheep. *Ultrasound in Medicine and Biology*, **16**, 19–27.

Alexander, G. (1974). Birthweight of lambs: Influences and consequences. In *Size at birth* (ed. K. Elliot and J. Knight), pp. 215–54. Elsevier, Amsterdam.

Barcroft, J. and Kennedy, J. A (1939). The distribution of blood between the foetus and the placenta in sheep. *Journal of Physiology* (London), **95**, 173–86.

Boddy, K. and Robinson, J. S. (1971). External method for detection of fetal breathing *in utero*. *Lancet*, **ii**, 1231.

Daffos, F., Capella-Pavlovsky, M., and Forestier, F. (1985). Fetal blood sampling during pregnancy with use of a needle guided by ultrasound: A study of 606 consecutive cases *American Journal of Obstetrics and Gynecology*, **153**, 655–60.

Dawes, G. S. (1962). The umbilical circulation. *American Journal of Obstetrics and Gynecology*, **84**, 1634–48.

Deas, D. W. (1977). Pregnancy diagnosis in the ewe by an ultrasonic rectal probe. *Veterinary Record*, **101**, 113–15.

Erskine, R. L. A. and Ritchie, J. W. K. (1985). Quantitative measurement of fetal blood flow using Doppler ultrasound. *British Journal of Obstetrics and Gynaecology*, **92**, 600–4.

Fitzgerald, D. E. and Drumm, J. E. (1977). Non-invasive measurement of human fetal circulation using ultrasound: A new method. *British Medical Journal*, **2**, 1450–1.

Fouron, J. C., Teyssier, G., Marato, E., Lessard, M., and Marquette, G. (1991). Diastolic circulatory dynamics in the presence of elevated placental resistance and retrograde diastolic flow in the umbilical artery: A Doppler echographic study in lambs. *American Journal of Obstetrics and Gynecology*, **164**, 195–203.

Fowler, D. G. and Wilkins, J. F. (1980). The identification of single and multiple bearing ewes by ultrasound imaging. *Proceedings of the Australian Society of Animal Production*, **13**, 492.

Fowler, D. G. and Wilkins, J. F. (1984). Diagnosis of pregnancy and number of foetuses in sheep by real-time ultrasound imaging 1. Effects of number of foetuses, stage of gestation, operator and breed of ewe on accuracy of diagnosis. *Livestock Production Science*, **11**, 437–50.

Giles, W., Trudinger, B., and Baird, P. (1985). Fetal umbilical artery flow velocity waveforms and placental resistance: Pathological correlation. *British Journal of Obstetrics and Gynaecology*, **92**, 31–8.

Giles, W. B., Trudinger, B. J., Stevens, D., Alexander, G., and Bradley, L. (1989). Umbilical artery flow velocity waveform analysis in normal ovine pregnancy and after carunculectomy. *Journal of Developmental Physiology*, **11**, 135–8.

Gill, R. W. (1979). Pulsed Doppler with B-mode imaging for quantitative blood flow measurement. *Ultrasound in Medicine and Biology*, **5**, 222–35.

Hecker, J. F. (1983). The sheep as an experimental animal In *The sheep as an experimental animal* (ed. J. F. Hecker), pp. 1–5. Academic Press, London.

Irion, G. L. and Clark, K. E. (1990). Direct determination of the ovine fetal umbilical artery blood flow waveform. *American Journal of Obstetrics and Gynecology*, **162**, 541–9.

Joubert, D. M. (1956). A study of pre-natal growth and development in the sheep. *Journal of Agricultural Science (Cambridge)*, **47**, 382–427.

Kelly, R. W. and Newnham, J. P. (1989). Estimation of gestational age in Merino ewes by ultrasound measurement of fetal head size. *Australian Journal of Agricultural Research*, **40**, 1293–9.

Kelly, R. W. and Newnham, J. P. (1990). Nutrition of the pregnant ewe. In *Reproductive physiology of Merino sheep, concepts and consequences* (ed. C. M. Oldham, G. B. Martin, and I. W. Purvis), pp. 161–8. School of Agriculture, University of Western Australia.

Kelly, R. W., Newnham, J. P., Johnson, T., and Speijers, E. J. (1987). An ultrasound technique to measure placental growth in ewes. *Australian Journal of Agricultural Research*, **38**, 757–64.

Kelly, R. W., Wilkins, J. F., and Newnham, J. P. (1989). Fetal mortality from day 30 of pregnancy in Merino ewes offered different levels of nutrition. *Australian Journal of Experimental Agriculture*, **29**, 339–42.

Mellor, D. (1980). Investigations of fluid spaces of the sheep conceptus In *Animal models in fetal medicine* (ed. P. W. Nathanielsz), pp. 59–106. Elsevier/North Holland Biochemical Press, Amsterdam.

Meschia, G., Cotter, J. R., Breathnach, C. S., and Barrow, D. H. (1965). Haemoglobin, oxygen, carbon dioxide and hydrogen concentrations in the umbilical bloods of sheep and goats as sampled via indwelling plastic catheters. *Quarterly Journal of Experimental Physiology*, **50**, 185–95.

Mires, G., Dempster, J., Patel, N. B., and Crawford, J. W. (1987). The effect of fetal heart rate on umbilical artery flow velocity waveforms. *British Journal of Obstetrics and Gynaecology*, **94**, 665–9.

Mollison, P. L. (1983). *Blood transfusion in clinical medicine*, (7th edn), pp. 558–626. Blackwell Scientific Publications, Oxford.

Moore, T. R. (1990). Superiority of the four-quadrant sum over the single-deepest pocket technique in ultrasonographic identification of abnormal amniotic fluid volume. *American Journal of Obstetrics and Gynecology*, **163**, 762–7.

Moore, T. R. and Brace, R. A. (1989). Amniotic fluid index (AFI) in the term ovine pregnancy: A predictable relationship between AFI and amniotic fluid volume.

Proceedings of 36th Annual meeting of Society for Gynecologic Investigation, San Diego, Abstract 286.

Morrow, R. J., Adamson, S. L., Bull, S. B., and Ritchie, J. W. K. (1989). Effect of placental embolization on the umbilical arterial velocity waveform in fetal sheep. *American Journal of Obstetrics and Gynecology*, **161**, 1055–60.

Newnham, J. P., Lam, R. W., Hobel, C. J., Padbury, J. F., Polk, D. H., and Fisher, D. A. (1986). Differential response of ovine placental lactogen levels in maternal and fetal circulations following single umbilical artery ligation in fetal sheep. *Placenta*, **7**, 51–64.

Newnham, J. P., Kelly, R. W., Roberts, R. V., Macintyre, M., Speijers, J., Johnson, T., *et al.* (1987). Fetal and maternal Doppler flow velocity waveforms in normal sheep pregnancy. *Placenta*, **8**, 467–76.

Newnham, J. P., Kelly, R. W., Boyne, P., and Reid, S. E. (1989). Ultrasound guided blood sampling from fetal sheep. *Australian Journal of Agricultural Research*, **40**, 401–7.

Nimrod, C., Clapp, J. III, Larrow, R., D'Alton, M., and Persaud, D. (1989). Simultaneous use of Doppler ultrasound and electromagnetic flow probes in fetal flow assessment. *Journal of Ultrasound in Medicine*, **8**, 201–5.

Russel, A. J. F. (1985). Sheep scanning. *The Sheep Farmer*, **5**, 31–2.

Thompson, R. S., Trudinger, B. J., and Cook, C. M. (1986). A comparison of Doppler ultrasound waveform indices in the umbilical artery — 1. Indices derived from the maximum velocity waveform. *Ultrasound in Medicine and Biology*, **12**, 835–44.

Trudinger, B. J., Stevens, D., Connelly, A., Hales, J. R. S. , Alexander, G., Bradley, L., *et al.* (1987). Umbilical artery flow velocity waveforms and placental resistance: The effects of embolization of the umbilical circulation. *American Journal of Obstetrics and Gynecology*, **157**, 1443–8.

Tyrrell, R. N. and Plant, J. W. (1979). Rectal damage in ewes following pregnancy diagnosis by rectal–abdominal palpation. *Journal of Animal Science*, **48**, 348–50.

van Huisseling, H., Hasaart, T. H. M., Ruissen, C. J., Muijsers, G. J. J. M., and de Haan, J. (1989). Umbilical artery flow velocity waveforms during acute hypoxaemia and the relationship with hemodynamic changes in the fetal lamb. *American Journal of Obstetrics and Gynecology*, **161**, 1061–4.

White, I. R., Russel, A. J. F., and Fowler, D. G. (1984). Real-time ultrasonic scanning in the diagnosis of pregnancy and the determination of fetal numbers in sheep. *The Veterinary Record*, **115**, 140–3.

Wittmann, B. K., Rurak, D. W., Gruber, N., and Brown, S. (1981). Real-time ultrasound observation of breathing and movements in the fetal lamb. *American Journal of Obstetrics and Gynecology*, **141**, 807–10.

11

Symposium: Thromboembolic disease in the peripartum woman
A   Clinical background
Ian A. Greer

Incidence

Although it is clear that pregnancy substantially increases the risk of thrombo-embolism (Royal College of General Practitioners 1967), there are wide variations in the reported incidence of thromboembolic complications during pregnancy. This reflects diagnostic difficulties and the inclusion of various clinical entities within the disease classification. However, the thorough and detailed reports of the Confidential Enquiries into Maternal Deaths in England and Wales, which more recently have also included data from Scotland and Northern Ireland, have given us reliable data on fatal thromboembolic complications in pregnancy. Since 1952, when these data were first collected, the incidence of fatal pulmonary thromboembolism (PTE) has fallen dramatic-ally (Table 11.1), but PTE remains the most common cause of maternal death in the United Kingdom today (Department of Health *et al.* 1991). Fatal PTE is more common following Caesarean section, and although the rate fell by almost 90 per cent between the 1955–57 Report and the 1978–81 Report, the relative risk of fatal PTE following Caesarean section increased compared to vaginal delivery, where the reduction has been greater (Table 11.1). While the majority of these deaths occur in the first two weeks after delivery almost 40 per cent occur between 15–42 days following delivery (Table 11.2), thus most of these fatalities will occur after the initial discharge from hospital and those practi-tioners caring for women in the puerperium must be aware of, and alert to, the possibility of PTE occurring in this period. The ratio of fatal PTE occurring postpartum to those occurring antepartum has also decreased so that they now have similar frequencies. It is also of concern that many of these antepartum deaths occur in the first and second trimesters. In the most recent Confidential Enquiries Report, six deaths occurred in the first trimester and four in the second trimester with all but two of the 17 deaths occurring by 32 weeks' gestation. Furthermore, eight of these antepartum deaths were associated with early pregnancy problems such as hyperemesis.

Table 11.1 Incidence of death from pulmonary thromboembolism in England and Wales 1952–1987. (Source: Departments of Health. *Report on confidential enquiries into maternal deaths in England and Wales (1989) 1952–1984 and United Kingdom (1991) 1985–87.* London, HMSO)

Triennium	Total deaths	Post-abortion or ectopic pregnancy	Antenatal and intrapartum (rate*)	Postpartum vaginal delivery (rate*)	Postpartum Caesarean section (rate*)	Death ratio of Caesarean: vaginal delivery
1985–1987	25	1	16	5 (N/A)	3 (N/A)	N/A
1982–1984	29	4	9	4 (2.4)	12 (64.6)	26:1
1979–1981	28	5	12	4 (2.4)	7 (41.9)	16:1
1976–1978	45	2	14	20 (12.7)	9 (74.6)	6:1
1973–1975	36	3	14	13 (7.7)	6 (59.2)	8:1
1970–1972	61	10	14	22 (11.6)	15 (145.2)	12:1
1967–1969	82	6	22	36 (20.0)	18 (180.0)	9:1
1964–1966	95	4	23	43 (20.0)	25 (270.0)	13:1
1961–1963	140	11	36	66 (40.0)	27 (360.0)	9:1
1958–1960	138	6	30	80 (60.0)	22 (370.0)	6:1
1955–1957	164	7	17	114 (90.0)	26 (530.0)	6:1
1952–1954	138	N/A	4	104	30	

*Rates per million vaginal deliveries or Caesarean section
N/A: data not available

Table 11.2 Time between delivery and fatal pulmonary embolism following vaginal delivery and Caesarean section (Data for England and Wales 1970–87)

	Vaginal delivery	Caesarean section
Up to 7 days	27 (39.7%)	19 (36.5%)
8–14 days	14 (20.6%)	12 (23.1%)
15–42 days	27 (39.7%)	21 (40.4%)

Source: Department of Health *et al.* (1991). *Report on confidential enquiries into maternal deaths in the United Kingdom 1985–87*. London, HMSO.

In contrast to the reliable figures for fatal PTE, the reported incidence of deep venous thrombosis (DVT) and non-fatal PTE varies considerably. The most reliable diagnostic techniques of venography and radio-iodine labelled fibrinogen are unsuitable for screening an obstetric population. In the past, figures generated using only clinical diagnostic criteria put the incidence of DVT during pregnancy between 0.05–1.8 per cent, increasing to between 0.08–1.2 per cent following a vaginal delivery, and to 2.2–3.0 per cent following Caesarean section. The clinical diagnosis of DVT is notoriously inaccurate (Genton and Turpie 1980) and there has only been one sizeable study using ^{125}I-labelled fibrinogen (Friend and Kakkar 1970), which reported an incidence of 2.6 per cent following vaginal delivery suggesting that, using clinical criteria alone, underdiagnosis was occurring. A more recent Swedish study which confirmed the clinical diagnosis by objective means — plethysmography, thermography, and venography — found an incidence of 0.07 per cent during pregnancy in their population (Bergqvist *et al.* 1983). The same group, using plethysmography, screened 169 women following Caesarean section and found an incidence of DVT of 1.8 per cent (Bergqvist *et al.* 1979). The diagnosis of DVT is of course crucial as PTE will occur in 16 per cent of patients with untreated DVT resulting in a 13 per cent mortality (Villa Santa 1965). Anticoagulation substantially reduces the risk of PTE and subsequent mortality, the latter being reduced to 0.7 per cent (Villa Santa 1965).

Long-term morbidity from DVT associated with pregnancy

DVT during pregnancy increased the risk of a future thrombosis both during and after pregnancy, with a 15 per cent risk of recurrence during pregnancy and the puerperium and a 33 per cent risk of DVT not associated with pregnancy over a median follow-up time of over 10 years (Bergqvist *et al.* 1991). However, prospective studies (de Swiet *et al.* 1987) suggest that this may be an over-estimate with regard to recurrence in pregnancy as will be discussed later in this chapter.

In addition to the risk of recurrent DVT, there is the risk of developing deep venous insufficiency. This occurs secondary to the damage and destruction of the valves in the deep veins during the thrombotic process and manifests as pain, leg swelling, varicose veins, pigmentation, and ulceration. The frequency of objectively diagnosed deep venous insufficiency has been studied in women with a history of proven DVT in pregnancy after a median follow-up period of 7 years (Lindhagen *et al.* 1986). The frequency of deep venous insufficiency in the previously thrombosed leg was 65 per cent compared to 22 per cent in the healthy leg, the latter acting as a control. There was no correlation between the size of the thrombosis and development of venous insufficiency. Venous insufficiency occurred despite all patients being treated by anticoagulants during the acute episode. Furthermore, this frequency of 65 per cent is significantly greater (Bergqvist *et al.* 1991) than found after post-operative DVT diagnosed by radiolabelled fibrinogen uptake testing (32 per cent) or after clinically suspected acute DVT confirmed by venography (49 per cent) (Lindhagen *et al.* 1984, 1985). In view of the young age of the pregnant group relative to the other groups studied, DVT in pregnancy, with subsequent deep venous insufficiency, is likely to pose a significant health problem for these women. This is supported by a questionnaire study following up a group of women who had developed DVT in pregnancy or the puerperium (Bergqvist *et al.* 1991). This study, with a median follow-up time of around 10 years, examined the frequency of subjective complaints associated with deep venous insufficiency. Only 24 per cent were asymptomatic, while 55 per cent complained of leg swelling, 34 per cent of varicose veins, 27 per cent of skin discoloration, 15 per cent required the regular use of a compression bandage, and 4 per cent had leg ulceration. Thus DVT in pregnancy is not simply associated with a risk of PTE and mortality, but also from a risk of deep venous insufficiency and further DVT.

Risk factors for thrombosis in pregnancy

Physiological adaptation of the coagulation system in pregnancy

In normal pregnancy the balance between the coagulation and fibrinolytic systems changes in favour of coagulation. Along with increased blood volume these changes are required to cope with the haemostatic challenge of delivery and placental separation. There is an increase in several of the coagulation factors including fibrinogen, and factors VII, VIII, X, and XII during pregnancy (Stirling *et al.* 1984; Hathaway and Bonnar 1987; Forbes and Greer 1991), with the largest increase occurring in the fibrinogen concentration which increases almost two-fold by term. Prothrombin and factor IX levels remain normal or are slightly increased.

The endogenous inhibitor of coagulation anti-thrombin III (ATIII) was thought initially to decrease in pregnancy, however more recent studies have shown normal levels throughout pregnancy (Stirling *et al.* 1984). Other important inhibitors of coagulation are proteins C and S. Protein C levels appear to remain constant (Mannucci *et al.*1984) or to increase (Malm *et al.* 1988); protein S activity appears to be significantly reduced (Comp *et al.* 1986). These changes in coagulation factors are accompanied by suppression of fibrinolysis. The mechanism underlying the suppressed fibrinolysis appears to be mainly a placentally derived inhibitor of plasminogen activator, hence the rapid return of the fibrinolytic system to normal following delivery (Hathaway and Bonnar 1987).

The overall effect of these changes is an increased thrombotic potential which is most marked around term and the immediate postpartum period.

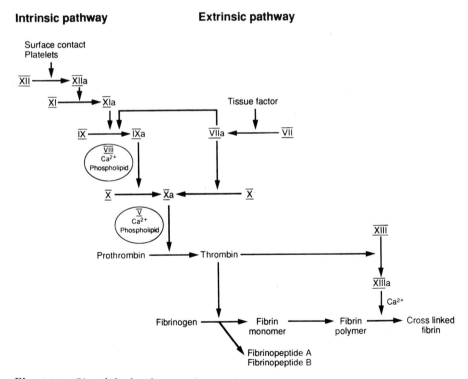

Fig. 11.1. Simplified scheme of coagulation cascade. Coagulation factors indicated with Roman numerals; 'a' denotes an activated coagulation factor.

Mode of delivery

As can be seen from Table 11.1 the risk of fatal PTE following Caesarean section, between 1982–84, was around 26 times greater than after vaginal delivery and the risk appears greater after an emergency procedure. This may be due to reduced mobility, and trauma to pelvic veins at the time of operation. It is also likely that there is an increased risk following forceps deliveries since one study showed that 25 per cent of cases of thromboembolism occurred in complicated pregnancies which included difficult forceps deliveries and prolonged labour (Aaro and Juergens 1971, 1974).

Age and parity

The Confidential Enquiries into Maternal Deaths for England and Wales show that age and parity are important, with risk increasing more sharply with age, especially in those over 35 years old, than with increasing parity. The risk of fatal PTE in a 40-year-old para 4 woman is 263.6 per million maternities compared to 11.3 per million maternities in a 20–24-year-old para 4 woman (Department of Health 1989).

Obesity

Obesity is undoubtedly an important risk factor for DVT/PTE as obese patients have impaired fibrinolytic activity and increased likelihood of venous stasis and poor mobility.

Immobilization

Restricted activity, often associated with hospitalization and bed rest for complications of pregnancy, such as hypertension, is also an important risk factor especially when the patient may have an increased likelihood of other risk factors, such as operative delivery.

Suppression of lactation by oestrogens

The relationship between suppression of lactation with oestrogen (stilboestrol) and thromboembolism was first highlighted by Daniel *et al.* (1967). There is no place in modern obstetrics for such therapy.

Venous flow in pregnancy

The venous tone appears to be reduced in pregnancy resulting in diminished flow prior to physical obstruction by the gravid uterus, although physical obstruction of the inferior vena cava also occurs later in pregnancy due to uterine size and is exacerbated by engagement of the fetal head (Flessa *et al.* 1974).

Surgical procedures in pregnancy

If a surgical procedure is carried out during pregnancy or the puerperium, such as postpartum sterilization, then there is an increased risk of thrombotic problems.

Previous thrombotic episode

If the patient has a history of a previous thrombotic problem then the risk of a further problem is increased. The risk has been estimated from retrospective studies at 12–15 per cent (Badaracco and Vessey 1974; Bergqvist *et al.* 1991). In a prospective randomized study of anticoagulant therapy in pregnancy in such patients, only one patient in the control group of 20 developed a DVT (Howell *et al.* 1983). More recently, de Swiet's group have reported 59 pregnancies in women with a history of thrombosis who received no antepartum anticoagulant therapy (although intrapartum and postpartum prophylaxis was given). None of these women had any thromboembolic complication (de Swiet *et al.* 1987). These figures suggest that the risk is much lower than had been thought previously.

Other risk factors

Other risk factors include a hypertensive problem in pregnancy, excessive blood loss (Department of Health 1989), sickle cell anaemia (Thomas *et al.* 1982, Van Dinh *et al.* 1982), dehydration, and to have a blood group other than O (Jick *et al.* 1969; Bergqvist *et al.* 1983). Hereditary thrombotic problems, such as ATIII or protein C deficiency, and acquired thrombotic problems, such as lupus anticoagulant, also place the patient at increased risk.

Diagnosis of DVT

The diagnosis of DVT is crucial as the presence of a DVT places the woman at substantial risk of PTE, while without a firm diagnosis the woman may be subjected to unnecessary and potentially dangerous anticoagulant therapy. The clinical diagnosis of DVT, however, is notoriously unreliable. The most common symptoms and signs are pain, tenderness, swelling, oedema, Homan's sign, a change in leg colour and temperature, and a palpable thrombosed vein. It is of interest that over 80 per cent of DVT in pregnancy are left sided

(Lindhagen *et al.* 1986). However, clinical examination has both a low sensitivity and a low specificity for DVT diagnosis. Less than 50 per cent of cases of DVT, including those involving major proximal veins, are recognizable clinically, while venography substantiates the diagnosis in only about 40 per cent of patients with clinical findings compatible with DVT (Genton and Turpie 1980; Ramsey 1983). It is also noteworthy that the majority of women dying from PTE had no clinical evidence of DVT, yet thrombus was found in leg and pelvic veins post-mortem (Department of Health *et al.* 1991). An objective assessment of the diagnosis is, therefore, required. Despite this, a survey among general physicians in Scotland in 1982 showed that 47 per cent were diagnosing (and presumably treating) DVT on clinical diagnosis alone (Prentice *et al.* 1982), and one might presume that obstetricians may be no different. Ramsay (1983) has estimated, by using clinical diagnosis criteria alone, that two patients out of every three would receive anticoagulants unnecessarily. The causes of 'pseudothrombophlebitis' include ruptured Bakers cyst, muscular injury, and cellulitis, although the presence of such diagnoses does not exclude DVT; a Bakers cyst and DVT not uncommonly coexist (Belch *et al.* 1981). In view of the low sensitivity and specificity of clinical diagnosis outlined above it is crucial that an objective assessment of DVT is performed, and this is discussed in this volume by Dr Paul Allan in the second part to this chapter. However, perhaps the biggest contribution the clinician can make is to be aware of the presence of risk factors and to be alert to the possibility of the diagnosis. He should not depend on clinical examination alone to exclude thrombosis.

Diagnosis of PTE

The signs and symptoms of PTE depend on the number and size of the emboli and arise from mismatching ventilation and perfusion, reduced cardiac output due to arterial obstruction, and infarction or collapse of lung segments. Clinical features are non-specific and include dyspnoea, pleurisy, haemoptysis, chest pain, abdominal pain, hypertension, fever, collapse, and sudden death. The differential diagnosis will include chest infection, pneumothorax, aspiration, amniotic fluid embolism, and myocardial infarction. Like DVT, the bedside diagnosis of PTE is unreliable. The classic triad of dyspnoea, pleuritic pain, and haemoptysis is present in only a fifth of patients with major PTE (Wenger *et al.* 1972) and pulmonary embolus is diagnosed in less than one-third of episodes (Windebank 1987). In view of these non-specific symptoms the clinician must remain vigilant to the possibility of PTE. Traditionally, initial investigations include ECG, chest X-ray, and blood gases. However, these tests are of no diagnostic value for PTE (Robin 1977). They may be normal initially and the ECG may show changes resulting from the effects of pregnancy itself on the heart in the absence of PTE. The main use of these tests is in helping to exclude other pathology. Chest X-rays, ECG, and arterial blood gases not in keeping with the diagnosis of PTE were the principal reasons for treatment not being given in many of the cases reported in the Confidential Enquiries (Department of Health *et al.* 1991), yet symptoms or signs such as dyspnoea, chest pain, hyperventilation, and cyanosis were present. A ventilation–perfusion isotope lung scan should be obtained if PTE is suspected. The radiation dose to the fetus is low. Perfusion is assessed by intravenous administration of ^{99}[Tc] microspheres. This is best performed in the supine position to increase apical perfusion, and imaged erect for good visualization of the bases. Ventilation is assessed with radioactive xenon or krypton. A ventilation perfusion mismatch is suggestive of PTE. A normal result effectively excludes the possibility of PTE. An abnormal result showing normal ventilation and a perfusion defect which is segmental or larger in size is diagnostic of PTE (Windebank 1987). With smaller defects the diagnosis is far from certain (McBride *et al.* 1986; Hull *et al.* 1986*b*) as other conditions can cause sub-segmental mismatch. In addition, matched defects do not always indicate a chest problem other than PTE, as one-third of patients with matched defects have been shown to have PTE (Windebank 1987).

Pulmonary angiography is the 'gold standard' for PTE diagnosis. It is highly invasive, involving injection of contrast media into the pulmonary artery, but it does give accurate imaging of the pulmonary circulation. In patients in whom the ventilation–perfusion scan shows sub-segmental mismatching angiography should be considered. If this is unavailable, or the patient is too ill for the procedure, then venography should be performed as this may help to reach a decision regarding treatment (Genton and Turpie 1980), although it must be remembered that one-third of patients with PTE have no evidence of DVT (Hull *et al.* 1986*b*).

Techniques other than imaging may also have a role in the diagnosis of DVT and PTE. D-Dimer, which can be readily measured in plasma using monoclonal antibodies, may provide a useful test to exclude the presence of DVT or PTE or aid the diagnosis where other investigations, such as the ventilation–perfusion lung scan, are equivocal. Although this technique has not been assessed in the pregnant population, it is still likely to provide assistance with the diagnosis in this situation, or at least in the absence of other complications, such as severe pre-eclampsia or major haemorrhage, or disseminated intravscular coagulation.

Treatment of DVT and pulmonary embolism

The treatment of DVT and PTE is anticoagulation. This will not remove the clot already present but prevents further deposition of a fresh clot which is likely to embolize. The two anticoagulants relevant to clinical practice in the UK are heparin and warfarin. Both these agents have special considerations regarding their hazards and safety during pregnancy which must be taken into account prior to their use.

Heparin

Heparin acts by enhancing the action of ATIII. The more recently developed low-molecular weight heparins appear to have a more specific antithrombotic effect and are associated with less haemorrhagic risk. Neither unfractionated standard heparin nor the low-molecular weight heparins cross the placenta (Flessa *et al.* 1965; Forestier *et al.* 1984, 1987; Omri *et al.* 1989) or the breast. Heparin is thus particularly suited in this respect for use in pregnancy. Although it might increase the risk of haemorrhage in the mother and in the uteroplacental bed, because it does not cross the placenta there is no risk of fetal haemorrhage *per se* or of any teratogenic effect. There are, however, other risks associated with the use of heparin in pregnancy. Perhaps the most worrying of these is heparin-induced osteoporosis. This was first described in 1965 in non-pregnant patients on long-term subcutaneous (s.c.) heparin for ischaemic heart disease (Griffith *et al.* 1965). There have been several reports of heparin-induced osteoporosis in patients on long-term heparin therapy during pregnancy with resultant problems, such as vertebral collapse (Squires and Pinch 1979; Wise and Hall 1980). This was initially thought to be an idiosyncratic phenomenon. However, de Swiet *et al.* (1983) have shown objectively that the effects are dose related and that significant bone demineralization occurs in women taking s.c. heparin 20 000 IU daily in pregnancy and 16 000 IU daily after delivery for longer than 22 weeks compared to women on short-term therapy (< 7 weeks). In a small randomized study of prophylactic heparin therapy during pregnancy compared to no prophylaxis during pregnancy, one of the 20 therapy patients developed severe debilitating osteopenia (Howell *et al.* 1983).

Heparin can also cause thrombocytopenia, allergic reactions, and alopecia, but these appear to be uncommon.

It has been reported that heparin is associated with an adverse fetal outcome in up to one-third of pregnancies (Hall *et al.* 1980). This is surprising as heparin does not cross the placenta and bleeding complications are not common enough to explain it. However, this finding was based on a literature survey which did not control for the presence of other conditions which could be associated with fetal loss independently of heparin therapy. For example, many of the patients in this study were given heparin for treatment of hypertension in pregnancy. A recent literature review of 186 studies which reported 1325 pregnancies associated with anticoagulant therapy and which took into account factors such as maternal co-morbid conditions, found that heparin therapy was not associated with any adverse fetal or infant outcome (Ginsberg *et al.* 1989; Ginsberg 1991).

Warfarin

Warfarin is a coumarin derivative which acts by antagonizing vitamin K. Because of its high degree of protein binding warfarin does not significantly cross the breast (Orme *et al.* 1977) and is, therefore, safe to use during lactation. However, it is a small molecule and does cross the placenta. Warfarin is a known teratogen. It produces a specific warfarin embryopathy which may occur following exposure to the drug in the first trimester, with the period between 6–9 weeks' gestation (Hall *et al.* 1980) being the most vulnerable time. It is difficult to estimate the incidence of warfarin embryopathy as most studies have been retrospective, however, an extensive recent literature review has placed the incidence at 4.6 per cent (45 of 970 pregnancies associated with oral anticoagulant therapy) (Ginsberg *et al.* 1989; Ginsberg 1991). The only prospective study of coumarin anticoagulation in pregnancy was performed in patients with valvular heart disease (Iturbe-Alessio *et al.* 1986). This study showed an incidence of fetal abnormality of almost 30 per cent in infants exposed to a coumarin between 6–12 weeks' gestation. Furthermore, when heparin was substituted for warfarin between the 6th–12th weeks, none of the infants were found to have warfarin embryopathy. Thus, warfarin embryopathy appears to be a significant, but potentially preventable, problem for mothers requiring anticoagulation in pregnancy.

The warfarin embryopathy takes the form of abnormal bone and cartilage formation — chrondrodysplasia punctata. This is characterized by nasal and midface hypoplasia, frontal bossing, short stature, and stippled chondral calcification. Other abnormalities have also been documented in association with warfarin therapy, including microcephaly, central nervous system abnormalities, optic atrophy, cardiac defects, and the asplenia syndrome (Cox *et al.* 1977; Hall *et al.*1980; Stevenson *et al.* 1980; Ginsberg 1991). It should be noted however, that central nervous system abnormalities may occur after warfarin exposure at any stage of pregnancy (Hall *et al.* 1980; Ginsberg 1991). The mechanism behind central nervous system abnormalities is thought to be related to small intracerebral bleeds and subsequent scarring *in utero.* As the fetal liver enzyme systems are immature, the levels of vitamin K-dependent coagulation factors are low. Consequently, warfarin therapy, maintained in the therapeutic range in the mother, is likely to be associated with excessive anticoagulation and subsequent bleeding in the fetus. The incidence of CNS abnormalities has been estimated at around 3 per cent from retrospective studies (Hall *et al.* 1980; Ginsberg 1991) based on literature reviews. A recent study has shown no intellectual or developmental difference between a group of 22 infants whose mothers took warfarin during the second and third trimesters compared to matched controls (Chong *et al.* 1984). This is also supported by a study by Chen *et al.* (1982) which found no developmental problems in infants exposed to warfarin in the second and third trimester except in one infant with congenital hydrocephalus. These latter two studies suggest that the incidence of CNS abnormalities may be much lower than previously thought. The outcome of affected infants is variable due to varying severity of the warfarin embryopathy syndrome. However, around 50 per cent of survivors with the embryopathy appear to do well, while those with haemorrhages or CNS abnormalities do poorly (Hall *et al.* 1980).

The use of warfarin also places both mother and fetus at increased risk of haemorrhagic complications in later pregnancy, during delivery, and in the early postpartum period (de Swiet *et al.* 1977). Early reports found a high incidence of fetal intracerebral haemorrhage in late pregnancy (Villa Santa 1965). There is a substantial risk of major haemorrhagic complications for both mother and fetus during delivery, especially if this is carried out by operative means, even with optimal anticoagulant control. As warfarin has such a long duration of action it will take several hours for any reversal of anticoagulation to occur following parenteral vitamin K administration, and fresh frozen plasma will be required to correct the haemostatic defect in an emergency situation.

Warfarin has also been associated with an increase in spontaneous abortion rates when administered in the first trimester, ranging from 28–44 per cent (Lutz *et al.* 1978; Chen *et al.* 1982; Salazar *et al.* 1984). There is some evidence to suggest that if heparin is substituted for coumarin derivatives the spontaneous abortion rate may be lessened. Larrea *et al.* (1983) found an abortion rate of 34.6 per cent in women who received a coumarin the first trimester compared with 9.5 per cent of women treated with heparin over the same period. However, the study of Iturbe-Alessio *et al.* (1986) found no significant difference in spontaneous abortion rates for women who received a coumarin throughout the first trimester compared to those who were changed to heparin before six weeks' gestation. Clearly, more information is required to confirm or refute this possibility.

The management of established thrombosis

Anticoagulant therapy aims to prevent further thromboembolic complications and the extension of any existing thrombus. The effectiveness of such therapy is evidenced by the study of Villa Santa (1965) which showed a substantial reduction in mortality from 13 per cent to 0.7 per cent with the use of anticoagulants.

The acute therapy for DVT/PTE is heparin. Many regimes exist for its use and most are satisfactory, provided that monitoring of heparin activity and adjustment of the dose is carried out to establish and maintain therapeutic levels. Most regimes employ intravenous administration of a bolus of 5000–10 000 IU followed by a continuous infusion of 1000–1600 IU per hour for 5–10 days. Continuous intravenous administration is safer than intermittent intravenous injections in terms of major haemorrhagic complications (Salzman *et al.* 1975; Glazier and Crowel 1976). However, subcutaneous therapy may be a satisfactory alternative as it is a more practicable treatment regime for patients and staff alike, by avoiding continuous intravenous infusion. The efficacy and risk of haemorrhagic complications with subcutaneous therapy does not appear to be any greater than with continuous intravenous infusion (Bentley *et al.* 1980; Andersson *et al.* 1982; Hull *et al.* 1986a).

A variety of tests are available for monitoring heparin therapy. These include the activated partial thromboplastin time (APTT), the heparin level measured by the protamine sulphate neutralization test (PSNT), the thrombin clotting time, and factor Xa inhibitory activity (anti-Xa). The most commonly used of these is the APTT. This should be maintained in the range of 1.5–2 times the normal result. In some patients with venous thrombosis, very high doses of heparin are required — in excess of 50 000 IU/day, to prolong the APTT by 1.5–2 times the normal mean. Such patients are often termed heparin resistant. However, this may be a laboratory phenomenon, especially in late pregnancy, related to high concentrations of procoagulant factors particularly of factor VIII (Hirsh 1986). The anticoagulant effect of heparin is markedly decreased in late pregnancy with approximately 1.5 times as much heparin being required in pregnancy to double the APTT compared to the non-pregnant situation (Whitfield *et al.* 1983). In addition, a 5000 IU subcutaneous dose of heparin at 14 weeks' gestation is equivalent to a 10 000 IU dose at 35 weeks in terms of plasma heparin concentration (Bonnar 1976), and this may be related to the increased plasma volume of pregnancy. True heparin resistance may also occur and is usually seen in the early stages of treatment of patients with large venous thrombosis or PTE, due to increased heparin clearance (Hirsh 1986) related to the size of the thrombus.

Following the acute phase of therapy, chronic anticoagulation is required. The options lie between subcutaneous heparin and warfarin. In view of the problems of warfarin in pregnancy (see above) the former is clearly preferable. This is given as 10 000 IU heparin, twice daily, subcutaneously. Since such low-dose heparin does not affect the conventional coagulation tests, therapy is monitored by anti-Xa activity (Denson and Bonnar 1973), and levels should be maintained at less than 0.4 IU/ml. This is rarely exceeded with a dose of 20 000 IU a day in pregnancy. It is unnecessary to employ any more than this in pregnancy (de Swiet 1985) and there appears to be no excess risk of bleeding in labour if anti-Xa levels are less than 0.4 IU/ml (Howell *et al.* 1983; Hathaway and Bonnar 1987). Blood loss during Caesarean section performed following subcutaneous low-dose heparin has been shown to be no different from that following placebo (Hill *et al.* 1988). As heparin is cleared by the kidney, care should be taken in patients with renal impairment or pre-eclampsia as high heparin levels and haemorrhagic complications may occur. In the puerperium, the heparin dosage can be reduced to 7500 IU twice daily subcutaneously as recommended by de Swiet (1985) or 5000 IU three times daily. In view of the risk of haemorrhage if warfarin is employed in the early puerperium, heparin should be continued for at least 7–10 days. After this time warfarin may safely be used. The duration of anticoagulant therapy is quite arbitrary. In the case of an antenatal thrombosis, treatment should be continued throughout pregnancy and for at least six weeks following delivery as it takes some time for the 'physiological coagulopathy' of pregnancy to resolve. Six weeks' therapy seems satisfactory for a simple postpartum DVT, but a longer period of three months or more may be required in the case of a PTE or a very extensive DVT.

If warfarin is employed, it should be started approximately three days prior to stopping heparin, due to the time required for its maximal effect to occur. The prothrombin time is used to monitor the effect of warfarin. Heparin should not be stopped until the prothrombin time is in the therapeutic range (2.0–4.0 times the normal control plasma).

Thrombolytic therapy with streptokinase has been employed in pregnancies complicated by major PTE (Pfeiffer 1970; Hall *et al.* 1972; Ludwig 1973; McTaggart and Ingram 1977) with some success. However, major haemorrhagic problems may be encountered, especially from the placental site or any surgical wounds. It should only be employed after due consideration of these major risks, in the most life-threatening situations. Recently, recombinant tissue plasminogen activator tPA has become available and has been successfully employed in thrombolysis. It is superior to streptokinase and urokinase both in terms of its specific activity and lack of systemic fibrinolytic activation (Collen 1985). It has not been assessed in pregnancy but may be a possible therapeutic option in the future.

Should heparin therapy fail to prevent recurrent thromboembolism despite adequate anticoagulation, surgical interruption of the vena cava may be required. Open ligation or plication can, for the most part, be avoided by the use of filters which can be inserted into the inferior vena cava via the femoral vein and lodged below the renal veins.

Surgical embolectomy under cardiopulmonary bypass may be required in patients with severe life-threatening PTE associated with sustained hypotension and hypoxia. Prompt surgical referral and pulmonary angiography are required.

Prophylaxis

Until recently, long-term administration of anticoagulants was employed in the antenatal period as prophylaxis for women with a past history of thrombo-embolism occurring during or outside pregnancy. This was because the incidence of recurrence of this potentially lethal complication was thought to be around 12–15 per cent (Badaracco and Vessey 1974; Bergqvist *et al.* 1991) and the risks of long-term anticoagulants in pregnancy were not appreciated. Nonetheless, 52 per cent of UK obstetricians would still use prophylaxis antenatally in women with a previous DVT outside a pregnancy, rising to 81 per cent if the previous DVT had occurred during pregnancy (Greer and de Swiet, unpublished data).

This view of routine prophylaxis has, justifiably, been challenged in the last few years, principally by de Swiet's group at Queen Charlotte's Hospital,

London. They have published two studies where anticoagulant therapy was not used in the antenatal period. The first was a randomized study of 40 women with a history of previous thromboembolic problems. They were randomized to receive heparin 10 000 IU subcutaneously, twice daily, antenatally or no anti-coagulant therapy antenatally. Both groups were given heparin postpartum. One DVT occurred in the control group and none in the treatment group, while one patient in the treatment group developed severe debilitating osteopenia (Howell *et al.* 1983). The second study involved 26 patients with a past history of thromboembolism (Lao *et al.* 1985). None received anticoagulants antenatally, but Dextran was used intrapartum and heparin or heparin followed by warfarin was used postpartum for six weeks to cover the increased risk associated with the puerperium. Only one patient had a possible thromboembolic event antenatally and none had any problems postnatally. There were no significant problems from the therapy. These figures have recently been updated (de Swiet *et al.* 1987) and no thromboembolic problems have occurred either antenatally or postnatally in 59 patients with this regime. These studies clearly suggest that the risk of antenatal thromboembolism in these women is much lower than previously thought. When this is balanced against the hazards of anticoagulation, prophylactic therapy is questionable and perhaps is best reserved for those with recurrent severe problems, congenital or acquired thrombophilia, or those with post-phlebitic insufficiency. Additionally, pregnancy is not contraindicated in women with such a history. Some authorities, however, still advise prophylactic anticoagulant therapy if the previous problem occurred in pregnancy, starting four to six weeks before the gestation time when the previous thromboembolic problem occurred (Rutherford and Phelan 1986; Hathaway and Bonnar 1987). If subcutaneous heparin prophylaxis is employed, then it should be used in a similar manner as chronic therapy following a thromboembolic problem, as discussed above. As thromboembolism is a potentially fatal condition and prophylaxis is not without hazard, it seems prudent to discuss the various risks of these problems, with the patient, pre-pregnancy, or at least in early pregnancy, no matter which prophylactic philosophy is taken, especially since neither approach has been fully evaluated in a large controlled clinical study. All authorities do agree, however, on postnatal prophylactic therapy in patients with a past history of thromboembolism.

Increasingly, short-term prophylactic heparin is being used postpartum in patients with significant risk factors, such as operative delivery, obesity, age over 35 years old, and restricted activity prior to delivery. Such prophylaxis must be encouraged if we wish to make an impact upon the morbidity and mortality associated with DVT and PTE in the puerperium.

The role of low molecular weight heparins in thromboprophylaxis in pregnancy has yet to be established. However, their efficacy in the non-pregnant situation, potentially a lower risk of haemorrhagic complications and better bioavailability, suggest that they will be of value. There are anecdotal reports of the use of these compounds in pregnancy (Priollet *et al.* 1986), and in our own practice we have found that the low molecular weight heparin, enoxaparine (Rhone–Poulenc–Rorer, UK), has better bioavailability than unfractionated heparin as determined by anti-Xa levels (unpublished data). While low molecular weight heparin may only need to be given once a day in the non-pregnant situation, we have noted that twice daily administration may be required in pregnancy to provide satisfactory anti-Xa levels over a 24-hour period (unpublished observation). Thus, if low molecular weight heparin is employed in pregnancy for thromboprophylaxis, we would recommend, at least until more experience is gained, that anti-Xa levels are monitored and dosage adjusted to achieve a satisfactory anti-Xa level. In the puerperium once daily administration may provide adequate thromboprophylaxis, but again anti-Xa levels should be monitored to determine if this is sufficient.

Dextran may also be considered for intrapartum or intraoperative prophylaxis. Its precise mode of action is unknown but may be due to haemodilution and improved flow as well as its effects on the haemostatic system which include anti-platelet effects, a fall in factor VIII and possibly enhanced plasminogen activators (Bergqvist 1983). Its disadvantage is the small risk of anaphylactoid reaction, but this can be markedly reduced by pre-treatment with the low molecular weight hapten Dextran (Bergqvist 1983), which is widely used in Europe. There is also evidence to suggest that heparin and Dextran may be associated with haemorrhagic problems if used together (Bergqvist 1983). Physical methods of prophylaxis such as intermittent calf compression are also useful intraoperatively.

Conclusions

Thromboembolism contributes substantially to maternal mortality and morbidity. The clinician must be aware of the risk factors for thromboembolism as these are often present in patients who go on to develop DVT or PTE. The risk can be reduced by thromboprophylaxis with agents such as low-dose heparin, and the wider use of such prophylaxis in high- and moderate-risk situations associated with pregnancy should be encouraged. Furthermore, the clinician must be alert to the possible diagnosis of DVT or PTE in pregnancy or the puerperium. In view of the poor reliability of clinical diagnosis objective investigations, such as ultrasound examination, should be employed to confirm or refute the presence of thrombosis and guide further management. Such an increased awareness and greater use of prophylaxis may allow us to reduce the mortality from PTE in pregnancy and the puerperium.

References

Aaro, L. A. and Juergens, J. L. (1971). Thrombophlebitis associated with pregnancy. *Am. J. Obstet. Gynecol.*, **109**, 1128–33.

Aaro, L. A. and Juergens, J. L. (1974). Thrombophlebitis and pulmonary embolism as a complication of pregnancy. *Medical Clinics of North America*, **58**, 829.

Andersson, G., Fagrell, B., Holmgren, K., Johnsson, H., Ljungberg, B., Nilsson, E., *et al.* (1982). Subcutaneous administration of heparin. A randomized comparison with intravenous administration of heparin to patients with deep-vein thrombosis. *Thromb. Res*, **27**, 631–9.

Badaracco, M. A. and Vessey, M. (1974). Recurrence of venous thromboembolism disease and use of oral contraceptives. *Br. Med. J.*, **1**, 215–17.

Belch, J. J. F., McMillan, N. C., Fogelman, I., Capell, H., and Forbes, C. D. (1981). Combined phlebography and arthrography in patients with painful swollen calf. *Br. Med. J.*, **282**, 949.

Bentley, P. G., Kakkar, V. V., Scully, M. F., MacGregor, I. R., Webb, P., Chan, P., *et al.* (1980). An objective study of alternative methods of heparin administration. *Thromb. Res.*, **18**, 177–87.

Bergqvist, A., Bergqvist, D., and Hallbrook, T. (1979). Acute deep venous thrombosis after caesarean section. *Acta Obstet. Gynecol. Scand.*, **58**, 473–6.

Bergqvist, A., Bergqvist, D., and Hallbrook, T. (1983). Deep vein thrombosis during pregnancy. *Acta Obstet. Gynecol. Scand.*, **62**, 443–8.

Bergqvist, D. (1983). *Post-operative thromboembolism*, pp. 106–7. Springer Verlag, New York.

Bergqvist, D., Bergqvist, A., Lindhagen, A., and Matzsch, T. (1991). Long term outcome of patients with venous thromboembolism during pregnancy. In *Haemostasis and thrombosis in obstetrics and gynaecology*, (ed. I. A. Greer, A. G. G., Turpie, and C. D. Forbes), pp. 349–360. Chapman and Hall, London.

Bonnar, J. (1976). Long-term self-administered heparin therapy for prevention of thromboembolic complications in pregnancy. In *Heparin: chemistry and clinical usage.* (ed. V. V. Kakkar and D. P. Thomas), pp. 247–60. Academic Press, London.

Chen, W. C. C., Chan, C. S., Lee, P. K., Wang, R. Y. C., and Wong, V. C. W. (1982). Pregnancy in patients with prosthetic heart valves: an experience with 45 pregnancies. *Quart. J. Med., **L1**, 358–65.

Chong, M. K. B., Harvey, D., and de Swiet, M. (1984). Follow up of children whose mothers were treated with warfarin during pregnancy. *Br. J. Obstet. Gynaecol.*, **91**, 1070–3.

Collen, D. (1985). Fibrinolysis: mechanism and clinical aspects. In *Haemostasis and thrombosis* (ed. E. J. W. Bowie and A. A. Sharp), pp. 237–58, Butterworths, London.

Comp, P. C., Thurneau, G. R., Welsh, J., and Esmon, C. T. (1986). Functional and immunologic protein S levels are decreased during pregnancy. *Blood*, **68**, 881–5.

Cox, D. R., Martin, L. and Hall, B. D. (1977). Asplenia syndrome after fetal exposure to warfarin. *Lancet*, **ii**, 1134.

Daniel, D. G., Campbell, H., and Turnbull, A. C. (1967). Puerperal thromboembolism and suppression of lactation. *Lancet*, **ii**, 287–9.

de Swiet, M. (1985). Thromboembolism. *Clinics in Haematology*, **14**, 643–61.

de Swiet, M., Letsky, E., and Mellows, H. (1977). Drug treatment and prophylaxis of thromboembolism in pregnancy. In *Therapeutic problems in pregnancy* (ed. P. J. Lewis), pp. 81–9. MTP, Lancaster.

de Swiet, M., Dorrington, Ward, P., Fidler, J., Horsman, A., Katz, D., *et al.* (1983). Prolonged heparin therapy in pregnancy causes bone demineralisation (heparin-induced osteopenia). *Br. J. Obstet Gynaecol*, **90**, 1129–34.

de Swiet, M., Floyd, E. and Letsky, E. (1987). Low risk of recurrent thromboembolism in pregnancy. *Br. J. Hosp. Med*, **38**, 264.

Denson, K. W. E. and Bonnar, J. (1973). The measurement of heparin: a method based on the potentiation of anti-factor Xa. *Thrombosis et Diathesis Haemorrhagica*, **30**, 471–9.

Department of Health (1989). *Confidential enquiries into maternal deaths in England and Wales 1982–84*. HMSO, London.

Department of Health, Welsh Office, Scottish Home and Health Departments, and Department of Health and Social Services, Northern Ireland (1991). *Confidential enquiries into maternal deaths in the United Kingdom 1985–87*. HMSO, London.

Flessa, H. C., Kapstrom, A. B., Glueck, H. I., and Will, J. J. (1965). Placental transport of heparin. *Am. J. Obstet Gynaecol.*, **93**, 570–3.

Flessa, H. C., Glueck, H. I., and Dritschilo, A. (1974). Thromboembolic disorders in pregnancy. *Clin. Obstet. Gynaecol.*, **17**, 195–235.

Forbes, C. D. and Greer, I. A. (1991). Physiology of haemostasis and the effect of pregnancy. In *Haemostasis and thrombosis in obstetrics and gynaecology.* (ed. I. A., Greer, A. G. G. Turpie, and C. D. Forbes), pp. 1–26. Chapman and Hall, London.

Forestier, F., Daffos, F., and Capella-Pavlovsky, M. (1984). Low molecular weight heparin (PK 10169) does not cross the placenta during the second trimester of pregnancy: Study by direct fetal blood sampling under ultrasound. *Thromb. Res.*, **34**, 557–60.

Forestier, F., Daffos, F., Rainaux, M., and Toulemonde, F. (1987). Low molecular weight heparin (CY216) does not cross the placenta during the third trimester of pregnancy. *Thromb. Haemostas.* **57**, 234.

Friend, J. F. and Kakkar, V. V. (1970). The diagnosis of deep venous thrombosis in the puerperium. *J. Obstet & Gynaecol. Br. Commonw.* **77**, 820–3.

Genton, E. and Turpie, A. G. G. (1980). Venous thromboembolism associated with gynaecologic surgery. *Clin. Obstet. Gynaecol.*, **23**, 209–41.

Ginsberg, J. S. (1991). Fetal abnormalities and anticoagulants. In *Haemostasis and thrombosis in obstetrics and gynaecology.* (ed. I. A. Greer, A. G. G. Turpie, and C. D. Forbes), pp. 361–9. Chapman and Hall, London.

Ginsberg, J. S. Hirsh, J., Turner, D. C., *et al.* (1989). Risks to the fetus of anticoagulant therapy during pregnancy. *Thromb. Haemostas*, **61**, 197–203.

Glazier, R. L. and Crowel, E. B. (1976). Randomized prospective trial of continuous versus intermittent heparin therapy. *Journal of the American Medical Association,* **236**, 1365–7.

Griffith, G. C., Nichols, G., Asher, J. D., and Flanagan, B. (1965). Heparin osteoporosis. *Journal of the American Medical Association*, **193**, 85–8.

Hall, J. G., Pauli, R. M., and Wilson, K. M. (1980). Maternal and fetal sequelae of anticoagulation during pregnancy. *Am. J. Med.*, **68**, 122–40.

Hall, R. J., Young, C., Sutton, G. C., and Campbell, S. (1972). Treatment of acute massive pulmonary embolism by streptokinase during labour and delivery. *Br. Med. J.*, **4**, 647–9.

Hathaway, W. E. and Bonnar, J. (1987). *Haemostatic disorders of the pregnant woman and newborn infant*. Elsevier, New York.

Hill, N. S. W., Hill, J. G., Sargent, J. M., Taylor, C. G., and Bush, P. V. (1988). Effect of low dose heparin on blood loss at caesarean section. *Br. Med. J.*, **296**, 1505–6.

Hirsh, J. (1986). Mechanism of action and monitoring of anticoagulants. *Sem. Thromb. Haemostas*, **12**, 1–11.

Howell, R., Fidler, J., Letsky, E., and de Swiet, M. (1983). The risks of antenatal subcutaneous heparin prophylaxis; a controlled trial. *Br. J. Obstet. Gynaecol.*, **90**; 1124–8.

Hull, R. D., Raskob, G. E., Hirsh, J., Tay, R. M., Leclerc, J. R., Geerts, W. H., *et al.* (1986*a*) Continuous intravenous heparin compared with intermittent subcutaneous heparin in the initial treatment of proximal-vein thrombosis. *N. Engl. J. Med.*, **315**, 1109–14.

Hull, R. D., Roskob, G. E., and Hirsh, J. (1986*b*). The diagnosis of clinically suspected pulmonary embolism. *Chest*, **89**, (suppl) 417–25.

Iturbe-Alessio, I., del Carmen Fonseca, M., Mutchinik, O., Santos, M. A., Zajarias, A., and Salazar, E. (1986). Risks of anticoagulant therapy in pregnant women with artificial heart valves. *N. Engl. J. Med.*, **315**, 1390–3.

Jick, H., Slone, D., Westerholm, B., Inman, W. H. W., Vessey, M. P., Shapiro, S., *et al.* (1969). Venous thromboembolic disease and ABO blood type. A co-operative study, *Lancet*, **i**, 539–42.

Lao, T. T., de Swiet, M., Letsky, E., and Walters, B. N. J. (1985). Prophylaxis of thromboembolism in pregnancy: an alternative. *Br. J. Obstet. Gynaecol.*, **92**, 202–6.

Larrea, J. L., Nunez, L., Reque, J. A., Gil Aguado, M., Matarros, R., and Minguez, J. A. (1983). Pregnancy and mechanical valve prostheses: A high risk situation for the mother and the fetus. *Ann. Thorac. Surg.*, **36**, 459–63.

Lindhagen, A., Bergqvist, D., and Hallbook, T. (1984). Deep venous insufficiency after postoperative thrombosis diagnosed with 125I-labelled fibrinogen uptake test. *Br.J. Surg.*, **71**, 511–15.

Lindhagen, A., Bergqvist, D. Hallbook, T., and Elsing, H. O. (1985). Venous function five to eight years after clinically suspected deep venous thrombosis. *Acta Med. Scand.,* **217**, 389–95.

Lindhagen, A., Bergqvist, A., Bergqvist, D., and Hallbook, T. (1986). Late venous function in the leg after deep venous thrombosis occurring in relation to pregnancy. *Br. J. Obstet. Gynaecol.*, **93**, 348–52.

Ludwig, H. (1973). Results of streptokinase therapy in deep vein thrombosis during pregnancy. *Postgraduate Med. J.*, (Suppl 5) **49**, 65–7.

Lutz, D. J., Noller, K. L., Spittell, J. A., Danielson, G. K., and Fish, C. R. (1978). Pregnancy and its complications following cardiac value prostheses. *Am. J. Obstet. Gynecol.*, **131**, 460–8.

McBride, K., La Morte, W. W., and Menzoian, J. O. (1986). Can ventilation–perfusion scans accurately diagnose pulmonary embolism. *Arch. Surg.*, **121**, 754–7.

McTaggart, D. R. and Ingram, T. G. (1977). Massive pulmonary embolism during pregnancy treated with streptokinase. *Med. J. Aust.* **1**, 18–20.

Malm, J., Laurell, M., and Dahlback, B. (1988). Changes in the plasma levels of Vitamin K-dependent proteins C and S and of C4b-binding protein during pregnancy and oral contraception. *Br. J. Haematol*, **68**, 437–43.

Mannucci, P. M., Canciani, M. T., Mari, D., *et al.* (1979). The varied sensitivity of partial thromboplastin and prothrombin reagents in the demonstration of the lupus-like anticoagulant. *Scand. J. Haematol.*, **22**, 423–32.

Mannucci, P. M., Vigano, S., Bottasso, B. *et al.* (1984). Protein C antigen during pregnancy delivery and the puerperium. *Thromb. Haemostas.* **52**, 217–20.

Omri, A., Delaloye, J. F. Anderson, H., and Bachman, F. (1989). Low molecular weight heparin Novo (LHN-1) does not cross the placenta during the second trimester of pregnancy. *Thromb. Haemostas*, **61**, 55–6.

Orme, M., L' E Lewis, P. J., de Swiet, M. J., Sibeon, R., Baty, J. D., and Breckenbridge, A. M. (1977). May mothers given warfarin breast-feed their infants? *Br. Med. J.*, **1**, 1564–5.

Pfeiffer, G. W. (1970). The use of thrombolytic therapy in obstetrics and gynaecology. *Aust. Ann. Med.*, (Suppl) 28–31.

Prentice, A. G., Lowe, G. D. O., and Forbes, C. D. (1982). Diagnosis and treatment of venous thromboembolism by consultants in Scotland. *Br. Med. J.*, **285**, 630–2.

Priollet, P., Roncato, M., Aiach, M., Housset, E., Poissonnier, M. H., and Chavinie, J. (1986). Low molecular weight heparin in venous thrombosis during pregnancy. *Br. J. Haematol*, **63**, 605–6.

Ramsey, L. E. (1983). Impact of venography on the diagnosis and management of deep venous thrombosis. *Br. Med. J.*, **286**, 698–9.

Robin, E. D. (1977). Overdiagnosis and over-treatment of pulmonary embolism: The emperor may have no clothes. *Ann. Intern. Med.*, **87**, 775–81.

Royal College of General Practitioners (1967). Oral contraception and thromboembolic disease. *Journal of the Royal College of General Practitioners*, **13**, 267–79.

Rutherford, S. E. and Phelan, J. P. (1986). Thromboembolic disease in pregnancy. *Clinics in Perinatology*, **13**, 719–39.

Salazar, E., Zajarias, A., Gutierrez, N., and Iturbe, I. (1984). The problem of cardiac valve prostheses anticoagulants and pregnancy. *Circulation*, **70** (Suppl 1), 169–77.

Salzman, E. W., Deykin, D., Shapiro, R. M., and Rosenberg, R. (1975). Management of heparin therapy. *N. Engl. J. Med.*, **292**, 1046–50.

Squires J. W. and Pinch, L. W. (1979). Heparin induced spinal fractures. *Journal of the American Medical Association*, **241**, 2417–18.

Stevenson, R. E., Burton, M., Ferlauto, G. J., and Taylor, H. A. (1980). Hazards of oral anticoagulants during pregnancy. *Journal of the American Medical Association* **243**, 1549–51.

Stirling, Y., Woolf, L., North, W. R. S., Seghatchian, M. J., and Meade, T. W. (1984). Haemostasis in normal pregnancy. *Thromb. Haemostas*, **52**, 176–82.

Thomas, A. N., Pattison, C., and Serjeant, G. R. (1982) Causes of death in sickle-cell disease in Jamaica. *Br. Med. J.*, **285**, 633–5.

Van Dinh, T., Boor, P. J., and Gazra, J. R. (1982). Massive pulmonary embolism following delivery of a patient with sickle cell trait. *Am. J. Obstet. Gynecol.*, **143**, 722–40.

Villa Santa, U. (1965). Thromboembolic disease in pregnancy. *Am. J. Obstet. Gynecol*, **93**, 142.

Wenger, N. K., Stein, P. D., and Willis, P. W. (1972). Massive acute pulmonary embolism. The deceivingly non-specific manifestations. *Journal of the American Medical Association*, **220**, 843–4.

Whitfield, L. R., Lele, A. S., and Levy, G. (1983). Effect of pregnancy on the relationship between concentration and anticoagulant action of heparin. *Clin. Pharmacol. Ther.*, **34**, 23–8.

Windebank, W. J. (1987). Diagnosing pulmonary thromboembolism. *Br. Med. J.*, **294**, 1369–70.

Wise, P. H. and Hall, A. J. (1980). Heparin induced osteopenia in pregnancy. *Br. Med. J.* **281**, 110–11.

11

Symposium: Thromboembolic disease in the peripartum woman
B   Ultrasound diagnosis
P. L. Allan

Diagnosis of deep vein thrombosis

Pulmonary thromboembolism secondary to deep vein thrombosis remains a major source of maternal morbidity and mortality. Clinical diagnosis is unreliable and imaging techniques are of major importance in establishing or excluding the diagnosis of deep vein thrombosis. For many years contrast venography was the only method available for imaging the deep leg veins and demonstrating thrombus. Various other techniques have been tried including thermography, plethysmography, and isotope studies. However, it is only since the arrival of duplex ultrasound, and more recently colour Doppler, that a viable alternative diagnostic method has become available which can play a useful role in the management of suspected deep vein thrombosis in pregnant, as well as non-pregnant patients (Greer *et al.* 1990).

Both venography and ultrasound have advantages and disadvantages. Venography is still the 'gold standard' for demonstrating thrombus in the deep veins of the leg or pelvis. Contrast can be injected through a foot vein or directly into the femoral vein to get a better image of the pelvic veins. However, it does have some disadvantages which include exposure to the small risks from radiation (Ginsberg *et al.* 1989) and contrast agents. Neither of these factors makes venography absolutely contra-indicated in pregnancy, but these small risks must be weighed carefully against the likely benefits from establishing an accurate diagnosis. In addition, the technique is sometimes unpleasant and painful for the patient, often making her less keen to undergo a repeat study if necessary. There is a small risk (5 per cent) of actually inducing thrombophlebitis in the leg after the injection of contrast, although this is less likely with modern, non-ionic agents. Finally the profunda femoris and internal iliac veins are difficult or impossible to demonstrate clearly and significant thrombus in these may be overlooked.

Ultrasound has been shown to give good results in the diagnosis of thrombus in the veins of the femoropopliteal segment. White *et al.* (1989) reviewed 15 studies which showed a mean sensitivity of 95 per cent (range 88–98 per cent) and a specificity of 99 per cent (97–100 per cent). Initial reports for the detection of calf vein thrombosis were a little less encouraging with accuracies of 78–90 per cent being reported. Rose *et al.* (1990) used colour Doppler and reported overall accuracies of 99 per cent for thrombus in the femoropopliteal segment but only 81 per cent in the calf. However 40 per cent of their calf studies were judged to be technically inadequate for various reasons; when these studies were excluded the accuracy for detection of calf vein thrombosis rose to 98 per cent compared with only 57 per cent in the technically inadequate studies. Ultrasound is non-invasive and painless, and patients will therefore tolerate repeat examinations. It does not require the use of contrast agents or ionizing radiation. A further advantage of ultrasound is that it may identify other causes of a painful leg, such as a Baker's cyst or muscle haematoma. At the levels used for diagnostic imaging ultrasound has been shown, over the years, to have no significant deleterious effects *in vivo*. Doppler machines can have higher outputs and this must be borne in mind when using Doppler near the uterus, especially during early pregnancy. Current research performed on the theoretical, physical, and biological effects of ultrasound has not yet shown any significant adverse effects at the levels of exposure which would normally be considered adequate for diagnostic Doppler examinations (McDicken 1991).

There are, however, disadvantages of ultrasound and these must be borne in mind if it is being used to confirm or exclude a diagnosis of deep vein thrombosis. The iliac veins may not be well seen, especially in the later stages of pregnancy when deep vein thrombosis in these veins is more common but the uterus impairs access. The calf veins are more difficult to assess and segmental thrombus confined to one or two of the calf veins can be difficult to detect, especially in obese, swollen, or oedematous legs. Obesity and oedema can also significantly affect the adequate demonstration of the thigh veins. Finally, and most importantly, the accuracy of any ultrasound examination is dependent on the skill, knowledge, and experience of the operator performing the examination. This relates not only to the operator's ability to pick up signs of thrombosis but also to recognize when an inadequate examination has been performed so that further imaging/investigation is required to confirm or exclude the diagnosis.

Examination technique

The deep veins of the lower limbs are best examined when the couch is tilted with a head-up angle of some 20–25°. Alternatively, the patient can lie on a horizontal couch but with her head and chest elevated into a sitting position.

The reason for this is that these positions will produce some pooling of blood in the leg veins, thereby making them easier to assess. Towards term some mothers may find it uncomfortable to lie on their backs as the large uterus impedes venous return; if this is the case then they should be positioned lying at 45° on their side, as this is less uncomfortable and will also improve blood flow in the deep veins of the higher leg by reducing the pressure from the uterus.

Starting at the groin, with the transducer positioned transversely, the femoral vessels are identified as they enter the leg with the common femoral vein lying medial to the artery. The long saphenous vein can be seen entering the medial aspect of the common femoral vein and the profunda femoris vein will be seen a little lower down. Gentle pressure is applied to the transducer in an attempt to compress and obliterate the vein lumen. The superficial femoral vein is then followed down the thigh to the adductor canal with the transducer transversely positioned in relation to the vein and with frequent applications of compression. The veins are then examined longitudinally looking for any visible evidence of thrombus and also to assess blood flow using colour or spectral Doppler.

When the thigh veins have been assessed the patient is asked to lie on her side so that the leg being examined is the lower one. This allows access to the popliteal veins and to the veins in the region of the adductor canal so that imaging and Doppler information can be obtained. The calf veins can be examined with the patient lying on the couch with her trunk elevated and the hip and knee partly flexed. Alternatively, she can be asked to sit on the side of the couch with her lower legs hanging down. If colour Doppler is being used the easiest way to locate the three major groups of calf veins is to locate the relevant artery and then assess the adjacent veins. The posterior tibial vessels are best located from a posteromedial approach in the mid or lower calf. In the first instance, transverse positioning of the transducer is of value in locating them, but variable positioning may be required for adequate assessment. Once located, their patency can be assessed by gently squeezing the foot and confirming the presence of blood flow in the veins. The anterior tibial vessels run down the anterior aspect of the interosseous membrane and are located using an anterio-lateral approach between the tibia and the fibula. Compression of the foot may be less successful in producing venous flow and squeezing the lower peroneal area may be more successful. Finally, the peroneal vessels run down the posterior aspect of the interosseous membrane and may be identified from a posteromedial approach, lying more deeply than the posterior tibial vessels. Alternatively, an anterolateral approach may reveal them lying deep to the interosseous membrane.

The iliac veins and inferior vena cava can be examined, especially in early pregnancies, but the uterus often makes adequate, direct assessment of these vessels impossible and indirect evidence of patency must be sought. For a complete examination both legs should be examined as there is a small, but significant, possibility that a clot will be found in the asymptomatic limb.

Equipment

Ultrasound examination of the leg veins requires assessment of both imaging information and Doppler blood flow information. Colour Doppler equipment makes the whole process easier, quicker, and more reliable, especially for the calf veins (Polak 1989). Ordinary spectral Doppler examinations will provide much of the blood flow information but they can be quite time-consuming. Some workers (Cronan 1987; Semrow 1988) have reported satisfactory results in the thigh and calf using imaging and compression alone, without any Doppler information. However, the additional information provided by Doppler, especially colour Doppler, makes the examination easier and quicker to perform, it also allows greater confidence in the results. Linear or convex array transducers with frequencies of 5 MHz or 7 MHz are adequate for most leg examinations but in many cases, lower frequencies are required for the pelvic veins. With the development of Doppler techniques in obstetric and gynaecological practice, an increasing number of obstetric departments will acquire machines that will be able to perform Doppler examinations. If these are equipped with satisfactory transducers then they may be capable of measuring venous flow; although the low flow capabilities of some machines may not be sufficient for reliable examinations.

In addition to the equipment, the experience of the operator is an important factor in obtaining satisfactory results. This experience takes some time to acquire but should not be beyond anyone performing obstetric Doppler examinations, although currently most examinations are performed by staff in radiology or vascular laboratory settings.

Normal and abnormal findings

An experienced operator, using satisfactory colour Doppler equipment can examine a normal leg in about 15 minutes. If thrombus is present, or colour Doppler is not available, it may take longer to adequately assess the veins in the

Table 11.3 Criteria for a normal examination

Imaging:	Compressible with mild/moderate pressure
	Anechoic lumen
	Complete colour fill in
	Thin, smooth vein walls
	Mobile, thin valve leaflets
Blood flow:	Spontaneous flow
	Respiratory variation
	Good augmentation response

Table 11.4 Criteria for an abnormal examination

Imaging:	Impaired or absent compressibility
	Static echoes in the lumen
	Absent or incomplete colour fill in
	Thickened, irregular vein walls
Blood flow:	No spontaneous flow
	No respiratory variation
	Absent or damped augmentation response
	Collateral flow

leg. The findings which indicate a normal, patent vein are shown in Table 11.3 and the findings which suggest an abnormal vein are shown in Table 11.4.

Compression

This is probably the single most useful criterion for thrombosis. A normal vein lumen can be obliterated by mild or moderate pressure from the transducer (Fig. 11.2), but if thrombus is present then this will hold the vein 'lumen' open when pressure is applied. It is important to remember that fresh thrombus is also compressible to some extent, especially if hard pressure is used. Conversely, the superficial femoral vein in the lower thigh, the popliteal vein, and the calf veins may be difficult to compress, particularly if the patient is obese or the leg is oedematous.

Echoes in the lumen of the vein

Fresh thrombus is anechoic and becomes increasingly echogenic with time as it organizes and contracts (Fig. 11.3). Although very fresh thrombus is anechoic its

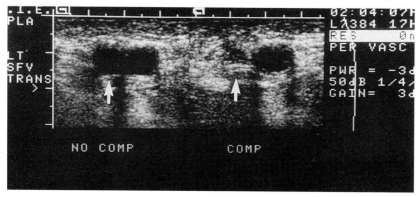

Fig. 11.2(a). The left femoral vein (arrows) and artery in a patient showing complete obliteration of the lumen on gentle compression.

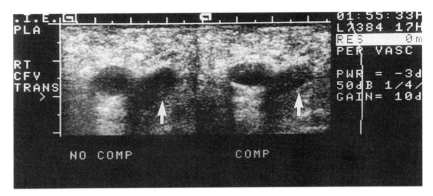

Fig. 11.2(b). The right femoral vein (arrows) and artery in the same patient showing failure of the lumen to collapse.

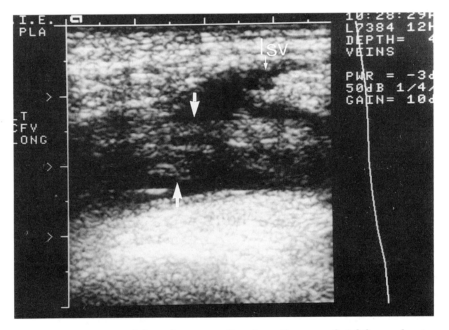

Fig. 11.3. A tongue of thrombus extending from the superficial femoral vein into the common femoral vein. The thrombus (arrows) shows moderate echogenicity but is not yet adherent to the vein wall. The inflow of the long saphenous vein is seen superiorly.

presence can be detected by lack of compression. Another clue to its presence is the appearance of the vein which often looks a little distended and rounded in cross section. Over a variable period of time the thrombus contracts and solidifies, this results in increased echogenicity and a reduction in the calibre of the vessel. If recanalization occurs this usually results in an asymmetrical, irregular lumen which is often best appreciated with colour Doppler. Mobile echoes may sometimes be seen in the vein lumen where the lumen is patent. This phenomenon is usually seen in conditions of low flow rates such as can occur with the pressure of the uterus on the iliac veins. The correct identification of these echoes usually presents little problem as they can be seen moving on the real-time display and they will accelerate on augmentation. A colour signal will also be observed with an adequately sensitive machine.

Colour flow

In a normal patient, using a machine with appropriate sensitivity and settings, the vein lumen should be completely filled in by the colour (Plate 6(a)). If the vein is not well seen, due to obesity, oedema, or location, then the colour may be patchy and difficult to assess due to the relatively low signal to noise ratio. In these cases some estimation of the likelihood of a structural filling defect can be obtained by gentle movement of the probe. A fixed colour void suggests thrombus (Plate 6(b)), whereas variable filling in will often be seen in cases due to a poor signal. In addition, augmentation will enhance the signal to noise ratio and improve the colour image. Colour is particularly useful in the detection and assessment of a non-occlusive thrombus which is only partly obliterating the lumen of the veins.

Vein walls and valves

The vein walls are normally smooth, thin, and easily compressed. In patients with established thrombus they are thicker and more irregular. Normal valves, if seen, are thin, mobile, linear structures which can be seen moving in response to changes in blood flow (Fig. 11.4) in patients with established thrombus they are not often identified. However, in patients with very early thrombus formation one of the first signs of a clot may be the fixation of a valve leaflet; a thrombus often starts to form in the small sinus above the valve and then propagates proximally. Fixation of a valve may, therefore, alert the sonologist to the presence of very early thrombus.

Spontaneous flow and respiratory variation

Even with the patient tilted head-up there should be a spontaneous flow of blood up the leg veins. This flow is modulated by the changes in abdominal pressure which occur during respiration (Fig. 11.5). As the diaphragm descends on inspiration the intra-abdominal pressure increases and flow into the abdomen from the legs is decreased. Conversely, when the diaphragm relaxes on expiration the intra-abdominal pressure decreases, allowing an

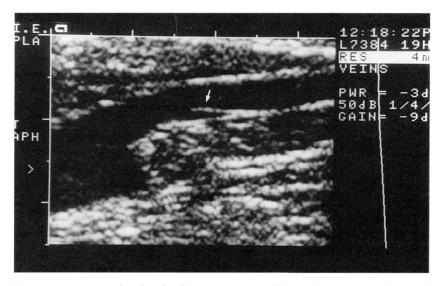

Fig. 11.4. A normal valve leaflet (arrow) just below the sapheno–femoral junction. On real-time ultrasound this can be seen to move with the normal respiratory variations in venous flow.

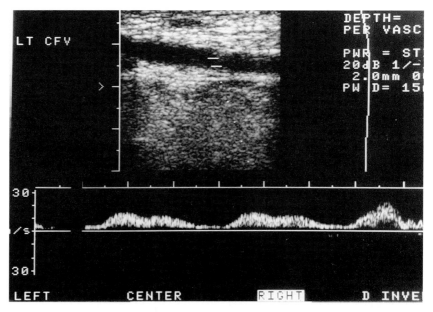

Fig. 11.5. A fairly pronounced example of respiratory variation in the normal venous flow in the leg veins. The sample gate has been placed over the vein, the flow velocity waveform is displayed below

increased flow of blood into the abdomen. In a pregnant woman in the supine position, the uterus may impair or abolish this spontaneous, variable flow. It is, therefore, important to reassess the flow with the patient in the decubitus position. Failure to demonstrate normal flow in the decubitus position raises the possibility of a significant obstruction in the iliac veins and this warrants further investigation.

Augmentation

This refers to the increase in blood flow and velocity which occurs when the leg or foot is rapidly squeezed at a position below the transducer. This causes a surge of blood up normal veins which can be detected by Doppler (Plate 7). The same effect can be obtained by asking the patient to plantar-flex the relevant foot, preferably against some resistance such as a hand or the foot board of the couch, if there is one. An absent response or an abnormal, damped response is strongly suggestive of a degree of significant obstruction in the veins being examined. A careful search should be made, both proximally and distally, for the cause of this.

Unfortunately, a reasonable augmentation response may be obtained in patients with subtotal occlusion so that partial thrombus or recanalization may not be detected. Therefore, although an abnormal response is suggestive of thrombus, a normal response does not exclude partial thrombus.

Collaterals

Two forms of increased collateral flow may be detected in the presence of thrombus: firstly, increased flow may occur through 'normal' channels such as the long saphenous vein or the profunda femoris vein; secondly, in chronic cases, multiple abnormal venous collateral channels may be apparent in the muscles and subcutaneous tissues on colour Doppler. As with other abnormalities of blood flow these changes are not diagnostic but should alert the examiner to the likelihood of thrombus and stimulate a careful search for it.

Problems and pitfalls

Poor visualization of the veins

This may be due to the uterus in the pelvis, the adductor canal in the thigh, or to muscular, oedematous, or obese legs. The less well the veins are seen, the less adequate the examination, and the less confidence in the result. In addition, in these situations, it is often difficult to apply adequate compression, which results in a further impairment of the examination.

Double thigh veins

These occur in a small proportion of individuals (5–10 per cent). In some cases one of the paired superficial veins may be clear, producing good images and flow signals; whereas the other contains significant thrombus (Plate 8). This situation should be identified by scanning the thigh and popliteal regions transversely as well as longitudinally, but it can be a trap for the inexperienced, careless, or unwary sonographer.

Partial occlusion

This can be due to recanalization or, more importantly, to non-occlusive, fresh thrombus (Plate 9). This is of greater significance as it is these tails of thrombus which are more likely to break off and pass into the central circulation. Colour Doppler has made recognition of these thrombi easier, but if visualization is impaired they can still be easy to overlook.

Previous thrombosis

In patients with symptoms in a leg which has had a previous thrombus it can be very difficult to confirm or exclude the presence of fresh thrombus with any degree of certainty using either ultrasound or venography (Plate 10). If fresh, non-adherent, hypoechoic thrombus is positively identified then the diagnosis is relatively straightforward. However, in many cases this is not seen and the patient's management must depend on the clinical picture.

Inadequate equipment or machine settings

For many modern ultrasound machines their specifications and software are biased towards a particular group of examinations: cardiology, general purpose, obstetrics, etc. This means that a cardiac machine may be good at the high flow rates and volumes found in the heart but less good at detecting the low velocities and volumes found in peripheral venous work. Similarly, any particular machine requires setting up differently for assessment of high or low velocities. It is important to be aware of the capabilities of the equipment being used and the various parameters which have to be adjusted for different situations. Care must, therefore, be taken in setting up a machine for venous work, as a poorly calibrated machine will give inadequate, misleading, or erroneous results.

The place of ultrasound

The value of ultrasound in any particular institution for the investigation of possible deep venous thrombosis will depend on the equipment available and the experience of the people using it. However, assuming that there is satisfactory equipment and suitably experienced staff, it is reasonable to suggest a basic scheme for the assessment of patients with possible deep venous thrombosis (Fig. 11.6).

In many cases ultrasound will confirm a positive diagnosis, or confidently exclude a significant thrombosis. In some cases it will be equivocal; in White's review of 15 series the rate of equivocal examinations was between 2–10 per cent for femoral and popliteal disease (White *et al.* 1989). Rose *et al.* (1990) found that 40 per cent of calf vein examinations were technically inadequate. If, for whatever reason, an examination is considered to be inadequate to confirm, or to reliably exclude, the presence of a significant clot then it is important to recognize the fact and consider the necessity for further investigation, namely venography. The decision to proceed will depend on many factors including the specific clinical situation and the reason for an inadequate examination. If there is sufficient doubt and concern then it is reasonable to proceed directly to

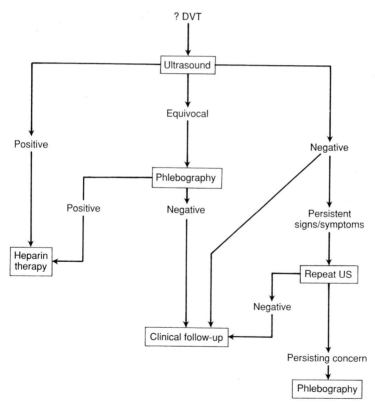

Fig. 11.6. A suggested schema for investigating patients with possible venous thrombosis, providing adequate equipment and suitably trained staff are available (with thanks to Mr M. J. Callam).

venography. Most of the patients will be in the second and third trimester, when the risks from radiation and contrast agents will be negligible.

If there is a lesser degree of concern then it may be appropriate to wait a day or two and then re-examine the patient if symptoms persist or deteriorate. Should this second examination also turn out to be inadequate then again, venography should be considered.

Using this approach the majority of patients will be spared venography, but in those patients who do require venography the radiologist can concentrate on the areas which were not adequately seen on ultrasound, such as the pelvic veins, or calf veins, and can thus limit the examination and radiation dose.

Conclusion

Venous thrombosis in pregnancy has some features which distinguish it from venous thrombosis in other patient groups. Ultrasound, particularly colour Doppler, provides a satisfactory method for assessing many of these patients and should be the initial examination, always providing that there is adequate equipment and suitably experienced staff to perform the examination.

References

Cronan, J. J., Dorfman, G. S., Scola, F. H., Schepps, B. and Alexander, J. (1987). Deep venous thrombosis: US assessment using vein compression. *Radiology*, **162**, 191–4.

Ginsberg, J. S., Hirsch, J., Rainbo, A. J., and Coates, G. (1989). Risks to the fetus of radiologic procedures used with diagnosis of maternal venous thromboembolic disease. *Thromb. Haemostas.*, **61**, 189–96.

Greer, I. A., Barry, J., Mackou, N., and Allan, P. L. (1990). Diagnosis of deep venous thrombosis in pregnancy: a new role for diagnostic ultrasound. *Br. J. Obstet. Gynaecol.*, **97**, 53–7.

McDicken, W. N. (1991). The safety factor in diagnostic ultrasonics. In *Diagnostic ultrasonics: principles and use of instrument* (3rd edn) (ed. W. N. McDicken), pp. 1–102. Churchill Livingstone, Edinburgh.

Polak, J. F., Culter, S. S., and O'Leary, D. H. (1989). Deep veins of the calf, assessment with colour Doppler flow imaging. *Radiology*, **171**, 481–5.

Rose, S. C., Zwiebel, W. J., Nelson, B. D., Priest, D. L., Knighton, B. A., Brown, J. W., *et al.* (1990). Symptomatic lower extremity deep venous thrombosis: accuracy, limitations and role of colour duplex flow imaging in diagnosis. *Radiology*, **175**, 636–44.

Semrow, C. M., Friedell, M. L., Buchbinder, D., and Rollins, D. L. (1988). The efficiency of ultrasound venography in the detection of calf vein thrombosis. *J. Vasc. Technol.*, **12**, 240–4.

White, R. H., McGahan, J. P., Daschback, M. M., and Hartling, R. P. (1989). Diagnosis of deep venous thrombosis using duplex ultrasound. *Ann. Intern. Med.*, **111**, 297–304.

12
Compendium of prenatal diagnoses using ultrasound
J. M. Connor

This compendium aims to provide, in tabular form, details of prenatal diagnoses which have been achieved using ultrasound. In addition to diagnosis using ultrasound (342 entries) it also includes prenatal diagnoses accomplished using other imaging modalities (fetoscopy, radiography, magnetic resonance imaging, and fetal echocardiography — 21 entries).

The current status of prenatal diagnosis is indicated under each subheading using +, (+), or (–). The symbol + indicates that successful prenatal diagnosis has been widely reported with a high degree of reliability in the second trimester or earlier. The symbol (+) indicates that prenatal diagnosis has been reported but with a limitation: (+)E = limited world experience (under 5–10 cases); (+)R = known reduced sensitivity or specificity or suspected limited reliability (see references); and (+)L = diagnosis may not be possible until the third trimester. The symbol (–) indicates that prenatal diagnosis should be possible but as yet has not been reported. For some conditions (for example hypophosphatasia and osteogenesis imperfecta) alternative approaches to prenatal diagnosis are available and these are indicated in the references for those entries.

If conditions are included in McKusick's *Mendelian inheritance in man* (McKusick 1990) then the appropriate MIM number is given. This has advantages in providing consistency of nosology, and in allowing direct access to a summary and bibliography, but it does have the potentially confusing limitation that inclusion does not mean that the condition is always or even usually inherited as a single gene disorder. Hence the Table should be used as a guide to the prenatal diagnostic situation for the condition and other data will be required to determine appropriate risks for genetic counselling.

For each entry one to five references are cited. These aim to be recent, easily accessible, and to give good coverage of relevant previously published work. Currently, there are over 500 publications each year in the field of prenatal diagnosis and hence selection of a limited number of key references is bound to generate some controversy. I look to the generosity of users to accept this limitation and also to help identify misconceptions and omissions.

256 *Compendium of prenatal diagnoses using ultrasound*

References

McKusick, V. A. (1990). *Mendelian inheritance in man. Catalogs of autosomal dominant, autosomal recessive and X-linked Traits* (9th edn). Johns Hopkins University Press, Baltimore.
Whittle, M. J. and Connor, J. M. (1989). *Prenatal diagnosis in obstetric practice*. Blackwell Scientific Publications, Oxford.

References to Table 12.1

Abbitt, P. L. and McIhenny, J. (1990). Prenatal detection of gallstones. *Journal of Clinical Ultrasound*, **18**, 202–4.
Abrams, S. L. and Filly, R. A. (1985). Congenital vertebral malformations: prenatal diagnosis using ultrasonography. *Radiology*, **155**, 762.
Abrams, S. L., Callen, P. W., and Filly, R. A. (1985). Umbilical vein thrombosis: sonographic detection *in utero. Journal of Ultrasound in Medicine*, **4**, 283–5.
Abu-Yousef, M. M., Wray, A. B., Williamson, R. A., and Bonsib, S. M. (1987). Antenatal ultrasound diagnosis of variant of pentalogy of Cantrell. *Journal of Ultrasound in Medicine*, **6**, 535–8.
Achiron, R., Malinger, G. Zaidel, L., and Zakut, H. (1988). Prenatal sonographic diagnosis of endocardial fibroelastosis secondary to aortic stenosis. *Prenatal Diagnosis*, **8**, 73–7.
Adams, A. H., Robinson, H. P., Pont, M., Hood, V. D., and Gibson, A. A. M. (1979). Prenatal diagnosis of fetal lymphatic system abnormalities by ultrasound. *Journal of Clinical Ultrasound*, **7**, 361–4.
Albright, E. R., *et al.* (1988). Prenatal diagnosis of a bronchogenic cyst. *Journal of Ultrasound in Medicine*, **7**, 91–5.
Alexander, E. Jr and Davis C. H. (1969). Intrauterine fracture of the infant's skull. *Journal of Neurosurgery*, **30**, 446–54.
Allan, L. D. (1987). Prenatal diagnosis of congenital heart disease. *Hospital Update*, **13**, 553–60.
Allan, L. D., Desai, G., and Tynan, M. J. (1982). Prenatal echocardiographic screening for Ebstein's anomaly for mothers on lithium therapy. *Lancet*, **ii**, 875–6.
Allan, L. D., Crawford, D. C., Handerson, R., and Tynan, M. (1985). Spectrum of congenital heart disease detected echocardiographically in prenatal life. *British Heart Journal*, **54**, 523–6.
Allan, L. D. *et al.* (1986). Pulmonary atresia in prenatal life. *Journal of the American College of Cardiology*, **8**, 1131–6.
Ambrosino, M. M., Hernanz-Schulman, M., Horii, S. C., Raghavendra, B. N., and Genieser, N. B. (1990). Prenatal diagnosis of nephroblastomatosis in two siblings. *Journal of Ultrasound Medicine*, **9**, 49–51.
Andersen, P. E. Jr, *et al.* (1988). Dyssegmental dysplasia in siblings: prenatal ultrasonic diagnosis. *Skeletal Radiology*, **17**, 29–31.
Anyane-Yeboa, K., Kasznila, J., Malin, J., and Maidman, J. (1987). Herrmann-Opitz syndrome: report of an affected fetus. *American Journal of Medical Genetics*, **27**, 467–70.

Table 12.1

Disease	MIM	US	Other	Reference
Abruption, placental	0	(+)R		Gottesfeld (1978)
Absent cerebellum	0	(+)E		Campbell and Pearce (1983), see also Joubert syndrome
Absent pulmonary valve	121000	(+)E		Kleinman *et al.* (1982)
Acardius	0	(+)E		Wexler *et al.* (1985); Zanke (1986)
Achondrogenesis Type 1A (Parenti–Fraccaro syndrome)	200600	(+)E		Glenn and Teng (1985); Benacerraf *et al.* (1984); Mahony *et al.* (1984*a*)
Achondrogenesis Type 1B (Langer–Saldino syndrome)	200610	(+)E		Wenstrom *et al.* (1989)
Achondroplasia	100800	(+)L		Kurtz *et al.* (1986)
Acrorenal syndrome	102520	(+)E		Meizner *et al.* (1986*a*)
Adrenal haemorrhage	0	(+)E		Gotoh *et al.* (1989); Marino *et al.* (1990)
Adult polycystic kidney disease	173900	(+)E		Journel *et al.* (1989); Ceccherini *et al.* (1989); Novelli *et al.* (1989)
Agnathia–holoprosencephaly syndrome	202650	(+)E		Rolland *et al.* (1991)
Agnathia–microstomia–synotia syndrome	0	(+)E		Cayea *et al.* (1985)
Allantoic cyst	0	(+)E		Fink and Filly (1983)
Ambiguous genitalia	0	(+)E		Cooper *et al.* (1985)
Amelia	104400	+		Campbell and Pearce (1983)
Amniotic bands	104400	(+)E		Herbert *et al.* (1985); Mahony *et al.* (1985*a*); Hill *et al.* (1988)
Anal atresia (imperforate anus)	207500	(+)E		Shalev (1983)
Androgen insensitivity (testicular feminization)	313700	(+)E		Stephens (1984); Wieacker *et al.* (1987) Brown *et al.* (1988)
Anencephaly	182940	+		Goldstein *et al.* (1989)
Aneurysm, left ventricular	0	(+)E		Gembruch *et al.* (1990*c*)
Aneurysm, vein of Galen	0	(+)E		Jeanty *et al.* (1990); Ordorica *et al.* (1990)
Annular pancreas	0	(+)E		Boomsa *et al.* (1982)

Table 12.1 (*cont.*):

Disease	MIM	US	Other	Reference
Anophthalmia	206900	(+)E		Pilu *et al.* (1986*a*)
Antley–Bixler syndrome	207410	(+)E		Savoldelli and Schnizel (1983); Schinzel *et al.* (1983)
Aortic atresia	121000	(+)E		Allan *et al.* (1985); Silverman *et al.* (1981); Gembruch *et al.* (1990*b*)
Aortic stenosis	121000	(+)E		Allan *et al.* (1985)
Apert syndrome (Acrocephalosyndactyly Type I)	101200	(+)E	(+)E	Hill *et al.* (1987); Narayan and Scott (1991)
Arachnoid cyst	0	(+)E		Chervenak *et al.* (1983)
Arnold–Chiari malformation	207950	+		Johnson *et al.* (1980)
Arterial calcification, idiopathic infantile	208000	(+)E		Spear *et al.* (1990)
Arteriovenous fistula (brain)	0	(+)E		Mao and Adams (1983)
Arteriovenous fistula (lung)	0	(+)E		Kalugdan *et al.* (1989)
Arteriovenous malformation of the vein of galen	0	(+)E		Reiter *et al.* (1986)
Arthrogryposis	108110	(+)E		Baty *et al.* (1988); Gorczyca *et al.* (1989)
Asphyxiating thoracic dysplasia (Jeune syndrome)	208500	(+)E		Elejalde *et al.* (1985); Schinzel *et al.* (1985)
Asymmetric septal hypertrophy (hypertrophic obstructive cardiomyopathy)	192600	(+)E		Allan *et al.* (1985); Stewart *et al.* (1986)
Atelencephalic microcephaly	0	(+)E		Siebert *et al.* (1986)
Atelosteogenesis	108720	(+)E		Chervenak *et al.* (1986)
Atrial bigeminal rhythm	0	(+)E	+	Steinfeld *et al.* (1986)
Atrial flutter	0	(+)E	+	Kleinman *et al.* (1983)
Atrial haemangioma	0	(+)E		Leithiser *et al.* (1986)
Atrial septal defect	108800	(+)E		Allan *et al.* (1985)
Atrioventricular canal defect	0	(+)E		Kleinman *et al.* (1983); Gembruch *et al.* (1990*a*)
Bartter syndrome	241200	(+)E		Steck and Ohlsson (1984)
Beckwith–Wiedemann syndrome (EMG syndrome)	130650	(+)E		Cobellis *et al.* (1988); Shah and Metlay (1990)

Table 12.1 (*cont.*):

Disease	MIM	US	Other	Reference
Blackfan–Diamond syndrome	205900	(–)		Visser *et al.* (1988)
Bladder exstrophy	0	(+)E		Jaffe *et al.* (1990); Barth *et al.* (1990)
Blagowidow syndrome	0	(+)E		Blagowidow *et al.* (1986)
Blighted ovum	0	+		Kurjak and Latin (1979)
Body stalk anomaly	0	+		Abu-Yousef *et al.* (1987); Jauniaux *et al.* (1990)
BOR syndrome (Branchio–Oto–Renal dysplasia)	113650	(+)E		Greenberg *et al.* (1988)
Bradycardia, sinus	0	(+)E	+	Kleinman *et al.* (1983)
Bronchial atresia	0	(+)		McAlister *et al.* (1987)
Bronchogenic cyst	0	(+)E		Young *et al.* (1989*a*), see also pulmonary cyst
Calcification, ectopic	0	(+)E		Corson *et al.* (1983)
Campomelic dysplasia	211970	(+)E		Cordone *et al.* (1989)
Cardiac rhabdomyoma	0	(+)E		Schaffer *et al.* (1986); Stanford *et al.* (1987), see also tuberous sclerosis
Cardiomyopathy	0	(+)E		Schmidt *et al.* (1989)
Caudal regression syndrome	0	(+)E		Loewy *et al.* (1987): Baxi *et al.* (1990)
Cerebrocostomandibular dysplasia	117650	(+)E		Merlob *et al.* (1987)
Choledochal cyst	0	(+)E		Elrad *et al.* (1985) Wiedeman *et al.* (1985); Schroeder *et al.* (1989)
Chondrodysplasia punctata (Conradi–Hunerman type)	118650	(+)E		Tuck *et al.* (1990); Holmes *et al.* (1987)
Chondrodysplasia punctata (rhizomelic type)	215100	(+)E		Duff *et al.* (1990); Schutgens *et al.* (1989); Connor *et al.* (1985)
Chondroectodermal dysplasia (Ellis–van Creveld syndrome)	225500	(+)E	(+)E	Mahoney and Hobbins (1977); Bui *et al.* (1984)
Chordae tendinae, thickening	0	(+)E		Schechter *et al.* (1987)
Choroid plexus cyst	0	+		Khouzam and Hooker (1989); Gabrielli *et al.* (1989)
Choroid plexus haemorrhage	0	(+)E		Chambers *et al.* (1988)

Table 12.1 (*cont.*):

Disease	MIM	US	Other	Reference
Chylothorax	0	(+)E		Meizner *et al.* (1986*b*); Schmidt *et al.* (1985); Petres *et al.* (1982)
Cleft lip/palate	119530	(+)E		Chervenak *et al.* (1984*b*); Saltzman *et al.* (1986)
Cleidocranial dysostosis	119600	(+)E		Campbell and Pearce (1983)
Cloacal dysgenesis	0	(+)E		Petrikovsky *et al.* (1988)
Cloverleaf skull (Kleeblattschadel anomaly)	148800	(+)E		Stamm *et al.* (1987); Salvo (1981); see also thanatophoric dysplasia with cloverleaf skull
Coarctation of the aorta	120000	(+)E		Benacerraf *et al.* (1989*a*)
Congenital bowing, isolated	0	(+)E		Kapur and Van Vloten (1986)
Congenital chloridorrhoea (congenital chloride diarrhoea)	214700	(+)E		Patel *et al.* (1989)
Congenital coxa vara	122750	(+)E		Russell (1973)
Congenital dislocation of the knee	0		(+)E	McFarland (1929)
Congenital heart block	140400	(+)E	+	Moodley *et al.* (1986)
Congenital muscular dystrophy	158810	(+)E		Socol *et al.* (1985)
Congenital short femur (proximal focal femoral deficiency)	0	(+)E		Graham (1985); Jeanty and Kleinman
Conjoined twins	0	+		Lituania *et al.* (1988); Apuzzio *et al.* (1988); Filly *et al.* (1990)
Coronal cleft vertebra	0		(+)E	Rowley (1955)
Corpus callosum, agenesis	217900	(+)E		Mulligan and Meier (1989); Meizner et. al. (1987); Hilpert et.al. (1990)
Corpus callosum, lipoma	0	(+)E		Mulligan and Meier (1989)
Craniopharyngioma	0	(+)E	(+)	Snyder *et al.* (1986); Bailey *et al.* (1990)
Craniosynostosis, sagittal suture	123100	(+)E		Campbell and Pearce (1983)
Cranium bifidum	0	(+)E		Barr *et al.* (1986)

Table 12.1 (*cont.*):

Disease	MIM	US	Other	Reference
Crossed renal ectopia	0	(+)E		Greenblatt *et al.* (1985)
Crouzon craniofacial dysostosis	123500	(+)E		Menashe *et al.* (1989)
Cryptophthalmia syndrome	219000	(+)E		Feldman *et al.* (1985)
Cystic adenomatoid malformation	0	(+)E		Fitzgerald and Toi (1986); Rempen *et al.* (1987)
Cystic hygroma	257350	+		Macken *et al.* (1989)
Dandy–Walker syndrome	220200	(+)		Russ *et al.* (1989)
De la Chapelle dysplasia (neonatal osseous dysplasia I)	256050	(+)E		Whitley *et al.* (1986)
Diaphragmatic hernia/eventration	222400	(+)E		Thiagarajah *et al.* (1990); Benaceraff and Adzick (1987); Comstock (1986)
Diastematomyelia	222500	(+)E		Winter *et al.* (1989); Caspi *et al.* (1990)
Diastrophic dysplasia	222600	(+)E		Gembruch *et al.* (1988); Hastbacka *et al.* (1990)
Diverticulum, left ventricular	0	(+)E		Kitchiner *et al.* (1990)
Double outlet right ventricle	121000	(+)E		Stewart *et al.* (1985)
Duodenal atresia	223400	+		Miro and Bard (1988)
Dyssegmental dwarfism	224400	(+)E		Andersen *et al.* (1988); Izquierdo *et al.* (1990)
Ebstein anomaly	224700	(+)E		Allan *et al.* (1982); Robertson *et al.* (1989)
Ectopia cordis	0	(+)E		Klingensmith *et al.* (1988)
Ectopic beat	0	+	+	Steinfeld *et al.* (1986)
Ectopic fetal liver	0	(+)E		Mack *et al.* (1978)
Ectopic pregnancy	0	(+)R		Smith *et al.* (1981)
Ectrodactyly	183600	(+)E		Henrion *et al.* (1980)
Ectrodactyly, Ectodermal dysplasia, Cleft palate (EEC) syndrome	129900	(+)E		Kohler *et al.* (1989)
Encephalocele	182940	+		Chatterjee *et al.* (1985); Cullen *et al.* (1990)
Endocardial fibroelastosis	226000	(+)E		Ben-Ami *et al.* (1986); Achiron *et al.* (1988)
Exencephaly	0	(+)E		Hendricks *et al.* (1988); Kennedy *et al.* (1990)

Table 12.1 (*cont.*):

Disease	MIM	US	Other	Reference
Exomphalos	164750	+		Gray *et al.* (1989); Brown *et al.* (1989); Pagliano *et al.* (1990)
Extralobar pulmonary sequestration	0	(+)E		Mariona *et al.* (1986); Thomas *et al.* (1986)
Femoral hypoplasia — unusual facies syndrome	134780	(+)E		Gamble *et al.* (1990)
Femur–Fibula–Ulna (FFU) syndrome	228200	(+)E		Hirose *et al.* (1988)
Fetal toxoplasmosis infection	0	(+)R		Desmonts *et al.* (1985); Blaakaer (1986)
Fetal varicella infection	0	(+)E		Cutherbertson *et al.* (1987); Byrne *et al.* (1990)
Fetofetal transfusion syndrome	0	(+)E		Filly *et al.* (1990); Pretorius *et al.* (1988); Brennan *et al.* (1982); see also twin embolizatin syndrome
Fetus *in fetu*	0	(+)E		Sada *et al.* (1986)
Fetus papyraceous	0	(+)E		Kurjak and Latin (1979)
Foramen ovale, premature closure	0	(+)E		Buiss-Liem *et al.* (1987); Fraser *et al.* (1989)
Fraser syndrome	219000	(+)E		Schauer *et al.* (1990); Ramsing *et al.* (1990)
Fryns syndrome	229850			Samueloff *et al.* (1987)
Gallstones (fetal)	0	(+)E		Heijne *et al.* (1985); Abbitt and McIlhenny (1990)
Gastric obstruction	0	(+)E		Zimmerman (1978)
Gastroenteric cyst	0	(+)E		Newnham *et al.* (1984)
Gastroschisis	230750	+		Bair *et al.* (1986); Lindfors *et al.* (1986); Guzman (1990); Kushnir *et al.* (1990)
Glioblastoma	137800	(+)E		Geraghty *et al.* (1989)
Goitre	274600	(+)E		Kourides *et al.* (1984)
Growth retardation	0	(+)R		Bruinse *et al.* (1989); Deter *et al.* (1989)

Table 12.1 (*cont.*):

Disease	MIM	US	Other	Reference
Haemangioma/teratoma	0	(+)E		McGahan and Schneider (1986); Pennel and Baltarowich (1986); Grundy *et al.* (1985); Trecet *et al.* (1984); Sabbagha *et al.* (1980)
Haematoma, extracranial	0	(+)E		Harper *et al.* (1989)
Haematoma, retroplacental	0	+		Spirt *et al.* (1987)
Hemifacial microsomia (Goldenhar syndrome)	164210	(+)E		Benacerraf and Frigoletto (1988)
Hemivertebra	0	(+)E		Abrams and Filly (1985); Benacerraf *et al.* (1986*a*)
Hepatic adenoma	0	(+)E		Marks *et al.* (1990)
Hepatic cyst	0	(+)E		Chung (1986)
Hepatic hamartoma	0	(+)E		Foucar *et al.* (1983)
Hepatic hemangioma	0	(+)E		Nakamoto *et al.* (1983)
Hepatic necrosis	0	(+)E		Nguyen and Leonard (1986)
Hereditary enlarged parietal foramina	168500	(+)E		Rasore-Quartin$_2$o *et al.* (1985)
Herrmann–Opitz syndrome	10	(+)E		Anyane-Yeboa *et al.* (1987)
Hirschsprung disease	249200	(+)E		Vermesh *et al.* (1986)
Holoprosencephaly	236100	(+)E		Toma *et al.* (1990), McGahan *et al.* (1990)
Holoprosencephaly with hypokinesia	306990	(+)E		Morse *et al.* (1987*b*)
Holt–Oram syndrome	142900	(+)E		Brons *et al.* (1988)
Horseshoe kidney	0	(+)E		Sherer *et al.* (1990)
Hydatidiform mole	236500	+		Spirt *et al.* (1987)
Hydranencephaly	236500	(+)E		Hadi *et al.* (1986)
Hydrocele	0	(+)E		Cacchio *et al.* (1983)
Hydrocephalus	236600	(+)L		Benacerraf and Birnholz (1987); Dreazen *et al.* (1989)
Hydrocephalus and cystic renal disease	0	(+)E		Reuss *et al.* (1989)

Table 12.1 (*cont.*):

Disease	MIM	US	Other	Reference
Hydrocephalus X-linked	307000	(+)L		Van Egmond-Linden *et al.* (1983); Friedman and Santos-Ramos (1984)
Hydrolethalus syndrome	236680	(+)E		Hartikainen-Sorri *et al.* (1983); Siffring *et al.* (1991)
Hydrometrocolpos	0	(+)E		Hill and Hirsch (1985)
Hydrometrocolpos, postaxial polydactyly, congenital heart malformation syndrome (Kauffman–McKusick syndrome)	236700	(+)E		Chitayat *et al.* (1987)
Hydronephrosis	143400	+		Grignon *et al.* (1986*a*); Quinlan *et al.* (1986)
Hydrops fetalis	0	+		Barss *et al.* (1985); Mahony *et al.* (1984*b*)
Hydrosyringomyelia	0	(+)E		Toma *et al.* (1991)
Hydrothorax	0	(+)E		Peleg *et al.* (1985); Bovicelli *et al.* (1981)
Hydroureter	0	(+)E		Grignon *et al.* (1986*b*)
Hypertelorism	145400	(+)E		Pilu *et al.* (1986*a*); see also Opitz–G syndrome
Hypochondrogenesis	0	(+)E		Donnenfeld *et al.* (1986)
Hypochondroplasia	146000	(+)E		Stoll *et al.* (1985); Jones *et al.* (1990)
Hypophosphatasia (severe autosomal recessive variant)	241500	(+)E		De Lange *et al.* (1990); Kishi *et al.* (1991); Brock and Barron (1991)
Hypoplastic left heart	241550	(+)E		Sahn *et al.* (1982); Allan *et. al.* (1985); Yagel *et. al.* (1986)
Hypoplastic right ventricle	121000	(+)E		De Vore and Hobbins (1979)
Hypotelorism	0	(+)E		Pilu *et al.* (1986*a*)
Ileal atresia	0	(+)E		Filkins *et al.* (1985); Kjoller *et al.* (1985)
Infantile cortical hyperostosis (Caffey disease)	114000	(+)E		Langer and Kaufmann (1986)
Infantile polycystic disease	263200	+		Morin (1981); Romero *et al.* (1984); Argubright and Wicks (1987); Zerres *et al.* (1988); Reuss *et al.* (1990)

Table 12.1 (*cont.*):

Disease	MIM	US	Other	Reference
Iniencephaly	0	(+)E		Foderaro *et al.* (1987); Meizner and Bar-Ziv (1987)
Interrupted aortic arch	107550	(+)E		Allan *et al.* (1985)
Intestinal duplication	0	(+)E		Van Dam *et al.* (1984)
Intestinal perforation	0	(+)E		Shalev *et al.* (1982); Glick *et al.* (1983)
Intestinal volvulus	0	(+)E		Witter and Molteni (1986)
Intracerebral haemorrhage	0	(+)E		Mintz *et al.* (1985)
Intracranial arteriovenous fistula	0	(+)E		See arteriovenous fistula, brain
Intracranial calcification	0	(+)E		Ghidini *et al.* (1989); Koga *et al.* (1990)
Intracranial haemorrhage (including subdural haematoma)	0	(+)E		Fogarty *et al.* (1989)
Intracranial teratoma	0	(+)E		Vintners *et al.* (1982)
Intrauterine fetal death	0	+		Bass *et al.* (1986)
Intrauterine growth retardation	0	+		Rizzo *et al.* (1987)
Intrauterine membranous cyst	0	(+)E		Kirkinen and Jouppila (1986)
Intraventricular haemorrhage	0	(+)E		McGahan *et al.* (1984)
Ivemark syndrome (asplenia syndrome)	208530	(+)E		Chitayat *et al.* (1988a)
Jarcho–Levin syndrome	277300	(+)E		Apuzzio *et al.* (1987); Tolmie *et al.* (1987a); Romero *et al.* (1988)
Jejunal atresia	0	(+)E		Filkins *et al.* (1985)
Jejunal atresia (apple peel type)	243600	(+)E		Fletman *et al.* (1980)
Joubert syndrome	243910	(+)E		Campbell *et al.* (1984)
Klippel–Trenaunay–Weber syndrome	149000	(+)E		Hatjis *et al.* (1981); Lewis *et al.* (1986); Shalev *et al.* (1988)
Lacrimal duct cysts	0	(+)E		Davis *et al.* (1987)
Larsen-like syndrome, lethal type	245650	(+)E		Mostello *et al.* (1991)
Laryngeal atresia	0	(+)E		Arizawa *et al.* (1989)
Laurence–Moon–Biedl syndrome	245800	(+)E		Ritchie *et al.* (1988)
Lipomyelomeningocele	0	(+)E		Seeds and Powers (1988)
Lissencephaly (Miller–Dieker syndrome)	247200	(+)L		Saltzman *et al.* (1991)

Table 12.1 (*cont.*):

Disease	MIM	US	Other	Reference
Lymphangiomatosis	0	(+)E		Haeusler *et al.* (1990)
Lymphoedema	153100	(+)E		Adam *et al.* (1979)
Macrocephaly, benign familial	153470	(+)E		Derosa *et al.* (1989)
Mandibulofacial dysostosis (Treacher–Collins syndrome)	154500	(+)E	(+)E	Nicolaides *et al.* (1984); Crane and Beaver (1986)
Meckel–Gruber syndrome	249000	(+)E		Johnson and Holzwarth (1984); Pachi *et al.* (1989); Nyberg *et al.* (1990*a*)
Meconium ileus	0	(+)E		Denholm *et al.* (1984); Nyberg *et al.* (1987)
Meconium peritonitis	0	(+)E		McGahan and Hanson (1983); Nancarrow *et al.* (1985)
Meconium plug syndrome	0	(+)E		Samuel *et al.* (1986)
Median cleft face syndrome	136760	(+)E		Chervenak *et al.* (1984*b*)
Megacystis–microcolon–intestinal hypoperistalsis syndrome	249210	(+)E		Young *et al.* (1989); Garber *et al.* (1990)
Megalourethra	0	(+)E		Fisk *et al.* (1990)
Megaureters	0	(+)E		Dunn and Glasier (1985)
Mesoblastic nephroma	0	(+)E		Apuzzio *et al.* (1986)
Mesomelic dwarfism, Langer type	249700	(+)E		Quigg *et al.* (1985); Evans *et al.* (1988)
Microcephaly	251200	(+)L		Chervenak *et al.* (1984*a*); Tolmie *et al.* (1987*b*)
Microcephaly–micromelia syndrome	251230	(+)E		Ives and Houston (1980)
Micrognathia	0	(+)E		Pilu *et al.* (1986*a*); Majoor-Krakauer *et al.* (1987)
Microphthalmia	251600	(+)E		Feldman *et al.* (1985)
Mitral atresia	121000	(+)E		Allan (1987)
Mucoid degeneration of cord	0	(+)E		Iaccarino *et al.* (1986)
Multiple contracture syndrome, Finnish type	253310	(+)E		Herva *et al.* (1985); Kirkinen *et al.* (1987)
Multiple gestation	0	+		Neilson *et al.* (1989); Winn *et al.* (1989); Filly *et al.* (1990)

Table 12.1 (*cont.*):

Disease	MIM	US	Other	Reference
Multiple pterygium syndrome	253290	(+)E		Lockwood *et al.* (1988); Zeitune *et al.* (1988)
Multiple pterygium syndrome with concentric bone fusion	0	(+)E		Van Regemorter *et al.* (1984)
Multiple pterygium syndrome with spinal fusion	252390	(+)E		Chen *et al.* (1984); Zeitune *et al.* (1988)
Multiple pterygium syndrome, X-linked variant	312150	(+)E		Tolmie *et al.* (1987*d*)
Myasthenia gravis	254200	(+)E		Stoll *et al.* (1991)
Nager acrofacial dysostosis	154400	(+)E		Benson *et al.* (1988)
Nephroblastomatosis	267000	(+)E		Ambrosino *et al.* (1990)
Neuroblastoma, adrenal	256700	(+)E		Ferraro *et al.* (1988)
Neuroblastoma, thoracic	0	(+)E		De Filippi *et al.* (1986)
Neu–Laxova syndrome	256520	(+)E		Tolmie *et al.* (1987*c*); Mennuti *et al.* (1990)
Noonan syndrome	163950	(+)E		Benacerraf *et al.* (1989*b*)
Obstructive uropathy	0	+		Hobbins *et al.* (1984); Stiller (1989)
Occipital hair	0	(+)E		Petrikovsky *et al.* (1989)
OEIS complex (Omphalocele, Exstrophy of the bladder, Imperforate anus and Spinal defects)	0	(+)		Kutzner *et al.* (1988)
Oesophageal atresia	189960	+		Pretorius *et al.* (1987)
Ohdo syndrome	0	(+)E		Ohdo *et al.* (1987)
Oligodactyly	0	(+)E		Russell (1973)
Opitz–G syndrome (Opitz BBB syndrome)	145410	(+)E		Patton *et al.* (1986); Hogdall *et al.* (1989)
Oromandibular limb hypogenesis syndrome	0	(+)E		Shechter *et al.* (1990)
Oro–facial–digital syndrome Type I	311200	(+)E		Iaccarino *et al.* (1985)
Osteogenesis imperfecta Type I (Milder-autosomal dominant variant)	166200	(+)E		Tsipouras *et al.* (1987); Pope *et al.* (1989)
Osteogenesis imperfecta Type II (severe congenital form)	166210	+		Pope *et al.* (1989); Grange *et al.* (1990); Munoz *et al.* (1990); Constantine *et al.* (1991)

Table 12.1 (*cont.*):

Disease	MIM	US	Other	Reference
Osteogenesis imperfecta — other types	259400	(+)E		Carpenter *et al.* (1986); Robinson *et al.* (1987); Pope *et al.* (1989)
Osteopetrosis (milder autosomal dominant variant)	166600	(+)E		Jenkinson *et al.* (1943); Camera *et al.* (1989)
Osteopetrosis (severe autosomal recessive variant)	259700	(+)E		El Khazen *et al.* (1986); Camera *et al.* (1989)
Osteopoikilosis	166700	(+)E		Martincic (1952)
Otocephaly (synotia)	0	(+)E		Cayea *et al.* (1985)
Ovarian cyst	0	(+)E		Rizzo *et al.* (1989)
Patent urachus	0	(+)E		Persutte *et al.* (1988*b*)
Pelvic kidney	0	(+)E		Hill and Peterson (1987); Colley and Hooker (1989)
Pelvi–ureteric obstruction	0	+		Grignon *et al.* (1986*b*); Kleiner *et al.* (1987)
Pena–Shokeir syndrome — Type I	208150	(+)E		Ohlsson *et al.* (1988); Persutte *et al.* (1988*a*); Genkins *et al.* (1989)
Pena–Shokeir syndrome — Type II	214150	(+)E		Preus *et al.* (1977)
Pentalogy of Cantrell	0	(+)E		Abu-Yousef *et al.* (1987); Ghidini *et al.* (1988*b*)
Pericardial effusion	0	(+)E		Shenker *et al.* (1989)
Pericardial tumour	0	(+)E		Cyr *et al.* (1988)
Persistent cloaca	0	(+)E		Holzgreve (1985)
Phocomelia	223340	(+)E		Campbell and Pearce (1983)
Pierre Robin sequence	261800	(+)E		Pilu *et al.* (1986*b*); Malinger *et al.* (1987)
Placenta praevia	0	+		Gottesfeld (1978)
Placental haemangioma	0	(+)E		Mann *et al.* (1983)
Placental tumour	0	(+)E		Kapoor *et al.* (1989*a*)
Placenta, succenturiate lobe	0	(+)C		Spirt *et al.* (1987)
Placentomegaly	0	+		Quagliarello *et al.* (1978)
Pleural effusion	0	(+)		Bruno *et al.* (1988); Lien *et al.* (1990)
Polysplenia syndrome	208530	(+)E		Chitayat *et al.* (1988*a*)

Table 12.1 (*cont.*):

Disease	MIM	US	Other	Reference
Porencephaly	175780	(+)E		Vintzileos *et al.* (1987); see also schizencephaly
Prune belly syndrome	100100	(+)E		Meizner *et al.* (1985)
Pulmonary atresia	178370	(+)E		Allan *et al.* (1986)
Pulmonary cyst	0	(+)E		Lebrun *et al.* (1985); see also bronchogenic cyst
Pulmonary lymphangiectasia	265300	(+)E		Wilson *et al.* (1985)
Pulmonary sequestration	0	(+)E		Davies *et al.* (1989)
Pulmonary vein atresia	121000	(+)E		Samuel *et al.* (1988)
Pyloric stenosis, congenital hypertrophic	179010	(+)E		Katz *et al.* (1988)
Radial aplasia	0	+		Brons *et al.* (1990); see also Holt–Oram syndrome and thrombocytopenia–absent radius syndrome
RAG syndrome	0	(+)E		Saal *et al.* (1986)
Renal agenesis	191830	+		Romero *et al.* (1985); Morse *et al.* (1987*a*)
Renal duplication	0	+		Sherer *et al.* (1989)
Renal multicystic dysplasia	0	(+)E		Rizzo *et al.* (1987); Stiller *et al.* (1988)
Renal vein thrombosis	0	(+)E		Patel and Connors (1988)
Roberts syndrome	268300	(+)E		Romke *et al.* (1987); Tomkins (1989)
Robinson's syndrome	180700	(+)E		Loverro *et al.* (1990)
Sacral agenesis	182940	(+)E		Fellous *et al.* (1982); Sonek *et al.* (1990)
Sacrococcygeal teratoma	0	+		Chervenak *et al.* (1985); Holzgreve *et al.* (1985); Gross *et al.* (1987)
Schizencephaly	269250	(+)E	(+)E	Lituania *et al.* (1989); Komarniski *et al.* (1990)
Schneckenbecken dysplasia	269250	(+)E		Laxova *et al.* (1973); Borochowitz *et al.* (1986)
Schwartz–Jampel syndrome	255800	(+)E		Hunziker *et al.* (1989)
Scoliosis	181800	(+)E		Henry and Norton (1987); see also Jarcho–Levin syndrome

Table 12.1 (*cont.*):

Disease	MIM	US	Other	Reference
Seckel syndrome	210600	(+)E		De Elejalde and Elejalde (1984)
Seizures	0	(+)E		Landy *et al.* (1989)
Short rib — polydactyly syndrome Type IV (Piepkorn)	0	(+)E		Piepkorn *et al.* (1977)
Short rib — polydactyly syndrome Type I (Saldino–Noonan syndrome)	263530	(+)E	(+)E	Toftager-Larsen and Benzie (1984); Meizner *et al.* (1989)
Short rib — polydactyly syndrome Type II (Majewski syndrome)	263520	(+)E	(+)E	Toftager-Larsen *et al.* (1984); Gembruch *et al.* (1985)
Short rib — polydactyly syndrome Type III (Spranger–Verma syndrome)	263510	(+)E		Verma *et al.* (1975); Meizner and Bar-Ziv (1985)
Simian Crease	0	(+)E		Jeanty *et al.* (1990); see also trisomy 21
Single umbilical artery	0	(+)E		Spirt *et al.* (1987); Jauniaux *et al.* (1989)
Sirenomelia	0	(+)E		Fitzmorris-Glass (1989), Sirtori *et al.* (1989)
Situs inversus	270100	(+)E		Stoker *et al.* (1983)
Skull deformation	0	(+)E		Romero *et al.* (1981)
Skull fracture	0	(+)E		Alexander and Davis (1969); McRae *et al.* (1982)
Smith–Lemli–Opitz syndrome	270400	(+)E		Curry *et al.* (1987)
Spina bifida	182940	+		Nicolaides *et al.* (1986); Chambers *et al.* (1989); Van Den Hof *et al.* (1990)
Splenic cyst	0	(+)E		Lichman and Miller (1988)
Spondyloepiphyseal dysplasia congenita	183900	(+)E		Donnefeld and Mennuti (1987); Kirk and Comstock (1990)
Spondylothoracic dysplasia	277300	(+)E		Marks *et al.* (1989); see also Jarcho–Levin syndrome
Stomach duplication	0	(+)E		Bidwell and Nelson (1986)
Subdural hygroma	0	(+)E		Ghidini *et al.* (1988*a*)
Supraventricular tachycardia	0	(+)E		Wiggins *et al.* (1986); Buiss-Liem *et al.* (1987)

Table 12.1 (*cont.*):

Disease	MIM	US	Other	Reference
Talipes	119800	(+)E		Bronshtein and Zimmer (1989)
Testicular torsion	0	(+)E		Hubbard *et al.* (1984)
Tetralogy of Fallot	185700	(+)E		Allan *et al.* (1985)
Thalidomide embryopathy	0	(+)E		Gollop *et al.* (1987)
Thanatophoric dysplasia	187600	(+)E		Pretorius *et al.* (1986)
Thanatophoric dysplasia with cloverleaf skull	273670	(+)E		Mahony *et al.* (1985*b*); Weiner *et al.* (1986)
Thoracic dysplasia — hydrocephalus syndrome	273730	(+)E		Winter *et al.* (1987)
Thoracic gastroenteric cyst	0	(+)E		Newnham *et al.* (1984); Albright *et al.* (1988)
Thoraco–abdominal eventration	0	(+)E		Seeds *et al.* (1984)
Thrombocytopenia–Absent Radius syndrome (TAR syndrome)	274000	(+)E	(+)E	Luthy *et al.* (1981); Filkins *et al.* (1984); Donnenfeld *et al.* (1990)
Trauma	0	(+)E		McRae *et al.* (1982)
Tricuspid atresia	121000	(+)E		De Vore *et al.* (1987)
Tricuspid incompetence	121000	(+)E		Brown *et al.* (1986)
Triploidy	0	(+)R		Pircon *et al.* (1989)
Trisomy 13	0	(+)R		Benacerraf *et al.* (1986*b*)
Trisomy 18	0	(+)R		Bundy *et al.* (1986); Benacerraf *et al.* (1986*b*)
Trisomy 21	0	(+)R		Benacerraf and Frigoletto (1987); Toi *et al.* (1987); Nyberg *et al.* (1990*b*)
Truncus arteriosus	121000	(+)E		Allan *et al.* (1985)
Tuberous sclerosis	191100	(+)E		Connor *et al.* (1987); Chitayat *et al.* (1988*b*)
Twin embolization syndrome	0	(+)E		Patten *et al.* (1989)
Uhl's anomaly	10790	(+)E		Wager *et al.* (1988)
Umbilical cord angiomyoxa	0	(+)E		Jauniaux *et al.* (1989)
Umbilical cord cyst	0	(+)E		Rempen (1989)
Umbilical cord haemangioma	0	(+)E		Ghidini *et al.* (1990)
Umbilical cord haematoma	0	(+)E		Sutro *et al.* (1984)
Umbilical cord thrombosis	0	(+)E		Abrams *et al.* (1985)

Table 12.1 (*cont.*):

Disease	MIM	US	Other	Reference
Umbilical cord, vesicoallantoic defect	0	(+)E		Donnenfeld *et al.* (1989)
Umbilical vein ectasia	0	(+)E		Vesce *et al.* (1987)
Univentricular heart	121000	(+)E		Allan *et al.* (1985)
Urachal cysts	0	(+)E		Hill *et al.* (1990)
Ureterocelle	191650	(+)E		Fitzsimons *et al.* (1986)
Ureteropelvic junction obstruction	0	(+)E		Campbell and Pearce (1983); Hobbins *et al.* (1984)
Urethral atresia	0	+		Hill *et al.* (1985); Hayden *et al.* (1988)
Urethral valves	0	+		Hill *et al.* (1985); Hayden *et al.* (1988)
Uterovesical junction obstruction	0	(+)E		Hobbins *et al.* (1984)
VATER syndrome	192350	(+)E		Claiborne *et al.* (1986); McGahan *et al.* (1988)
Ventricular septal defect	121000	(+)E		Allan *et al.* (1985)
Ventricular arrhythmia	0	(+)E	+	Lingman *et al.* (1986)
Walker–Warburg syndrome	236670	(+)E		Crowe *et al.* (1986); Farrell *et al.* (1987)
Weyers syndrome	193530	(+)E		Elejalde *et al.* (1983)
Wolffian duct cyst	0	(+)E		Kapoor *et al.* (1989*b*)
Wolf–Parkinson–White syndrome	194200	+		Wiggins *et al.* (1986)

Apuzzio, J. J., Unwin, W., Adhate, A., and Nichols, R. (1986). Prenatal diagnosis of fetal renal mesoblastic nephroma. *American Journal of Obstetrics and Gynecology*, **154**, 636–7.

Apuzzio, J. J., Diamond, N., Ganesh, V., and Desposito, F. (1987). Difficulties in the prenatal diagnosis of Jarcho–Levin syndrome. *American Journal of Obstetrics and Gynecology*, **156**, 916–18.

Apuzzio, J. J., Ganesh, V. V., Chervenak, J., and Sama, J. C. (1988). Prenatal diagnosis of dicephalous conjoined twins in a triplet pregnancy. *American Journal of Obstetrics and Gynecology*, **159**, 1214–15.

Argubright, K. F. and Wicks, J. D. (1987). Third trimester ultrasonic presentation of infantile polycystic kidney disease. *American Journal of Perinatology*, **4**, 1–4.

Arizawa, M., *et al.* (1989). Prenatal diagnosis of laryngeal atresia. *Nippon Sanka Fujinka Gakkai Zasshi*, **41**, 907–10.

Bailey, W., Freidenberg, G. R., James, H. E., Hesselink, J. R., and Jones, K. L. (199). Prenatal diagnosis of a craniopharyngioma using ultrasonography and magnetic resonance imaging. *Prenatal Diagnosis*, **10**, 623–9.

Bair, J. H., *et al.* (1986). Fetal omphalocele and gastroschisis: a review of 24 cases. *American Journal of Roentgenology*, **147**, 1047–51.

Barr, M. Jr, Heidelberger, K. P., and Dorovini-Zis, K. (1986). Scalp neoplasm associated with cranium bifidum in a 24-week human fetus. *Teratology*, **33**, 153–7.

Barss, V. A., Benacerraf, B. R., and Frigoletto, F. D. (1985). Antenatal sonographic diagnosis of fetal gastrointestinal malformations. *Paediatrics*, **76**, 445–9.

Barth, R. A., Filly, R. A., and Sondheimer, F. K. (1990). Prenatal sonographic findings in bladder exstrophy. *Journal of Ultrasound in Medicine*, **9**, 359–61.

Bass, H. N., Oliver, J. B., Srinivasan, M., Petrucha, R., Ng, W., and Lee, E. S. (1986). Persistently elevated AFP and AChE in amniotic fluid from a normal fetus following demise of its twin. *Prenatal Diagnosis*, **6**, 33–5.

Baty, B. J., Cubberley, D., Morris, C., and Carey, J. (1988). Prenatal diagnosis of distal arthrogryposis. *American Journal of Medical Genetics*, **29**, 501–10.

Baxi, L., Warren, W., Collins, M. H., and Timor-Tritsch, I. E. (1990). Early detection of caudal regression syndrome with transvaginal scanning. *Obstetrics and Gynaecology*, **75**, 486–9.

Benacerraf, B. R. and Adzick, N. S. (1987). Fetal diaphragmatic hernia: ultrasound diagnosis and clinical outcome in 19 cases. *American Journal of Obstetrics and Gynecology*, **156**, 573–6.

Benacerraf, B. R. and Birnholz, J. C. (1987). The diagnosis of fetal hydrocephalus prior to 22 weeks. *Journal of Clinical Ultrasound*, **15**, 531–6.

Benacerraf, B. R. and Frigoletto, F. D. (1987). Soft tissue nuchal fold in the second-trimester fetus: Standards for normal measurements compared with those in Down syndrome. *American Journal of Obstetrics of Gynecology*, **157**, 1146–9.

Benacerraf, B. and Frigoletto, F. D. (1988). Prenatal ultrasonographic recognition of Goldenhar's syndrome. *American Journal of Obstetrics and Gynecology*, **159**, 950–2.

Benacerraf, B. R., Osathanondh, R., and Bieber, F. R. (1984). Achondrogenesis type I: ultrasound diagnosis *in utero*. *Journal of Clinical Ultrasound*, **12**, 357–9.

Benacerraf, B. R., Greene, M. F., and Barss, V. A. (1986*a*). Prenatal sonographic diagnosis of congenital hemivertebra. *Journal of Ultrasound in Medicine*, **5**, 257–9.

Benacerraf, B. R., Frigoletto, F. D., and Greene, M. F. (1986*b*). Abnormal facial features and extremities in human trisomy syndromes: prenatal US appearance. *Radiology*, **159**, 243–6.

Benacerraf, B. R., Saltzman, D. H., and Sanders, S. P. (1989*a*). Sonographic sign suggesting the prenatal diagnosis of coarctation of the aorta. *Journal of Ultrasound in Medicine*, **8**, 65–9.

Benacerraf, B. R., Greene, M. F., and Holmes, L. B. (1989*b*). The prenatal sonographic features of Noonan's syndrome. *Journal of Ultrasound in Medicine*, **8**, 59–63.

Ben-Ami, A., Shalev, E., Romano, S., and Zuckerman, H. (1986). Midtrimester diagnosis of endocardial fibroelastosis and atrial septal defect: a case report. *American Journal of Obstetrics and Gynecology*, **155**, 662–3.

Benson, C. B., *et al.* (1988). Sonography of Nager acrofacial dysostosis syndrome *in utero*. *Journal of Ultrasound in Medicine*, **7**, 163–7.

Bidwell, J. K. and Nelson, A. (1986). Prenatal ultrasonic diagnosis of congenital duplication of the stomach. *Journal of Ultrasound in Medicine*, **5**, 589–91.

Blaakaer, J. (1986). Ultrasonic diagnosis of fetal ascites and toxomplasmosis. *Acta Obstetricia et Gynecologica Scandinavica*, **65**, 633–8.

Blagowidow, N., Mennuti, M. T., Huff, D. S., Eagle, R. C., and Zackai, E. H. (1986). A possible X-linked lethal disorder characterised by brain, eye and urogenital malformations. *American Journal of Human Genetics*, **39**, A53.

Boomsa, J. H., *et al.* (1982). Sonographic appearance of annular pancreas *in utero*: a case report. *Diagnostic Imaging*, **51**, 288–90.

Borochowitz, Z., Jones, K. L., Silbey, R., Adomian, G., Lachman, R., and Rimoin, D. L. (1986). A distinct lethal neonatal chondrodysplasia with snail-like pelvis: Schneckenbecken dysplasia. *American Journal of Medical Genetics*, **25**, 47–59.

Bovicelli, L., Rizzo, N., Orsini, L. F., and Calderoni, P. (1981). Ultrasonographic real-time diagnosis of fetal hydrothorax and lung hypoplasia. *Journal of Clinical Ultrasound*, **9**, 253–4.

Brennan, J. N., Diwan, R. J., Rosen, M. G., and Bellon, E. M. (1982). Fetofetal transfusion syndrome: a prenatal ultrasonographic diagnosis. *Radiology*, **143**, 535–6.

Brock, D. J. H. and Barron, L. (1991). First-trimester prenatal diagnosis of hypophosphatasia: experience with 16 cases. *Prenatal Diagnosis*, **11**, 387–92.

Brons, J. T. J., van Geijn, H. P., Wladimiroff, J. W., Van der Harten, J. J., Kwee, M. L., Sobotka-Blojhar, M., *et al.* (1988). Prenatal ultrasound diagnosis of the Holt–Oram syndrome. *Prenatal Diagnosis*, **8**, 175–82.

Brons, J. T. J., van der Harten, H. J., van Geijn, H. P., *et al.* (1990). Prenatal ultrasonographic diagnosis of radial-ray reduction malformations. *Prenatal Diagnosis*, **10**, 279–88.

Bronshtein, M. and Zimmer, E. Z. (1989). Transvaginal ultrasound diagnosis of fetal club feet at 13 weeks, menstrual age. *Journal of Clinical Ultrasound*, **17**, 518–20.

Brown, D. L., Emerson, D. S., Shulman, L. P., and Carson, S. A. (1989). Sonographic diagnosis of omphalocele during 10th week of gestation. *American Journal of Roentgenology*, **153**, 825–6.

Brown, J., *et al.* (1986). The prenatal diagnosis of cardiomegaly due to tricuspid incompetence. *Pediatric Radiology*, **16**, 440.

Brown, T. R., Lubahn, D. B., Wilson, E. M., *et al.* (1988). Deletion of the steroid-binding domain of the human androgen receptor gene in one family with complete androgen insensitivity syndrome: evidence for further genetic heterogeneity in this syndrome. *Proceedings of the National Academy of Science (USA)*, **85**, 8151–5.

Bruinse, H. W., Sijmons, E. A., and Reuwer, P. J. H. M. (1989). Clinical value of screening for fetal growth retardation by Doppler ultrasound. *Journal of Ultrasound in Medicine*, **8**, 207–9.

Bruno, M., Iskra, L., Dolfin, G., and Farina, D. (1989). Congenital pleural effusion: prenatal ultrasonic diagnosis and therapeutic management. *Prenatal Diagnosis*, **8**, 157–9.

Bui, T. H., Marsk, L., Eklof, O., and Theorell, K. (1984). Prenatal diagnosis of chondroectodermal dysplasia with fetoscopy. *Prenatal Diagnosis*, **4**, 155–9.

Buis-Liem, T. N., Ottenkamp, J., Meerman, R. H., and Verwey, R. (1987). The concurrence of fetal supraventricular tachycardia and obstruction of the foramen ovale. *Prenatal Diagnosis*, **7**, 425–31.

Bundy, A. L., Saltzman, D. H., Pober, B., Fine, C., Emerson, D., and Doubilet, P. M. (1986). Antenatal sonographic findings in trisomy 18. *Journal of Ultrasound in Medicine*, **5**, 361–4.

Byrne, J. L. B., Ward, K. Kochenour, N. K., and Dolcourt, J. L. (1990). Prenatal sonographic diagnosis of fetal varicella syndrome. *American Journal of Human Genetics*, **47**, A270.

Cacchio, M., *et al.* (1983). Anatomofunctional considerations and prenatal ultrasonic diagnosis of fetal cryptorchidism and hydrocele. *Minerva Ginecol.*, **35**, 483–8.

Camera, G., *et al.* (1989). Osteopetrosis: description of 2 cases, non-familial of the fatal infantile form and of a case of the mild adult form. Impossibility of performing early prenatal diagnosis. *Pathologica*, **81**, 617–25.

Campbell, S. and Pearce, J. M. (1983). The prenatal diagnosis of fetal structural anomalies by ultrasound. *Clinical Obstetrics and Gynaecology*, **10**, 475.

Campbell, S., Tsannatos, C., and Pearce, J. M. (1984). The prenatal diagnosis of Joubert's syndrome of familial agenesis of the cerebellar vermis. *Prenatal Diagnosis*, **4**, 391–5.

Carpenter, M. W., Abuelo, D., and Neave, C. (1986). Midtrimester diagnosis of severe deforming osteogenesis imperfecta with autosomal dominant inheritance. *American Journal of Perinatology*, **3**, 80–3.

Caspi, B., Gorbacz, S., Appelman, Z., and Elchalal, U. (1990). Antenatal diagnosis of diastematomyelia. *Journal of Clinical Ultrasound*, **18**, 721–5.

Cayea, P. D., Bieber, F. R., Ross, M. J., Davidoff, A., Osathanondh, R., and Jones, T. B. (1985). Sonographic findings in otocephaly (synotia). *Journal of Ultrasound in Medicine*, **4**, 377–9.

Ceccherini, I., Lituania, M., Cordone, M. S., Perfumo, F., Gusmano, R., Callea, F., *et al.* (1989). Autosomal dominant polycystic kidney disease: prenatal diagnosis by DNA analysis and sonography at 14 weeks. *Prenatal Diagnosis*, **9**, 751–8.

Chambers, S. E., Johnstone, F. D., and Laing, I. A. (1988). Ultrasound *in-utero* diagnosis of choroid plexus haemorrhage. *British Journal of Obstetrics and Gynaecology*, **95**, 1317–20.

Chambers, S. E., Muir, B. B., and Bell, J. E. (1989). 'Bullet'-shaped head in fetuses with spina bifida: a pointer to the spinal lesion. *Journal of Clinical Ultrasound*, **16**, 25–8.

Chatterjee, M. S., Bondoc, B., and Adhate, A. (1985). Prenatal diagnosis of occipital encephalocele. *American Journal of Obstetrics and Gynecology*, **153**, 646–7.

Chen, H., Immken, L., and Lachman, R. (1984). Syndrome of multiple pterygia, camptodactyly, facial anomalies, hypoplastic lungs and heart, cystic hygroma and skeletal anomalies: delineation of a new entity and review of lethal forms of multiple pterygium syndrome. *American Journal of Medical Genetics*, **17**, 809–26.

Chervenak, F. A., Berkowitz, R. L., Romero, R., *et al.* (1983). The diagnosis of fetal hydrocephalus. *American Journal of Obstetrics and Gynecology*, **147**, 703–16.

Chervenak, F. A., Jeanty, P., Cantraine, F., *et al.* (1984*a*). The diagnosis of fetal microcephaly. *American Journal of Obstetrics and Gynecology*, **149**, 512–17.

Chervenak, F. A., Tortora, M., Mayden, K., *et al.* (1984*b*). Antenatal diagnosis of median cleft face syndrome: sonographic demonstration of cleft lip and hypertelorism. *American Journal of Obstetrics and Gynecology*, **149**, 94–7.

Chervenak, F. A., Isaacson, G., Touloukian, R., *et al.* (1985). Diagnosis and management of fetal teratomas. *Obstetrics and Gynecology*, **66**, 666–71.

Chervenak, F. A., Isaacson, G., Rosenberg, J. C., and Kardon, N. B. (1986). Antenatal diagnosis of frontal cephalocele in a fetus with atelosteogenesis. *Journal of Ultrasound in Medicine*, **5**, 111–13.

Chitayat, D., Hahm, S. Y. E., Marion, R. W., *et al.* (1987). Further delineation of the McKusick–Kaufman hydrometrocolpos–polydactyly syndrome. *American Journal of Diseases of Childhood*, **141**, 1133–6.

Chitayat, D., Lao, A., Wilson, D., Fagerstrom, C., and Hayden, M. (1988*a*). Prenatal diagnosis of asplenia/polysplenia syndrome. *American Journal of Obstetrics and Gynaecology*, **158**, 1085–7.

Chitayat, D., McGillivray, B. C., Diamant, S., Wittmann, B. K., and Sandor, G. G. S. (1988*b*). Role of prenatal detection of cardiac tumours in the diagnosis of tuberous sclerosis — report of two cases. *Prenatal Diagnosis*, **8**, 577–84.

Chung, W. M. (1986). Antenatal detection of hepatic cyst. *Journal of Clinical Ultrasound*, **14**, 217–19.

Claiborne, A. K., Blocker, S. H., Martin, C. M., and McAllister, W. H. (1986). Prenatal and postnatal sonographic delineation of gastro-intestinal abnormalities in a case of the VATER sydrome. *Journal of Ultrasound in Medicine*, **5**, 45–7.

Cobellis, G., Iannoto, P., Stabile, M., Lonardo, F., Brunna, M. D., Caliendo, E., *et al.* (1988). Prenatal ultrasound diagnosis of macroglossia in the Wiedemann–Beckwith syndrome. *Prenatal Diagnosis,* **8**, 79–81.

Colley, N. and Hooker, J. G. (1989). Prenatal diagnosis of pelvic kidney. *Prenatal Diagnosis*, **9**, 361–3.

Comstock, C. M. (1986). The antenatal diagnosis of diaphragmatic anomalies. *Journal of Ultrasound in Medicine*, **5**, 391–6.

Connor, J. M., Connor, R. A. C., Sweet, E. M., Gibson, A. A. M., Patrick, W. J. A., McNay, M. B., *et al.* (1985). Lethal neonatal chondrodysplasias in the west of Scotland 1970–1983 with a description of a thanatophoric-like autosomal recessive disorder, Glasgow variant. *American Journal of Medical Genetics*, **22**, 243–53.

Connor, J. M., Loughlin, S. A. R., and Whittle, M. J. (1987). First trimester prenatal exclusion of tuberous sclerosis. *Lancet*, **i**, 269.

Constantine, G., McCormack, J., McHugo, J., and Fowlie, A. (1991). Prenatal diagnosis of severe osteogenesis imperfecta. *Prenatal Diagnosis*, **11**, 103–10.

Cooper, C., Mahony, B. S., Bowie, J. D., and Pope, I. I. (1985). Prenatal ultrasound diagnosis of ambiguous genitalia. *Journal of Ultrasound in Medicine* **4**, 433–6.

Cordone, M., Lituania, M., Zampatti, C., Passamonti, U., Magnano, G. M., and Toma, P. (1989). *In utero* ultrasonographic features of campomelic dysplasia. *Prenatal Diagnosis*, **9**, 745–50.

Corson, V. L., Sanders, R. C., Johnson, T. R. B. Jr., and Winn, K. J. (1983). Mid-trimester fetal ultrasound: diagnostic dilemmas. *Prenatal Diagnosis*, **3**, 47–51.

Crane, J. P. and Beaver, H. A. (1986). Midtrimester sonographic diagnosis of mandibulofacial dysostosis. *American Journal of Medical Genetics*, **25**, 251–5.

Crowe, C., Jassani, M., and Dickerman, L. (1986). The prenatal diagnosis of the Walker–Warburg syndrome. *Prenatal Diagnosis*, **6**, 177–85.

Cullen, M. T., Athanassiadis, A. P., and Romero, R. (1990). Prenatal diagnosis of anterior parietal encephalocele with transvaginal sonography. *Obstetrics and Gynaecology*, **75**, 489–91.

Curry, C. J. R., Carey, J. C., Holland, J. S., *et al.* (1987). Smith–Lemli–Opitz syndrome type II. Multiple congenital anomalies with male pseudohermaphroditism and frequent early lethality. *American Journal of Medical Genetics*, **26**, 45–57.

Cuthbertson, G., Weiner, C. P., Giller, R. H., and Grose, C. (1987). Prenatal diagnosis of second trimester congenital varicella syndrome by virus-specific immunoglobulin M. *Journal of Pediatrics*, **III**, 592–5.

Cyr, D. R., Gunteroth, W. G., Nyberg, D. A., Smith, J. R., Nudelman, S. R., and Ek, M. (1988). Prenatal diagnosis of an intrapericardial teratoma. A cause for non-immune hydrops. *Journal of Ultrasound in Medicine*, **7**, 87–90.

Davies, R. P., Ford, W. D. A., Lequesne, G. W., and Orell, S. R. (1989). Ultrasonic detection of subdiaphragmatic pulmonary sequestration *in utero* and post-natal diagnosis by fine needle aspiration biopsy. *Journal of Ultrasound in Medicine*, **8**, 47–9.

Davis, W. K., Mahony, B. S., Carroll, B. A., and Bowie, J. D. (1987). Antenatal sonographic detection of benign dacrocystoceles (lacrimal duct cysts). *Journal of Ultrasound in Medicine*, **6**, 461–5.

De Elejalde, M. M. and Elejalde, B. R. (1984). Visualisation of the fetal face by ultrasound. *Journal of Craniofacial Genetics and Developmental Biology*, **4**, 251.

De Filippi, G. Canestri, G., Bosio, U., Derchi, L. E., and Cospi, M. (1986). Thoracic neuroblastoma: antenatal detection in a case with unusual postnatal radiographic findings. *British Journal of Radiology*, **59**, 704–6.

De Lange, M. and Rouse, G. A. (1990). Prenatal diagnosis of hypophosphatasia. *Journal of Ultrasound in Medicine*, **9**, 115–17.

De Vore, G. R. and Hobbins, J. C. (1979). Diagnosis of structural abnormalities in the fetus. *Clinical Perinatology*, **6**, 293.

De Vore, G. R., Siassi, B., and Platt, L. D. (1987). Fetal echocardiography: The prenatal diagnosis of tricuspid atresia (type 1c) during the second trimester of pregnancy. *Journal of Clinical Ultrasound*, **15**, 317–24.

Denholm, T. A., Crow, H. C., Edwards, W. H., Simmons, G. M., Marin-Padilla, M., and Bartrum, R. J. (1984). Prenatal sonographic appearance of meconium ileus in twins. *American Journal of Roentgenology*, **143**, 371–2.

Derosa, R., Lenke, R. R., Kurczynski, T. W., Persutte, W. H., and Nemes, J. M. (1989). In utero diagnosis of benign fetal macrocephaly. *American Journal of Obstetrics and Gynecology*, **161**, 690.

Desmonts, G., Daffos, F., Forestier, F., Capella-Pavlovsky, M., Thulliez, P., and Chartier, M. (1985). Prenatal diagnosis of congenital toxoplasmosis. *Lancet*, **i**, 500–4.

Deter, R. L., Rossavik, I. K., and Carpenter, R. J. (1989). Development of individual growth standards for estimated fetal weight: II. Weight prediction during the third trimester and at birth. *Journal of Clinical Ultrasound*, **17**, 83–8.

Donnenfeld, A. E., Gussman, D., Mennuti, M. T., and Zackai, E. H. (1986). Evaluation of an unknown fetal skeletal dysplasia: prenatal findings in hypochondrogenesis. *American Journal of Human Genetics*, **39**, A252.

Donnenfeld, A. E. and Mennuti, M. T. (1987). Second trimester diagnosis of fetal skeletal dysplasias. *Obstetrics and Gynecology Survey*, **42**, 199–217.

Donnenfeld, A. E., Mennuti, M. T., Templeton, J. M., and Gabbe, G. G. (1989). Prenatal diagnosis of a vesico-allantoic abdominal wall defect. *Journal of Ultrasound in Medicine*, **8**, 43–5.

Donnenfeld, A. E., Wiseman, B., Lavi, E., and Weiner, S. (1990). Prenatal diagnosis of thrombocytopenia absent radius syndrome by ultrasound and cordocentesis. *Prenatal Diagnosis*, **10**, 29–35.

Dreazen, E., Tessler, F., Sarti, D., and Crandall, B. F. (1989). Spontaneous resolution of fetal hydrocephalus. *Journal of Ultrasound in Medicine*, **8**, 155–7.

Duff, P., Harlass, F. E., and Milligan, D. A. (1990), Prenatal diagnosis of chondrodysplasia punctata by sonography. *Obstetrics and Gynecology*, **76**, 497–500.

Dunn, V. and Glasier, C. M. (1985). Ultrasonographic antenatal demonstration of primary megaureters. *Journal of Ultrasound in Medicine*, **4**, 101–3.

Elejalde, B. R., De Elejalde, M. M., Booth, C., Kaye, C., and Hollison, L. (1983). Prenatal diagnosis of Weyers syndrome (deficient ulnar and fibular rays with bilateral hydronephrosis). *American Journal of Medical Genetics*, **21**, 439–44.

Elejalde, B. R., De Elejalde, M. M., and Pansch, D. (1985). Prenatal diagnosis of Jeune syndrome. *American Journal of Medical Genetics*, **21**, 433–8.

El Khazen, N., Faverley, D., Vamos, E., Van Regemorter, N., Flament-Durand, J., Carton, B., *et al.* (1986). Lethal osteopetrosis with multiple fractures *in utero*. *American Journal of Medical Genetics*, **23**, 811–19.

Elrad, H., Mayden, K. L., Ahart, S., Giglia, R., and Gleicher, N. (1985). Prenatal diagnosis of choledochal cyst. *Journal of Ultrasound in Medicine*, **4**, 533–5.

Evans, M. I., Zador, I. E., Qureshi, F., Budev, H., Quigg, M. H., and Nadler, H. L. (1988). Ultrasonographic prenatal diagnosis and fetal pathology of Langer mesomelic dwarfism. *American Journal of Medical Genetics*, **31**, 915–20.

Farrell, S. A., Toi, A., Leadman, M. L., Davidson, R. G., and Caco, C. (1987). Prenatal diagnosis of retinal detachment in Walker–Warburg syndrome. *American Journal of Medical Genetics*, **28**, 619–24.

Feldman, E., Shalev, E., Weiner, E., Cohen, H., and Zuckerman, H. (1985). Microphthalmia — prenatal ultrasonic diagnosis: a case report. *Prenatal Diagnosis*, **5**, 205–7.

Fellous, M., Boue, J., Malbrunot, C., *et al.* (1982). A five-generation family with sacral agenesis and spina bifida: possible similarities with the mouse T-locus. *American Journal of Medical Genetics*, **12**, 465–87.

Ferraro, E. M., Fakhry, J., Aruny, J. E., and Bracero, L. A. (1988). Prenatal adrenal neuroblastoma. Case report with review of the literature. *Journal of Ultrasound in Medicine*, **7**, 275–8.

Filkins, K., Russo, J., Bilinki, I., Diamond, N., and Searle, B. (1984). Prenatal diagnosis of thrombocytopenia-absent radius syndrome using ultrasound and fetoscopy. *Prenatal Diagnosis*, **4**, 139–42.

Filkins, K., *et al.* (1985). Third trimester ultrasound diagnosis of intestinal atresia following clinical evidence of polyhydramnios. *Prenatal Diagnosis*, **5**, 215–20.

Filly, R. A., Goldstein, R. B., and Callen, P. W. (1990). Monochorionic twinning: sonographic assessment. *American Journal of Roentgenology*, **154**, 459–69.

Fink, I. J. and Filly, R. A. (1983). Omphalocele associated with umbilical cord allantoic cyst: sonographic evaluation *in utero*. *Radiology*, **149**, 473–6.

Fisk, N. M., Dhillon, H. K., Ellis, C. E., Nicolini, U., Tannirandorn, Y., and Rodeck, C. H. (1990). Antenatal diagnosis of megalourethra in a fetus with the prune belly syndrome. *Journal of Clinical Ultrasound*, **18**, 124–8.

Fitzgerald, E. J., and Toi, A. (1986). Antenatal ultrasound diagnosis of cystic adenomatoid malformation of the lung. *Journal of the Canadian Association of Radiology*, **37**, 48–9.

Fitzmorris-Glass, R., Mattrey, R. F., and Cantrell, C. J. (1989). Magnetic resonance imaging as an adjunct to ultrasound in oligohydramnios. Detection of sirenomelia. *Journal of Ultrasound in Medicine*, **8**, 159–62.

Fitzsimons, P. J., *et al.* (1986). Prenatal and immediate postnatal ultrasonographic diagnosis of ureteocele. *Journal of the Canadian Association of Radiology*, **337**, 189–91.

Fletman, D., *et al.* (1980). 'Apple peel' atresia of the small bowel: prenatal diagnosis of the obstruction by ultrasound. *Pediatric Radiology*, **9**, 118–19.

Foderaro, A. E., Abu-Yousef, M. M., Benda, J. A., Williamson, R. A., and Smith, W. L. (1987). Antenatal ultrasound diagnosis of iniencephaly. *Journal of Clinical Ultrasound*, **15**, 550–4.

Fogarty, K., Cohen, H. L., and Haller, J. O. (1989). Sonography of fetal intracranial haemorrhage: unusual causes and a review of the literature. *Journal of Clinical Ultrasound*, **17**, 366–70.

Foucar, E., Williamson, R. A., Yiu-Chiu, V., Varner, M. W., and Kay, B. R. (1983). Mesenchymal hamartoma of the liver identified by fetal sonography. *American Journal of Roentgenology*, **140**, 970–2.

Fraser, W. D., Nimrod, C., Nicholson, S., and Harder, J. (1989). Antenatal diagnosis of restriction of the foramen ovale. *Journal of Ultrasound in Medicine*, **8**, 281–3.

Friedman, J. M. and Santos-Ramos, R. (1984). Natural history of X-linked aqueductal stenosis in the second and third trimesters of pregnancy. *American Journal of Obstetrics and Gynecology*, **150**, 104–6.

Gabrielli, S., Reece, E. A., Pilu, G., Perolo, A., Rizzo, N., Bovicelli, L., et al. (1989). The clinical significance of prenatally diagnosed choroid plexus cysts. *American Journal of Obstetrics and Gynecology*, **160**, 1207–10.

Gamble, C. N., Hershey, D. W., and Schaeffer, C. J. (1990). Femoral-facial syndrome detected in prenatal ultrasound. *American Journal of Human Genetics*, **47**, 274.

Garber, A., Shohat, M., and Sarti, D. (1990). Megacystis-microcolon-intestinal hypoperistalsis syndrome in two male siblings. *Prenatal Diagnosis*, **10**, 377–88.

Gembruch, U., Hansmann, M., and Fodisch, H. J. (1985). Early prenatal diagnosis of short rib–polydactyly (SRP) syndrome type II (Majewski) by ultrasound in a case at risk. *Prenatal Diagnosis*, **5**, 357–62.

Gembruch, U., Niesen, M., Kehrberg, G., and Hansmann, M. (1988). Diastrophic dysplasia: a specific prenatal diagnosis by ultrasound. *Prenatal Diagnosis*, **8**, 539–46.

Gembruch, U., Knople, G., Chatterjee, M., Bald, R., and Hansmann, M. (1990*a*). First-trimester diagnosis of fetal congenital heart disease by transvaginal two-dimensional and Doppler echocardiography. *Obstetrics and Gynaecology*, **75**, 496–8.

Gembruch, U., Chatterjee, M., Bald, R., Eldering, G., Gocke, H., Urban, A. E., et al. (1990*b*). Prenatal diagnosis of aortic atresia by colour Doppler flow mapping. *Prenatal Diagnosis*, **10**, 211–18.

Gembruch, U., Steil, E., Redel, D. A., and Hansmann, M. (1990*c*). Prenatal diagnosis of a left ventricular aneurysm. *Prenatal diagnosis*, **10**, 203–9.

Genkins, S. M., Hertzberg, B. S., Bowie, J. D., and Blow, O. (1989). Pena-Shokeir type I syndrome: *in utero* sonographic appearance. *Journal of Clinical Ultrasound*, **17**, 56–61.

Geraghty, A. V., Knott, P. O., and Hanna, H. M. (1989). Prenatal diagnosis of fetal glioblastoma multiforme. *Prenatal Diagnosis*, **9**, 613–16.

Ghidini, A., Vergani, P., Sirtori, M., Bozzo, G., Mariani, S., and Negri, R. (1988*a*). Prenatal diagnosis of subdural hygroma. *Journal of Ultrasound in Medicine*, **7**, 463–5.

Ghidini, A., Sirtori, M., Romero, R., and Hobbins, J. C. (1988*b*). Prenatal diagnosis of pentalogy of Cantrell. *Journal of Ultrasound in Medicine*, **7**, 567–72.

Ghidini, A., Sirtori, M., Vergani, P., Mariani, S., Tucci, E., and Scola, G. C. (1989). Fetal intracranial calcificaton. *American Journal of Obstetrics and Gynecology*, **160**, 86–7.

Ghidini, A., Romero, R., Eisen, R. N., Walker Smith, G. J., and Hobbins, J. C. (1990). Umbilical cord haemangioma. Prenatal identification and review of the literature. *Journal of Ultrasound in Medicine*, **9**, 297–300.

Glenn, L. W. and Teng, S. S. K. (1985). *In utero* sonographic diagnosis of achondrogenesis. *Journal of Clinical Ultrasound*, **13**, 195–8.

Glick, P. L., Harrison, M. R., and Filly, R. A. (1983). Antepartum diagnosis of meconium peritonitis. *New England Journal of Medicine*, **309**, 1392.

Goldstein, R. B., Filly, R. A., and Callen, P. W. (1989). Sonography of anencephaly: pitfalls in early diagnosis. *Journal of Clinical Ultrasound*, **17**, 397–402.

Gollop, T. R., Eigier, A., and Neto, J. G. (1987). Prenatal diagnosis of thalidomide syndrome. *Prenatal Diagnosis*, **7**, 295–8.

Gorczyca, D. P., McGahan, J. P., Lindfors, K. K., Ellis, W. G., and Grix, A. (1989). Arthrogryposis multiplex congenita: prenatal ultrasonographic diagnosis. *Journal of Clinical Ultrasound*, **17**, 40–4.

Gotoh, T., *et al.* (1989). Adrenal haemorrhage in the newborn with evidence of bleeding *in utero*. *Journal of Urology*, **141**, 1145–7.

Gottesfeld, K. R. (1978). Ultrasound in obstetrics. *Clinical Obstetrics and Gynecology*, **21**, 311.

Graham, M. (1985). Congenital short femur: prenatal sonographic diagnosis. *Journal of Ultrasound in Medicine*, **4**, 361–3.

Grange, D. K., Lewis, M. B., and Marini, J. C. (1990). Analysis of cultured chorionic villi in a case of osteogenesis imperfecta type II: implications for prenatal diagnosis. *American Journal of Medical Genetics*, **36**, 258–64.

Gray, D. L., Martin, C. M., and Crane, J. P. (1989). Differential diagnosis of first trimester ventral wall defect. *Journal of Ultrasound in Medicine*, **8**, 255–8.

Greenberg, C. R., Trevenen, C. L., and Evans, J. A. (1988). The BOR syndrome and renal agenesis—prenatal diagnosis and further clinical delineation. *Prenatal Diagnosis*, **8**, 103–8.

Greenblatt, A. M., Beretsky, I., Lankin, D. H., and Phelan, L. (1985). *In utero* diagnosis of crossed renal ectopia using high-resolution real time ultrasound. *Journal of Ultrasound in Medicine*, **4**, 105–7.

Grignon, A., Filion, R., Filiatrault, D., Robitaille, P., Homsy, Y., Boutin, H., *et al.* (1986*a*). Urinary tract dilatation *in utero*: classification and clinical applications. *Radiology*, **160**, 645–7.

Grignon, A., Filiatrault, D., Homsy, Y., Robitaille, P., Filion, R., Boutin, H., *et al.* (1986*b*). Ureteropelvic junction stenosis: antenatal ultrasonographic diagnosis, postnatal investigation and follow-up. *Radiology*, **160**, 649–51.

Gross, S. J., Benzie, R. J., Sermer, M., Skidmore, M. B., and Wilson, S. R. (1987). Sacrococcygeal teratoma: Pernatal diagnosis and management. *American Journal of Obstetrics and Gynecology*, **156**, 393–6.

Grundy, H., Glasmann, A., Burlbaw, J., Walton, S., Dannar, C., and Doan, L. (1985). Hemangioma presenting as a cystic mass in the fetal neck. *Journal of Ultrasound in Medicine*, **4**, 147–50.

Guzman, E. R. (1990). Early prenatal diagnosis of gastroschisis with transvaginal sonography. *American Journal of Obstetrics and Gynecology*, **162**, 1253–4.

Hadi, H. A., *et al.* (1986). Ultrasonographic prenatal diagnosis of hydranencephaly. A case report. *Journal of Reproductive Medicine*, **31**, 254–6.

Haeusler, M. C. H., Hofmann, H. M. H., Hoenigl, W., Karpf, E. F., and Rosenkranz, W. (1990). Congenital generalised cystic lymphangiomatosis diagnosed by prenatal ultrasound. *Prenatal Diagnosis*, **10**, 617–21.

Harper, A. K., Clark, J. A., Koontz, W. L., and Holmes, M. (1989). Sonographic appearance of fetal extracranial hematoma. *Journal of Ultrasound in Medicine*, **8**, 693–5.

Hartikainen-Sorri, A. L., Kirkinen, P., and Herva, R. (1983). Prenatal detection of hydrolethalus syndrome. *Prenatal Diagnosis*, **3**, 219–24.

Hastbacka, J., Kaitila, I., Sistonen, P., and de la Chapelle, A. (1990). Diastrophic dysplasia gene maps to the distal long arm of chromosome 5. *Proceedings of the National Academy of Science, USA*, **87**, 8056–9.

Hatjis, C. G., Philip, A. G., Anderson, G. G., and Mann, L. I. (1981). The *in-utero* ultrasonographic appearance of Klippel–Trenaunay–Weber syndrome. *American Journal of Obstetrics and Gynecology,* **139**, 972–4.

Hayden, S. A., *et al.* (1988). Posterior urethral obstruction. Prenatal sonographic findings and clinical outcome in fourteen cases. *Journal of Ultrasound in Medicine*, **7**, 371–5.

Heijne, L., *et al.* (1985). The development of fetal gallstones demonstrated by ultrasound. *Radiography*, **51**, 155–6.

Hendricks, S. K., Cyr, D. R., Nyberg, D. A., Raabe, R., and Mack, L. A. (1988). Exencephaly — clinical and ultrasonic correlation to anencephaly. *Obstetrics and Gynecology*, **72**, 898–901.

Henrion, R., Oury, J. F., Aubry, J. P., and Aubry, M. C. (1980). Prenatal diagnosis of ectrodactyly. *Lancet*, **ii**, 319.

Henry, R. J. W. and Norton, S. (1987). Prenatal ultrasound diagnosis of fetal scoliosis with termination of the pregnancy: Case report. *Prenatal Diagnosis*, **7**, 663–6.

Herbert, W. N., Seeds, J. W., Cefalo, R. C., and Bowes, W. A. (1985). Prenatal detection of intraamniotic bands: implications and management. *Obstetrics and Gynecology*, **65**, 36S–38S.

Herva, R., Leisti, J., Kirkinen, P., and Seppanen, U. (1985). A lethal autosomal recessive syndrome of multiple congenital contractures. *American Journal of Medical Genetics*, **20**, 431–9.

Hill, L. M., and Peterson, C. S. (1987). Antenatal diagnosis of fetal pelvic kidneys. *Journal of Ultrasound in Medicine*, **6**, 393–6.

Hill, L. M., *et al.* (1985). Prenatal detection of congenital malformations by ultrasonography: Mayo Clinic experience. *American Journal of Obstetrics and Gynecology*, **152**, 44–50.

Hill, L. M., Thomas, M. L., and Peterson, C. S. (1987). The ultrasonic detection of Apert syndrome. *Journal of Ultrasound in Medicine*, **6**, 601–4.

Hill, L. M., Kislak, S., and Jones, N. (1988). Prenatal ultrasound diagnosis of a forearm constriction band. *Journal of Ultrasound in Medicine*, **7**, 293–5.

Hill, L. M., Kislak, S., and Belfar, H. L. (1990). The sonographic diagnosis of urachal cysts *in utero*. *Journal of Clinical Ultrasound*, **18**, 434–7.

Hill, S. J. and Hirsch, J. H. (1985). Sonographic detection of fetal hydrometrocolpos. *Journal of Ultrasound in Medicine*, **4**, 323–5.

Hilpert, P. L., *et al.* (1990). Prenatal diagnosis of agenesis of the corpus callosum using transvaginal ultrasound. *Journal of Ultrasound in Medicine*, **9**, 363–5.

Hirose, K., Koyanagi, T., Hara, K., Inoue, M., and Nakano, H. (1988). Antenatal ultrasound diagnosis of the femur–fibula–ulna syndrome. *Journal of Clinical Ultrasound*, **16**, 199–203.

Hobbins, J. C., *et al.* (1984). Antenatal diagnosis of renal anomalies with ultrasound I. Obstructive uropathy. *American Journal of Roentgenology*, **148**, 868–77.

Hogdall, C., Siegl-Bartelt, J., Toi, A., and Ritchie, S. (1989). Prenatal diagnosis of Opitz (BBB) syndrome in the second trimester by ultrasound detection of hypospadias and hypertelorism. *Prenatal Diagnosis*, **9**, 783–93.

Holmes, R. D., Wilson, G. N., and Hajra, A. K. (1987). Peroxisomal enzyme deficiency in the Conradi–Hunerman form of chondrodysplasia punctata. *New England Journal of Medicine*, **316**, 1608.

Holzgreve, W. (1985). Prenatal diagnosis of persistent common cloaca with prune belly and anencephaly in the second trimester. *American Journal of Medical Genetics*, **20**, 729–32.

Holzgreve, W., Mahony, B. S., Glick, P. L., *et al.* (1985). Sonographic demonstration of fetal sacrococcygeal teratoma. *Prenatal Diagnosis*, **5**, 245–57.

Hubbard, A. E., Ayers, A. B., MacDonald, L. M., and James, C. E. (1984). *In utero* torsion of the testis: antenatal and postnatal ultrasonic appearances. *British Journal of Radiology*, **57**, 644–6.

Hunziker, U. A., Savoldelli, G., Bolthauser, E., Giedion, A., and Schinzel, A. (1989). Prenatal diagnosis of Schwartz–Jampel syndrome with early manifestation. *Prenatal Diagnosis*, **9**, 127–31.

Iaccarino, M., Lonardo, F., Giugliano, M., and Brunna, M. D. (1985). Prenatal diagnosis of Mohr syndrome by ultrasonography. *Prenatal Diagnosis*, **5**, 415–18.

Iaccarino, M., Baldi, F., Persico, O., and Palagiano, A. (1986). Ultrasonographic and pathologic study of mucoid degeneration of umbilical cord. *Journal of Clinical Ultrasound*, **14**, 127–9.

Ives, E. J. and Houston, C. S. (1980). Autosomal recessive microcephaly and micromelia in Cree Indians. *American Journal of Medical Genetics*, **7**, 351.

Izquierdo, L. A., Kushnir, O., Aase, J., Lantz, P., Castellano, T., and Curet, L. B. (1990). Antenatal ultrasonic diagnosis of dyssegmental dysplasia: a case report. *Prenatal Diagnosis*, **10**, 587–92.

Jaffe, R., Schoenfeld, A., and Ovadia, J. (1990). Sonographic findings in the prenatal diagnosis of bladder exstrophy. *American Journal of Obstetrics and Gynecology*, **162**, 675–8.

Jauniaux, E., Campbell, S., and Vyas, S. (1989). The use of color Doppler imaging for prenatal diagnosis of umbilical cord anomalies: report of three cases. *American Journal of Obstetrics and Gynaecology*, **161**, 1195–7.

Jauniaux, E., Vyas, S., Finlayson, C., Moscoso, G., Driver, M., and Campbell, S. (1990). Early sonographic diagnosis of body stalk anomaly. *Prenatal Diagnosis*, **10**, 127–32.

Jeanty, P. (1990). Prenatal detection of Simian Crease. *Journal of Ultrasound in Medicine*, **9**, 131–6.

Jeanty, P. and Kleinman, G. (1989). Proximal femoral focal deficiency. *Journal of Ultrasound in Medicine*, **8**, 639–42.

Jeanty, P., Kepple, D., Roussis, P., and Shah, D. (1990). *In utero* detection of cardiac failure from an aneurysm of the vein of Galen. *American Journal of Obstetrics and Gynecology*, **163**, 50–1.

Jenkinson, E. L., *et al.* (1943). A prenatal diagnosis of osteopetrosis. *American Journal of Roentgenology*, **49**, 455.

Johnson, M. L., Dunne, M. G., Mack, L. A., and Rashbaum, C. L. (1980). Evaluation of fetal intracranial anatomy by static and real-time ultrasound. *Journal of Clinical Ultrasound*, **8**, 311–12.

Johnson, V. P. and Holzwarth, D. R. (1984). Prenatal diagnosis of Meckel syndrome: case reports and literature review. *American Journal of Medical Genetics*, **18**, 699–711.

Jones, S. M., Robinson, L. K., and Sperrazza, R. (1990). Prenatal diagnosis of a skeletal dysplasia identified postnatally as hypochondroplasia. *American Journal of Medical Genetics*, **36**, 404–7.

Journel, H., Guyot, C., Barc, R. M., Belbeoch, P., Quemener, A., and Jouan, H. (1989). Unexpected ultrasonographic prenatal diagnosis of autosomal dominant polycystic kidney disease. *Prenatal Diagnosis*, **9**, 663–71.

Kalugdan, R. G., Satoh, S., Koyanagi, T., Shinzato, Y., and Nakano, H. (1989). Antenatal diagnosis of pulmonary arteriovenous fistula using real-time ultrasound and color Doppler flow imaging. *Journal of Clinical Ultrasound*, **17**, 607–14.

Kapoor, R., *et al.* (1989*a*). Antenatal sonographic diagnosis of chorioangioma of placenta. *Australian Radiol.*, **33**, 288–9.

Kapoor, R., Saha, M. M., and Mandal, A. K. (1989*b*). Antenatal sonographic detection of Wolffian duct cyst. *Journal of Clinical Ultrasound*, **17**, 515–17.

Kapur, S. and Van Vloten, A. (1986). Isolated congenital bowed long bones. *Clinical Genetics*, **29**, 165–7.

Katz, S., *et al.* (1988). Prenatal gastric dilatation and infantile hypertrophic pyloric stenosis. *Journal of Pediatric Surgery*, **23**, 1021–2.

Kennedy, K. A., Flick, K. J., and Thurmond, A. S. (1990). First trimester diagnosis of exencephaly. *American Journal of Obstetrics and Gynecology*, **162**, 461–3.

Khouzam, M. N. and Hooker, J. G. (1989). The significance of prenatal diagnosis of choroid plexus cysts. *Prenatal Diagnosis*, **9**, 213–16.

Kirk, J. S. and Comstock, C. H. (1990). Antenatal sonographic appearance of spondyl-oepiphyseal dysplasia congenita. *Journal of Ultrasound in Medicine*, **9**, 173–5.

Kirkinen, P. and Jouppila, P. (1986). Intrauterine membranous cyst: a report of antenatal diagnosis and obstetric aspects in two cases. *Obstetrics and Gynecology*, **67**, 265–305.

Kirkinen, P., *et al.* (1987). Early prenatal diagnosis of a lethal syndrome of multiple congenital contractives. *Prenatal Diagnosis*, **7**, 189–96.

Kishi, F., Matsuura, S., Murano, I., Akita, A., and Kajii, T. (1991). Prenatal diagnosis of infantile hypophosphatasia. *Prenatal Diagnosis*, **11**, 305–9.

Kitchiner, D., Leung, M. P., and Arnold, R. (1990). Isolated congenital left ventricular diverticulum: echocardiographic features in a fetus. *American Heart Journal*, **119**, 1435–7.

Kjoller, M., Holm-Nielsen, G., Meiland, H., Mauritzen, K., Berget, A., and Hancke, S. (1985). Prenatal obstruction of the ileum diagnosed by ultrasound. *Prenatal Diagnosis*, **5**, 427–30.

Kleiner, B., Callen, P. W., and Filly, R. A. (1987). Sonographic analysis of the fetus with ureteropelvic junction obstruction. *American Journal of Roentgenology*, **148**, 359–63.

Kleinman, C. S., Donnerstein, R. L., Devore, G. V., *et al.* (1982). Fetal echocardiography for evaluation of *in utero* congestive heart failure. *New England Journal of Medicine*, **306**, 568–75.

Kleinman, C. S., Donnerstein, R. L., Jaffe, C. C., *et al.* (1983). Fetal echocardiography. A tool for evaluation of *in utero* cardiac arrythmias and monitoring of *in utero* therapy: analysis of 71 patients. *American Journal of Cardiology*, **51**, 237–43.

Klingensmith, W. C., Cioffi-Ragan, D. T., and Harvey, D. E. (1988). Diagnosis of ectopia cordis in the second trimester. *Journal of Clinical Ultrasound*, **16**, 204–6.

Koga, Y., *et al.* (1990). Prenatal diagnosis of fetal intracranial calcifications. *American Journal of Obstetrics and Gynecology*, **163**, 1543–5.

Kohler, R., Sousa, P., and Jorge, C. S. (1989). Prenatal diagnosis of the ectodactyly, ectodermal dysplasia, cleft palate (EEC) syndrome. *Journal of Ultrasound in Medicine*, **8**, 337–9.

Komarniski, C. A., Cyr, D. R., Mack, L. A., and Weinberger, E. (1990). Prenatal diagnosis of schizencephaly. *Journal of Ultrasound in Medicine*, **9**, 305–7.

Kourides, L. A., Berkowitz, R. L., Pang, S., Van Natta, F. C., Barone, C. M., and Ginsberg-Fellner, F. (1984). Antepartum diagnosis of goitrous hypothyroidism by fetal ultrasonography and amniotic fluid thyrotrophin concentration. *Journal of Clinical Endocrinology and Metabolism*, **59**, 1016–18.

Kurjak, A. and Latin, V. (1979). Ultrasound diagnosis of fetal abnormalities in multiple pregnancy. *Acta Obstetrica et Gynaecologica Scandinavica*, **58**, 153.

Kurtz, A. B., Filly, R. A., Wapner, R. J., Golbus, M. S., Rifkin, M. R., Callen, P. W., *et al.* (1986). *In utero* analysis of heterozygous achondroplasia: variable time of onset as detected by femur length measurements. *Journal of Ultrasound in Medicine*, **5**, 137–40.

Kushnir, O., Izquierdo, L., Vigil, D., and Curet, L. B. (1990). Early transvaginal sonographic diagnosis of gastroschisis. *Journal of Clinical Ultrasound*, **18**, 194–7.

Kutzner, D. K., Wilson, W. G., and Hogge, W. A. (1988). OEIS complex (cloacal exstrophy): prenatal diagnosis in the second trimester. *Prenatal Diagnosis*, **8**, 247–53.

Landy, H. J., Khoury, A. N., and Heyl, P. S. (1989). Antenatal ultrasonographic diagnosis of fetal seizure activity. *American Journal of Obstetrics and Gynecology*, **161**, 308.

Langer, R., and Kaufmann, H. J. (1986). Case report 363. Infantile cortical hyperostosis (Caffey disease ICH) of iliac bones, femora, tibiae and left fibula. *Skeletal Radiology*, **15**, 377–82.

Laxova, R., *et al.* (1973). Family with probable achondrogenesis and lipid inclusions in fibroblasts. *Archives of Disease in Childhood*, **48**, 212.

Lebrun, D., *et al.* (1985). Prenatal diagnosis of a pulmonary cyst by ultrasonography. *European Journal of Pediatrics*, **144**, 399–402.

Leithiser, R. E. Jr, Fyfe, D., Weatherby, E., Sade, R., and Garvin, A. J. (1986). Prenatal sonographic diagnosis of atrial hemangioma. *American Journal of Roentgenology*, **147**, 1207–8.

Lewis, B. D., Doubilet, P. M., Heller, V. L., Bierre, A., and Bieber, F. R. (1986). Cutaneous and visceral hemangiomata in the Klippel–Trenaunay–Weber syndrome: antenatal sonographic detection. *American Journal of Roentgenology*, **147**, 598–600.

Lichman, J. P. and Miller, E. I. (1988). Prenatal ultrasonic diagnosis of a splenic cyst. *Journal of Ultrasound in Medicine*, **7**, 637–8.

Lien, J. M., Colmorgen, G. H. C., Gehret, J. F., and Evantash, A. B. (1990). Spontaneous resolution of fetal pleural effusion diagnosed during the second trimester. *Journal of Clinical Ultrasound*, **18**, 54–6.

Lindfors, K. K., McGahan, J. P., and Walter, J. P. (1986). Fetal omphalocele and gastroschisis: pitfalls in sonographic diagnosis. *American Journal of Roentgenology*, **147**, 797–800.

Lingman, G., *et al.* (1986). Fetal cardiac arrhythmia. Clinical outcome in 113 cases. *Acta Obstetrica et Gynaecologica Scandinavica*, **65**, 263–7.

Lituania, M., Cordone, M., Zampatti, C., Passimonti U., and Santi, F. (1988). Prenatal diagnosis of a rare heteropagus. *Prenatal Diagnosis*, **8**, 547–51.

Lituania, M., Passamonti, U., Cordone, M. S., Magnano, G. M., and Toma, P. (1989). Schizencephaly: prenatal diagnosis by computed tomography and magnetic resonance imaging. *Prenatal Diagnosis*, **9**, 649–55.

Lockwood, C., Irons, M., Troiani, I., Kawada, C., Chaudhury, A., and Cetrulo, C. (1988). The prenatal sonographic diagnosis of lethal multiple pterygium syndrome: a heritable cause of recurrent abortion. *American Journal of Obstetrics and Gynecology*, **159**, 474–6.

Loewy, J. A., Richards, D. G., and Toi, A. (1987). *In utero* diagnosis of the caudal regression syndrome: report of three cases. *Journal of Clinical Ultrasound*, **15**, 469–74.

Loverro, G., Guanti, G., Caruso, G., and Selvaggi, L. (1990). Robinow's syndrome: prenatal diagnosis. *Prenatal Diagnosis*, **10**, 121–6.

Luthy, D. A., Mack, I., Hirsch, J., *et al.* (1981). Prenatal ultrasound diagnosis of thrombocytopenia with absent radii. *American Journal of Obstetrics and Gynecology*, **141**, 3350–1.

McAlister, W. H., Wright, J. R. Jr, and Crane, J. P. (1987). Main-stem bronchial atresia: intrauterine sonographic diagnosis. *American Journal of Roentgenology*, **148**, 364–6.

McFarland, S. L. (1929). Congenital dislocation of the knee. *Journal of Bone and Joint Surgery*, 11, 281.

McGahan, J. P. and Hanson, J. (1983). Meconium peritonitis with accompanying pseudocyst: Prenatal sonographic diagnosis. *Radiology*, **148**, 125–6.

McGahan, J. P. and Schneider, J. M. (1986). Fetal neck hemangioendothelioma with secondary hydrops fetalis: sonographic diagnosis. *Journal of Clinical Ultrasound*, **14**, 384–8.

McGahan, J. P., Haesslein, H. C., Meyers, M., and Ford, K. B. (1984). Sonographic recognition of *in utero* intraventricular haemorrhage. *American Journal of Roentgenology*, **142**, 171–3.

McGahan, J. P., *et al.* (1988). Prenatal sonographic diagnosis of VATER association. *Journal of Clinical Ultrasound*, **16**, 588–91.

McGahan, J. P., Nyberg, D. A., and Mack, L. A. (1990). Sonography of facial features of alobar and semilobar holoprosencephaly. *American Journal of Roentgenology*, **154**, 143–8.

Mack, L., Gottesfeld, K., and Johnson, M. L. (1978). Antenatal detection of ectopic fetal liver by ultrasound. *Journal of Clinical Ultrasound*, **6**, 226–7.

Macken, M. B., Grantmyre, E. B., and Vincer, M. J. (1989). Regression of nuchal cystic hygroma *in utero*. Journal of Ultrasound in Medicine, **8**, 101–3.

McRae, S. M., *et al.* (1982). Intrauterine skull fracture diagnosed by ultrasound. *Australia and New Zealand Journal of Obstetrics and Gynecology*, **22**, 159–60.

Mahoney, M. J. and Hobbins, J. C. (1977). Prenatal diagnosis of chondroectodermal dysplasia (Ellis–van Creveld syndrome) with fetoscopy and ultrasound. *New England Journal of Medicine*, **297**, 258–60.

Mahony, B. S., *et al.* (1984*a*). Antenatal sonographic diagnosis of achondrogenesis. *Journal of Ultrasound in Medicine*, **3**, 333–5.

Mahony, B. S., Filly, R. A., Callen, P. W., Chinn, D. H., and Golbus, M. S. (1984*b*). Severe nonimmune hydrops fetalis: sonographic evaluation. *Radiology*, **151**, 757–61.

Mahony, B. S., Filly, R. A., Callen, P. W., and Golbus, M. S. (1985*a*). The amniotic band syndrome: Antenatal sonographic diagnosis and potential pitfalls. *American Journal of Obstetrics and Gynecology*, **152**, 63–8.

Mahony, B. S., Filly, R. A., Callen, P. W., and Golbus, M. S. (1985*b*). Thanatophoric dwarfism with the cloverleaf skull: a specific antenatal sonographic diagnosis. *Journal of Ultrasound in Medicine*, **4**, 151–4.

Majoor-Krakauer, D. F., *et al.* (1987). Microcephaly, micrognathia, and bird-headed dwarfism: Prenatal diagnosis of a Seckel-like syndrome. *American Journal of Medical Genetics*, **27**, 183–8.

Malinger, G., Rosen, N., Achiron, R., and Zakut, H. (1987). Pierre Robin sequence associated with amniotic band syndrome. Ultrasonographic diagnosis and pathogenesis. *Prenatal Diagnosis*, **7**, 455–9.

Mann, L., Alroomi, L., McNay, M., and Ferguson-Smith, M. A. (1983). Placental haemangioma: Case report. *British Journal of Obstetrics and Gynaecology*, **90**, 983–6.

Mao, K. and Adams, J. (1983). Antenatal diagnosis of intracranial arteriovenous fistula by ultrasonography. Case report. *British Journal of Obstetrics and Gynecology*, **90**, 872–3.

Marino, J., Martinez-Urrutia, M. J., Hawkins, F., and Gonzalez, A. (1990). Encysted adrenal haemorrhage. Prenatal diagnosis. *Acta Paediatrica Scandinavica*, **79**, 230–1.

Mariona, F., McAlpin, G., Zador, I., Philippart, A., and Jafri, S. Z. H. (1986). Sonographic detection of fetal extrathoracic pulmonary sequestration. *Journal of Ultrasound in Medicine*, **5**, 283–5.

Marks, F., Hernanz-Schulman, M., Horii, S., *et al.* (1989). Spondylothoracic dysplasia. Clinical and sonographic diagnosis. *Journal of Ultrasound in Medicine*, **8**, 1–5.

Marks, F., Thomas, P., Lustig, I., Greco, M. A., Raghavendra, B. N., and Wasserman, R. (1990). *In utero* sonographic description of a fetal liver adenoma. *Journal of Ultrasound in Medicine*, **9**, 119–22.

Martincic, N. (1952). Case reports: osteopoikilosis (spotted bones). *British Journal of Radiology*, **25**, 612.

Meizner, I. and Bar-Ziv, J. (1985). Prenatal ultrasonic diagnosis of short-rib polydactyly syndrome (SRPS) type III: a case report and a proposed approach to the diagnosis of SRPS and related conditions. *Journal of Clinical Ultrasound*, **13**, 284–7.

Meizner, I. and Bar-Ziv, J. (1987). Prenatal ultrasonic diagnosis of a rare case of iniencephaly apertus. *Journal of Clinical Ultrasound*, **15**, 200–3.

Meizner, I., Bar-Ziv, J., and Katz, M. (1985). Prenatal ultrasonic diagnosis of the extreme form of prune belly syndrome. *Journal of Clinical Ultrasound*, **13**, 581–3.

Meizner, I., Bar-Ziv, J., Barki, Y., and Abeliovich, D. (1986a). Prenatal ultrasonic diagnosis of radial-ray aplasia and renal anomalies (acrorenal syndrome). *Prenatal Diagnosis*, **6**, 223–5.

Meizner, I., Carmi, R., and Bar-Ziv, J. (1986b). Congenital chylothorax—prenatal ultrasonic diagnosis and successful post partum management. *Prenatal Diagnosis*, **6**, 217–21.

Meizner, I., Barki, Y., and Hertzanu, Y. (1987). Prenatal sonographic diagnosis of agenesis of corpus callosum. *Journal of Clinical Ultrasound*, **15**, 262–4.

Meizner, I., *et al.* (1989). Prenatal ultrasonic detection of short rib polydactyly syndrome type I. A case report. *Journal of Reproductive Medicine*, **34**, 668–72.

Menashe, Y., Baruch, G. B., Rabinovitch, O., Shalev, Y., Katzenlson, H. B. M., and Shalev, E. (1989). Exophthalmous—prenatal ultrasonic features for diagnosis of Crouzon syndrome. *Prenatal Diagnosis*, **9**, 805–8.

Mennuti, M. T., Zackai, E. H., Curtis, M. T., Giardine, R. M., and Driscoll, D. A. (1990). Early ultrasound diagnosis of Neu–Laxova syndrome. *American Journal of Human Genetics*, **47**, A281.

Merlob, P., Schonfeld, A., Grunebaum, M., Mor, N., and Reisner, S. H. (1987). Autosomal dominant cerebro–costo–mandibular syndrome: ultrasonographic and clinical findings. *American Journal of Medical Genetics*, **26**, 195–202.

Mintz, M. C., Arger, P. H., and Coleman, B. G. (1985). *In utero* sonographic diagnosis of intracerebral haemorrhage. *Journal of Ultrasound in Medicine*, **4**, 375–6.

Miro, J., and Bard, H. (1988). Congenital atresia and stenosis of the duodenum: the impact of a prenatal diagnosis. *American Journal of Obstetrics and Gynecology*, **158**, 555–9.

Moodley, T. R., *et al.* (1986). Congenital heart block detected *in utero*. A case report. *South African Medical Journal*, **70**, 433–4.

Morin, P. R. (1981). Prenatal detection of the autosomal recessive type of polycystic kidney disease by trehalase assay in amniotic fluid. *Prenatal Diagnosis*, **1**, 5–9.

Morse, R. P., Rawnsley, E., Crowe, H. C., Marin-Padilla, M., and Graham, J. M. (1987a). Bilateral renal agenesis in three consecutive siblings. *Prenatal Diagnosis*, **7**, 573–9.

Morse, R. P., Rawnsley, E., Sargent, S. K., and Graham, J. M. (1987b). Prenatal diagnosis of a new syndrome: holoprosencephaly with hypokinesia. *Prenatal Diagnosis*, **7**, 631–8.

Mostello, D., Hoechstetter, L., Bendon, R. W., *et al.* (1991). Prenatal diagnosis of recurrent Larsen syndrome: further definition of a lethal variant. *Prenatal Diagnosis*, **11**, 215–25.

Mulligan, G. and Meier, P. (1989). Lipoma and agenesis of the corpus callosum with associated choroid plexus lipomas. *In utero* diagnosis. *Journal of Ultrasound in Medicine*, **8**, 583–8.

Munoz, C., Filly, R. A., and Golbus, M. S. (1990). Osteogenesis imperfecta type II: prenatal sonographic diagnosis. *Radiology*, **174**, 181–5.

Nakamoto, S. K., *et al.* (1983). The sonographic appearance of hepatic hemangioma *in utero*. *Journal of Ultrasound in Medicine*, **2**, 239–41.

Nancarrow, P. A., Mattrey, R. F., Edwards, D. K., and Skram, C. (1985). Fibroadhesive meconium peritonitis: *in utero* sonographic diagnosis. *Journal of Ultrasound Medicine*, **4**, 213–15.

Narayan, H. and Scott, I. V. (1991). Prenatal ultrasound diagnosis of Apert's syndrome. *Prenatal Diagnosis*, **10**, 187–92.

Neilson, J. P., Danskin, F., and Hastie, S. J. (1989). Monozygotic twin pregnancy: diagnostic and Doppler ultrasound studies. *British Journal of Obstetrics and Gynaecology*, **96**, 1413–18.

Newnham, J. P., Crues, J. V. III, Vinstein, A. L., and Medearis, A. L. (1984). Sonographic diagnosis of thoracic gastroenteric cyst *in utero*. *Prenatal Diagnosis*, **4**, 467–71.

Nguyen, D. L. and Leonard, J. C. (1986). Ischemic hepatic necrosis: a cause of fetal liver calcification. *American Journal of Roentgenology*, **147**, 596–7.

Nicolaides, K. H., Johansson, D., Donnai, D., and Rodeck, C. H. (1984). Prenatal diagnosis of mandibulofacial dysostosis. *Prenatal Diagnosis*, **4**, 201–5.

Nicolaides, K. H., Campbell, S., Gabbe, S. G., and Guidetti, R. (1986). Ultrasound screening for spina bifida: cranial and cerebellar signs. *Lancet*, **ii**, 72–4.

Novelli, G., Frontali, M., Baldini, D., Bosman, C., Dallapiccola, B., Pachi, A., and Torcia, F. (1989). Prenatal diagnosis of adult polycystic kidney disease with DNA markers on chromosome 16 and the genetic heterogeneity problem. *Prenatal Diagnosis*, **9**, 759–67.

Nyberg, D. A., Hastrup, W., Watts, H., and Mack, L. A. (1987). Dilated fetal bowel. A sonographic sign of cystic fibrosis. *Journal of Ultrasound in Medicine*, **6**, 257–60.

Nyberg, D. A., *et al.* (1990*a*). Meckel–Gruber syndrome. Importance of prenatal diagnosis. *Journal of Ultrasound in Medicine*, **9**, 691–6.

Nyberg, D. A., Resta, R. G., Luthy, D. A., *et al.* (1990*b*). Prenatal sonographic findings of Down syndrome: review of 94 cases. *Obstetrics and Gynecology*, **76**, 370–7.

Ohdo, S., Madokoro, H., Sonoda, T., Takei, M., Yasuda, H., and Mori, N. (1987). Association of tetra-amelia, octodermal dysplasia, hypoplastic lacrimal ducts and sacs opening towards the exterior, peculiar face and developmental retardation. *Journal of Medical Genetics*, **24**, 609–12.

Ohlsson, A., Fong, K. W., Rose, T. H., and Moore D. C. (1988). Prenatal sonographic diagnosis of Pena–Shokeir syndrome type I or fetal akinesia deformation sequence. *American Journal of Medical Genetics*, **29**, 59–65.

Ordorica, S. A., Marks, F., Frieden, F. J., Hoskins, I. A, and Young, B. K. (1990). Aneurysm of the vein of Galen: a new cause for Ballantyne syndrome. *American Journal of Obstetrics and Gynecology*, **162**, 1166–7.

Pachi, A., Giancotti, A., Torcia, F., De Prosperi, V., and Maggi, E. (1989). Meckel–Gruber syndrome: ultrasonographic diagnosis at 13 weeks' gestational age in an at-risk case. *Prenatal Diagnosis*, **9**, 187–90.

Pagliano, M., Mossetti, M., and Ragno, P. (1990) Echographic diagnosis of omphalocele in the first trimester of pregnancy. *Journal of Clinical Ultrasound*, **18**, 658–60.

Patel, P. J., Kolawole, T. M., Ba'Aqueel, H. S., and Al-Jisi, N. (1989). Antenatal sonographic findings of congenital chloride diarrhoea. *Journal of Clinical Ultrasound*, **17**, 115–18.

Patel, R. B. and Connors, J. J. (1988). *In utero* sonographic findings in fetal renal vein thrombosis with calcifications. *Journal of Ultrasound in Medicine*, **7**, 349–52.

Patten, R. M., Mack, L. A., Nyberg, D. A., and Filly, R. A. (1989). Twin embolisation syndrome: prenatal sonographic detection and significance. *Radiology*, **173**, 685–9.

Patton, M. A., Baraitser, M., Nicolaides, K., Rodeck, C. H., and Gamsu, H. (1986). Prenatal treatment of fetal hydrops associated with the hypertelorism–dysphagia syndrome (Opitz-G syndrome). *Prenatal Diagnosis*, **6**, 109–15.

Peleg, D., *et al.* (1985). Fetal hydrothorax and bilateral pulmonary hypoplasia. Ultrasonic diagnosis. *Acta Obstetrica et Gynaecologica Scandinavica*, **64**, 451–3.

Pennel, R. G. and Baltarowich, O. H. (1986). Prenatal sonographic diagnosis of a fetal facial haemangioma. *Journal of Ultrasound in Medicine*, **5**, 525–8.

Persutte, W. H., Lenke, R. R., Kurczynski, T. W., and Brinker, R. A. (1988*a*). Antenatal diagnosis of Pena–Shokeir syndrome (type I) with ultrasonography and magnetic resonance imaging. *Obstetrics and Gynecology*, **72**, 472–5.

Persutte, W. H., *et al.* (1988*b*). Antenatal diagnosis of fetal patent urachus. *Journal of Ultrasound in Medicine*, **7**, 399–403.

Petres, R. E., Redwine, F. O., and Cruikshank, D. P. (1982). Congenital bilateral chylothorax. Antepartum diagnosis and successful intrauterine surgical management. *Journal of the American Medical Association*, **248**, 1360–1.

Petrikovsky, B. M., Walzak, M. P., and D'Addario, P. F. (1988). Fetal cloacal anomalies: prenatal sonographic findings and differential diagnosis. *Obstetrics and Gynecology*, **72**, 464–9.

Petrikovsky, B. M., Vintzileos, A. M. and Rodis, J. F. (1989). Sonographic appearance of occipital fetal hair. *Journal of Clinical Ultrasound*, **17**, 425–7.

Piepkorn, M., *et al.* (1977). A lethal neonatal dwarfing condition with short ribs, polysyndactyly, cranial synostosis, cleft palate, cardiovascular and urogenital anomalies and severe ossification defect. *Teratology*, **16**, 345.

Pilu, G., Reece, A., Romero, R., Bovicelli, L., and Hobbins, J. C. (1986*a*). Prenatal diagnosis of craniofacial malformations with ultrasonography. *American Journal of Obstetrics and Gynecology*, **155**, 45–50.

Pilu, G., Romero, R., Reece, A., Jeanty, P., and Hobbins, J. C. (1986*b*). The prenatal diagnosis of Robin anomalad. *American Journal of Obstetrics and Gynecology*, **154**, 630–2.

Pircon, R. A., Porto, M., Towers, C. V., Crade, M. L., and Gocke, S. E. (1989). Ultrasound findings in pregnancies complicated by fetal triploidy. *Journal of Ultrasound in Medicine* **8**, 507–11.

Pope, F. M., Daw, S. C. M., Narcisi, P., Richards, A. R., and Nicholls, A. C. (1989). Prenatal diagnosis and prevention of inherited disorders of collagen. *Journal of Inherited Metabolic Disease*, **12** (suppl 1), 135–73.

Pretorius, D. H., *et al.* (1986). Specific skeletal dysplasia *in utero*: sonographic diagnosis. *Radiology*, **159**, 237–42.

Pretorius, D. H., Drose, J. A., Dennis, M. A., Manchester, D. K., and Manco-Johnson, M.-L. (1987). Tracheoesophageal fistula *in utero*: Twenty-two cases. *Journal of Ultrasound in Medicine*, **6**, 509–13.

Pretorius, D., Manchester, D., Barkin, S., Parker, S., and Nelson, T. R. (1988). Doppler ultrasound of twin transfusion syndrome. *Journal of Ultrasound in Medicine*, **7**, 117–24.

Preus, M., Kaplan, P., and Kirkham, T. H. (1977). Renal anomalies and oligohydramnios in the cerebro–oculofacio–skeletal syndrome. *American Journal of Diseases of Children*, **131**, 62–4.

Quagliarello, J. R., Passalaqua, A. M., Greco, M. A., Zinberg, S., and Young, B. K. (1978). Ballantyne's triple colesia syndrome: prenatal diagnosis with ultrasound and maternal renal biopsy findings. *American Journal of Obstetrics and Gynecology*, **132**, 580–1.

Quigg, M. H., Evans, M. I., Zador, I., Budev, I., Belsky, R., Niederlueke, D., *et al.* (1985). Ultrasonographic prenatal diagnosis of Langer-type mesomelic dwarfism. *American Journal of Human Genetics*, **37**, A225.

Quinlan, R. W., Cruz, A. C., and Huddleston, J. F. (1986). Sonographic detection of fetal urinary tract anomalies. *Obstetrics and Gynecology*, **67**, 558–65.

Ramsing, M., Rehd, H., Holzgreve, W., Meinecke, P., and Lenz, W. (1990). Fraser syndrome (crytophthalmos with syndactyly) in the fetus and newborn. *Clinical Genetics*, **37**, 84–96.

Rasore-Quartino, A., *et al.* (1985). Hereditary enlarged parietal foramina (foramina parietalia permagna). Prenatal diagnosis, evolution and family study. *Pathologica*, **77**, 449–55.

Reiter, A. A., Hunta, J. C., Carpenter, R. J., Segall, G. K., and Hawkins, E. P. (1986). Prenatal diagnosis of arteriovenous malformation of the vein of Galen. *Journal of Clinical Ultrasound*, **14**, 623–8.

Rempen, A. (1989). Sonographic first-trimester diagnosis of umbilical cord cyst. *Journal of Clinical Ultrasound*, **17**, 53–5.

Rempen, A., Feige, A., and Wunsch, P. (1987). Prenatal diagnosis of bilateral cystic adenomatoid malformation of the lung. *Journal of Clinical Ultrasound*, **15**, 3–8.

Reuss, A., Den Hollander, J. C., Niermeijer, M. F., Wladimiroff, J. W., Van Diggelen, O. P., Lindhout, D., *et al.* (1989). Prenatal diagnosis of cystic renal disease with ventriculomegaly: a report of six cases in two related sibships. *American Journal of Medical Genetics*, **33**, 385–9.

Reuss, A., *et al.* (1990). Prenatal diagnosis by ultrasound in pregnancies at risk for autosomal recessive polycystic kidney disease. *Ultrasound in Medicine and Biology*, **16**, 355–9.

Ritchie, G., *et al.* (1988). Prenatal renal ultrasound of Laurence–Moon–Biedl syndrome. *Pediatric Radiology*, **19**, 65–6.

Rizzo, N., Gabrielli, S., Pilu, G., Perolo, A., Cacciari, A., Domini, R., *et al.* (1987). Prenatal diagnosis and obstetrical management of multicystic dysplastic kidney disease. *Prenatal Diagnosis*, **7**, 109–18.

Rizzo, N., Gabrielli, S., Perolo, A., Pilu, G., Cacciari, A., Domini, R., *et al.* (1989). Prenatal diagnosis and management of fetal ovarian cysts. *Prenatal Diagnosis*, **9**, 97–104.

Rizzo, G., Arduini, D., Pennestri, F., Romaninic, and Mancuso, S. (1987). Fetal behaviour in growth retardation: its relationship to fetal blood flow. *Prenatal Diagnosis*, **7**, 229.

Robertson, D. A., *et al.* (1989). Ebstein's anomaly: echocardiographic and clinical features in the fetus and neonate. *Journal of the American College of Cardiology*, **14**, 1300–7.

Robinson, L. P., Worthen, N. J., Lachman, R. S., Adomian, G. E., and Rimoin, D. L. (1987). Prenatal diagnosis of osteogenesis imperfecta type III. *Prenatal Diagnosis*, **7**, 7–15.

Rolland, M., Sarramon, M. F., and Bloom, M. C. (1991). Astomia–agnathia–holoprosencephaly association. Prenatal diagnosis of a new case. *Prenatal Diagnosis*, **11**, 199–203.

Romero, R., Chervenak, F. A., Devore, G., Tortora, M., and Hobbins, J. C. (1981). Fetal head deformation and congenital torticollii associated with a uterine tumour. *American Journal of Obstetrics and Gynaecology*, **141**, 839–40.

Romero, R., Cullen, M., Jeanty, P., Grannum, P., Reece, E. A., Venus, I., *et al.* (1984). The diagnosis of congenital renal anomalies with ultrasound. II. Infantile polycystic kidney disease. *American Journal of Obstetrics and Gynecology*, **150**, 259–62.

Romero, R., Cullen, M., Grannum, P., Jeanty, P., Reece, E. A., Venus, I., *et al.* (1985). Antenatal diagnosis of renal anomalies with ultrasound III. Bilateral renal agenesis. *American Journal of Obstetrics and Gynecology*, **151**, 38–43.

Romero, R., Ghidini, A., Eswara, M. S., Seashore, M. R., and Hobbins, J. C. (1988). Prenatal findings in a case of spondylocostal dysplasia type I (Jarcho–Levin syndrome). *Obstetrics and Gynecology*, **71**, 988–91.

Romke, C., Froster-Iskenius, U., Heyne, K., *et al.* (1987). Roberts syndrome and SC phocomelia: a single genetic entity. *Clinical Genetics*, **31**, 170–7.

Rowley, K. A. (1955). Coronal cleft vertebra. *Journal of the Faculty of Radiologists*, **6**, 267.

Russ, P. D., Pretorius, P. M., and Johnson, M. J. (1989). Dandy–Walker syndrome: a review of fifteen cases evaluated by prenatal sonography. *American Journal of Obstetrics and Gynecology*, **161**, 401–6.

Russell, J. G. B. (1973). *Radiology in obstetrics and antenatal paediatrics*, pp. 79–80. Butterworths, London.

Saal, H. M., Deutsch, L., Herson, V., Cassidy, S. B., Greenstein, R. M., and Poole, A. (1986). The RAG syndrome: a new autosomal recessive syndrome with Robin sequence, ancreolia and profound growth and developmental delays. *American Journal of Human Genetics*, **39**, A78.

Sabbagha, R. E., Tamura, R. K., Compo, S. D., Elias, S., Salvino, C., Shkolnik, A., *et al.* (1980). Fetal cranial and craniocervical masses: Ultrasound characteristics and differential diagnosis. *American Journal of Obstetrics and Gynecology*, **138**, 511–17.

Sada, I., *et al.* (1986). Antenatal diagnosis of fetus *in fetu*. *Asia Oceania Journal of Obstetrics and Gynecology*, **12**, 353–6.

Sahn, D. J., Shenker, L., Reed, K. L., Valdez-Cruz, L. M., Sobonya, R., and Anderson, C. (1982). Prenatal ultrasound diagnosis of hypoplastic left heart syndrome *in utero* associated with hydrops fetalis. *American Heart Journal*, **104**, 1368–72.

Saltzman, D. H., Benacerraf, B. R., and Frigoletto, F. D. (1986). Diagnosis and management of fetal facial clefts. *American Journal of Obstetrics and Gynecology*, **155**, 377–9.

Saltzman, D. H., Krauss, C. M., Goldman, J. M., and Benacerraf, B. R. (1991). Prenatal diagnosis of lissencephaly. *Prenatal Diagnosis*, **11**, 139–43.

Salvo, A. F. (1981). *In utero* diagnosis of Kleeblattschadel (cloverleaf skull). *Prenatal Diagnosis*, **1**, 141–5.

Samuel, N., Dicker, D., Landman, J., Feldberg, D., and Goldman, J. A. (1986). Early diagnosis and intrauterine therapy of meconium plug syndrome in the fetus: risks and benefits. *Journal of Ultrasound in Medicine*, **5**, 425–8.

Samuel, N., Sirotta, L., Bar-Ziv, J., Dicker, D., Feldberg, D., and Goldman, J. A. (1988). The ultrasonic appearance of common pulmonary vein atresia *in utero*. *Journal of Ultrasound in Medicine*, **7**, 25–8.

Samueloff, A., Navot, D., Bickenfeld, A., and Schenker, J. G. (1987). Fryns syndrome: a predictable, lethal pattern of multiple congenital anomalies. *American Journal of Obstetrics and Gynecology*, **156**, 86–8.

Savodelli, G. and Schinzel, A. (1983). Prenatal ultrasound detection of humero–radial synostosis in a case of Antley–Bixler syndrome. *Prenatal Diagnosis*, **2**, 219–33.

Schaffer, R. M., Cabbad, M., Minkoff, H., Schiller, M., Haller, J. O. and Shapiro, A. J. (1986). Sonographic diagnosis of fetal cardiac rhabdomyoma. *Journal of Ultrasound in Medicine*, **5**, 531–3.

Schauer, G. M., Dunn, L. K., Godmilow, L., *et al.* (1990). Prenatal diagnosis of Fraser syndrome at 18.5 weeks gestation with autopsy findings at 19 weeks. *American Journal of Medical Genetics*, **37**, 583–91.

Schechter, A. G., Fakhry, J., Shapiro, L. R., and Gewitz, M. H. (1987). *In utero* thickening of the chordae tendenae: a cause of intracardiac echogenic foci. *Journal of Ultrasound in Medicine*, **6**, 691–5.

Schinzel, A., Savoldelli, G., Briner, J., Sigg, P., and Massini, C. (1983). Antley–Bixler syndrome in sisters: a term newborn and a prenatally diagnosed fetus. *American Journal of Medical Genetics*, **14**, 139–47.

Schinzel, A., Savodelli, G., Briner, J., and Schubiger, G. (1985). Prenatal sonographic diagnosis of Jeune syndrome. *Radiology*, **154**, 777–8.

Schmidt, K. G., Birk, E., Silverman, N. H., and Scagnelli, S. A. (1989). Echocardiographic evaluation of dilated cardiomyopathy in the human fetus. *American Journal of Cardiology*, **63**, 599–605.

Schmidt, W., Harms, E., and Wolf, D. (1985). Successful prenatal treatment of non-immune hydrops fetalis due to congenital chylothorax. Case report. *British Journal of Obstetrics and Gynaecology*, **92**, 685–7.

Schroeder, D., *et al.* (1989). Antenatal diagnosis of choledochal cyst at 15 weeks' gestation: etiologic implications and management. *Journal of Pediatric Surgery*, **24**, 936–8.

Schutgens, R. B. H., Schrakamp, G., Wanders, R. J. A., Heymans, H. S. A., Tager, J. M., and Van den Bosch, H. (1989). Prenatal and perinatal diagnosis of peroxisomal disorders. *Journal of Inherited Metabolic Disease*, **12**(suppl 1), 118–34.

Seeds, J. W. and Powers, S. K. (1988). Early prenatal diagnosis of familial lipo-myelomeningocele. *Obstetrics and Gynecology*, **72**, 469–71.

Seeds, J. W., Cefalo, R. C., Lies, S. C., and Koontz, W. L. (1984). Early prenatal sonographic appearance of rare thoracoabdominal eventration. *Prenatal Diagnosis*, **4**, 437–41.

Shah, Y. G. and Metlay, L. (1990). Prenatal ultrasound diagnosis of Beckwith–Wiedemann syndrome. *Journal of Clinical Ultrasound*, **18**, 597–600.

Shalev, E. (1983). Prenatal ultrasound diagnosis of intestinal calcification with imperforate anus. *Acta Obstetrica et Gynaecologica Scandinavica*, **62**, 95–6.

Shalev, E., *et al.* (1988). Klippel–Trenaunay–Weber syndrome: ultrasonic prenatal diagnosis. *Journal of Clinical Ultrasound*, **16**, 268–70.

Shalev, J., Frankel, Y., Avigad, I., and Mashiach, S. (1982). Spontaneous intestinal perforation *in utero*: ultrasonic diagnostic criteria. *American Journal of Obstetrics and Gynecology*, **144**, 855–7.

Shechter, S. A., Sherer, D. M., Geilfuss, C. J., Metlay, L. A., and Woods, J. R. (1990).

Prenatal sonographic appearance and subsequent management of a fetus with oromandibular limb hypogenesis syndrome associated with pulmonary hypoplasia. *Journal of Clinical Ultrasound*, **18**, 661–5.

Shenker, L., Reed, K. L., Anderson, C. F., and Kern, W. (1989). Fetal pericardial effusion. *American Journal of Obstetrics and Gynaecology*, **160**, 1505–8.

Sherer, D. M., Menashe, M., Lebensart, P., Matoth, I., and Basel, D. (1989). Sonographic diagnosis of unilateral fetal renal duplication with associated ectopic ureterocele. *Journal of Clinical Ultrasound*, **17**, 371–3.

Sherer, D. M., Cullen, J. B. H., Thompson, H. O., Metlay, L. A., and Woods, J. R.(1990). Prenatal sonographic findings associated with a fetal horseshoe kidney. *Journal of Ultrasound in Medicine*, **9**, 477–9.

Siebert, J. R., Warkany, J., and Lemire, R. J. (1986). Atelencephalic microcephaly in a 21-week human fetus. *Teratology*, **34**, 9.

Sieck, U. V. and Ohlsson, A. (1984). Fetal polyuria and hydramnios associated with Bartter's syndrome. *Obstetrics and Gynecology*, **63**, 225.

Siffring, P. A., Forrest, T. S., and Frick, M. P. (1991). Sonographic detection of hydrolethalus syndrome. *Journal of Clinical Ultrasound*, **19**, 43–7.

Silverman, N. H., Enderlein, M. A., and Golbus, M. S. (1985). Ultrasonic recognition of aortic valve atresia *in utero*. *American Journal of Cardiology*, **53**, 391–2.

Sirtori, M., Ghidini, A., Romero, R., and Hobbins, J. C. (1989). Prenatal diagnosis of sirenomelia. *Journal of Ultrasound in Medicine*, **8**, 83–8.

Smith, H. J., *et al.* (1981). Ultrasound diagnosis of interstitial pregnancy. *Acta Obstetrica et Gynecologica Scandinavica*, **60**, 413.

Snyder, J. R., Lustig-Gillman, I., Milio, L., Morris, M., Pardes, J. G., and Young, B. K. (1986). Antenatal ultrasound diagnosis of an intracranial neoplasm (craniopharyngioma). *Journal of Clinical Ultrasound*, **14**, 304–6.

Socol, M. L., Sabbagha, R. E., Elias, S., Tamura, R. K., Simpson, J. L., Dooley, S. L., *et al.* (1985). Prenatal diagnosis of congenital muscular dystrophy producing arthrogryposis. *New England Journal of Medicine*, **313**, 1230.

Sonek, J. D., *et al.* (1990). Antenatal diagnosis of sacral agenesis syndrome in a pregnancy complicated by diabetes mellitus. *American Journal of Obstetrics and Gynecology*, **162**, 806–8.

Spear, R., Mack, L. A., Benedetti, T. J., and Cole, R. E. (1990). Idiopathic infantile arterial calcification: *in utero* diagnosis. *Journal of Ultrasound in Medicine*, **9**, 473–6.

Spirt, B. A., *et al.* (1987). *Prenatal ultrasound: a colour atlas with anatomic and pathologic correlation*. Churchill-Livingstone, Edinburgh.

Stamm, E. R., Pretorius, D. H., Rumack, C. M., and Manco-Johnson, M. L. (1987). Kleeblattschadel anomaly. *In utero* sonographic appearance. *Journal of Ultrasound in Medicine*, **6**, 319–24.

Stanford, W., Abu-Yousef, M., and Smith, W. (1987). Intracardiac tumour (rhabdomyoma) diagnosed by *in utero* ultrasound: a case report. *Journal of Clinical Ultrasound*, **15**, 337–41.

Steinfeld, L., *et al.* (1986). Diagnosis of fetal arrhythmias using echocardiographic and Doppler techniques. *Journal of the American College of Cardiology*, **9**, 1425.

Stephens, J. D. (1984). Prenatal diagnosis of testicular feminisation. *Lancet,* **ii**, 1038.

Stewart, P. A., Wladimiroff, J. W., and Becker, A. E. (1985). Early prenatal detection of double outlet right ventricle by echocardiography. *British Heart Journal*, **54**, 340–2.

Stewart, P. A., Buis-Liem, T., Verwey, R. A., and Wladimiroff, J. W. (1986). Prenatal ultrasonic diagnosis of familial asymmetric septal hypertrophy. *Prenatal Diagnosis*, **6**, 249–56.

Stiller, R. J. (1989). Early ultrasonic appearance of fetal bladder outlet obstruction. *American Journal of Obstetrics and Gynecology*, **160**, 584–5.

Stiller, R. J., Pinto, M., Heller, C., and Hobbins, J. C. (1988). Oligohydramnios associated with bilateral multicystic dysplastic kidneys: prenatal diagnosis at 15 weeks gestation. *Journal of Clinical Ultrasound*, **16**, 436–9.

Stoker, A. F., *et al.* (1983). Ultrasound diagnosis of situs inversus *in utero*. A case report. *South African Medical Journal*, **64**, 832–4.

Stoll, C., Willard, D., Czernichow, P., and Boue, J. (1985). Prenatal diagnosis of hypochondroplasia. *Prenatal Diagnosis*, **5**, 423–6.

Stoll, C., Ehret-Mentre, M. C., Treisser, A., and Tranchant, C. (1991). Prenatal diagnosis of congenital myasthenia with arthrogryposis in a myasthenic mother. *Prenatal Diagnosis*, **11**, 17–22.

Sutro, W. H., *et al.* (1984). Prenatal observation of umbilical cord hematoma. *American Journal of Roentgenology*, **142**, 801–2.

Thiagarajah, S., *et al.* (1990). Prenatal diagnosis of eventration of the diaphragm. *Journal of Clinical Ultrasound*, **18**, 46–9.

Thomas, C. S., Leopold, G. R., Hilton, S., Key, T., Coen, R., and Lynch, F. (1986). Fetal hydrops associated with extralobar pulmonary sequestration. *Journal of Ultrasound in Medicine*, **5**, 668–71.

Toftager-Larsen, K. and Benzie, R. J. (1984). Fetoscopy in prenatal diagnosis of the Majewski and the Saldino–Noonan types of the short rib–polydactyly syndromes. *Clinical Genetics*, **26**, 56–60.

Toi, A., Simpson, G. F., and Filly, R. A. (1987). Ultrasonically evident fetal nuchal skin thickening: is it specific for Down syndrome? *American Journal of Obstetrics and Gynecology*, **156**, 150–3.

Tolmie, J. L., McNay, M. B., and Connor, J. M. (1987*a*). Prenatal diagnosis of severe autosomal recessive spondylothoracic dysplasia (Jarcho–Levin type). *Prenatal Diagnosis*, **7**, 129–34.

Tolmie, J. L., McNay, M. B., Stephenson, J. B. P., Doyle, D., and Connor, J. M. (1987*b*). Microcephaly genetic counselling and antenatal diagnosis. *American Journal of Medical Genetics*, **27**, 583–94.

Tolmie, J. L., Mortimer, G., Doyle, D., McKenzie, R., McLaurin, J., and Neilson, J. P. (1987*c*). The Neu–Laxova syndrome in female sibs: clinical and pathological features with prenatal diagnosis in the second sib. *American Journal of Medical Genetics*, **27**, 175–82.

Tolmie, J. L., Patrick, A., and Yates, J. R. W. (1987*d*). A lethal multiple pterygium syndrome with apparent X-linked recessive inheritance. *American Journal of Medical Genetics*, **27**, 913–19.

Toma, P., Costa, A., Magnano, G. M., Cariati, M., and Lituania, M. (1990). Holoprosencephaly: prenatal diagnosis by sonography and magnetic resonance imaging. *Prenatal Diagnosis*, **10**, 429–36.

Toma, P., Dell'Acqua, A., Cordone, M., Passamonti, U., and Lituania, M. (1991). Prenatal diagnosis of hydrosyringomyelia by high resolution ultrasonography. *Journal of Clinical Ultrasound*, **19**, 51–4.

Tomkins, D. J. (1989). Premature centromere separation and the prenatal diagnosis of Roberts syndrome. *Prenatal Diagnosis*, **9**, 450–1.

Trecet, J. C., Claramunt, V., Larraz, J., Ruiz, E., Zuzuarregui, M., and Ugalde, F. J. (1984). Prenatal ultrasound diagnosis of fetal teratoma of the neck. *Journal of Clinical Ultrasound*, **12**, 509–11.

Tsipouras, P., Schwartz, R. C., Goldberg, J. D., Berkowitz, R. L., and Ramirez, F. (1987). Prenatal prediction of osteogenesis imperfecta (OI type IV): exclusion of inheritance using a collagen gene probe. *Journal of Medical Genetics*, **24**, 406–9.

Tuck, S. M., Slack, J., and Buckland, G. (1990). Prenatal diagnosis of Conradi's syndrome. Case report. *Prenatal Diagnosis*, **10**, 195–8.

Van Dam, L. J., *et al.* (1984). Case report. Intra-uterine demonstration of bowel duplication by ultrasound. *European Journal of Obstetrics, Gynecology and Reproductive Biology*, **18**, 229–32.

van den Hof, M. C., *et al.* (1990). Evaluation of the lemon and banana signs in one hundred and thirty fetuses with open spina bifida. *American Journal of Obstetrics and Gynecology*, **162**, 322–7.

Van Egmond-Linden, A., Wladimiroff, J. W., Jahoda, M. G. J., Niermeijer, M. F., Sachs, E. S., and Stefanko, S. (1983). Prenatal diagnosis of X-linked hydrocephaly. *Prenatal Diagnosis*, **3**, 245–8.

Van Regemorter, N., Wilkin, P., Englert, Y., *et al.* (1984). Lethal multiple pterygium syndrome. *American Journal of Medical Genetics*, **17**, 827–34.

Verma, I. C., *et al.* (1975). An autosomal recessive form of lethal chondrodystrophy with severe thoracic narrowing, rhizoacromelic type of micromelia, polydactyly, and genital anomalies. *Birth Defects*, **11**, 167.

Vermesh, M., Mayden, K. L., Confino, E., Giglia, R. V., and Gleicher, N. (1986). Prenatal sonographic diagnosis of Hirschsprung's disease. *Journal of Ultrasound in Medicine*, **5**, 37–9.

Vesce, F., Guerrini, P., Perri, G., Cavazzini, L., and Simonetti, V. (1987). Ultrasonographic diagnosis of ectasia of the umbilical vein. *Journal of Clinical Ultrasound*, **15**, 346–9.

Vintners, H. V., Murphy, J., Wittmann, B., and Norman, M. G. (1982). Intracranial teratoma: antenatal diagnosis at 31 weeks' gestation by ultrasound. *Acta Neuropathologica*, **58**, 233–6.

Vintzileos, A. M., *et al.* (1987). Congenital midline porencephaly: Prenatal sonographic findings and review of the literature. *American Journal of Perinatology*, **4**, 125.

Visser, G. H. A., Desmedt, M. C. H., and Meijboom, E. J. (1988). Altered fetal cardiac flow patterns in pure red cell anaemia (the Blackfan–Diamond syndrome). *Prenatal Diagnosis*, **8**, 525–9.

Wager, G. P., *et al.* (1988). Antenatal ultrasound findings in a case of Uhl's anomaly. *American Journal of Perinatology*, **5**, 164–7.

Weiner, C. P., Williamson, R. A., and Bonsib, S. M. (1986). Sonographic diagnosis of cloverleaf skull and thanatophoric dysplasia in the second trimester. *Journal of Clinical Ultrasound*, **14**, 463–5.

Wenstrom, K. D., Williamson, R. A., Hoover, W. W., and Grant, S. S. (1989). Achondrogenesis type II (Langer–Saldino) in association with jugular lymphatic obstruction sequence. *Prenatal Diagnosis*, **9**, 527–32.

Wexler, S., *et al.* (1985). An acardiac acephalic anomaly detected on sonography. *Acta Obstetrica et Gynecologica Scandandinavica*, **64**, 93–4.

Whitley, C. B., Burke, B. A., Granroth, G., and Gorlin, R. J. (1986). de la Chapelle dysplasia. *American Journal of Medical Genetics*, **25**, 29.

Wieacker, P., Griffin, J. E., Wienker, T., *et al.* (1987). Linkage analysis with RFLPs in families with androgen resistance syndromes: evidence for close linkage between the androgen receptor locus and the DXS1 segment. *Human Genetics*, **76**, 248–52.

Wiedeman, M. A., *et al.* (1985). Fetal sonography and neonatal scintigraphy of a choledochal cyst. *Journal of Nuclear Medicine*, **26**, 893–6.

Wiggins, J. W., Bowes, W., Clewell, W., *et al.* (1986). Echocardiographic diagnosis and intravenous digoxin management of fetal tachyarrhythmias and congestive heart failure. *American Journal of Diseases of Children*, **140**, 202–4.

Wilson, R. H. J. K., Duncan, A., Hume, R., and Bain, A. D. (1985). Prenatal pleural effusion associated with congenital pulmonary lymphangiectasia. *Prenatal Diagnosis*, **5**, 73–6.

Winn, H. N., Gabrielli, S., Reece, E. A., Roberts, J. A., Salafia, C., and Hobbins, J. C. (1989). Ultrasonographic criteria for the prenatal diagnosis of placental chorionicity in twin gestations. *American Journal of Obstetrics and Gynecology*, **161**, 1540–2.

Winter, R. K., *et al.* (1989). Diastematomyelia: prenatal ultrasonic appearances. *Clinical Radiology*, **40**, 291–4.

Winter, R. M., Campbell, S., Wigglesworth, J. S., and Nevrkla, E. J. (1987). A previously undescribed syndrome of thoracic dysplasia and communicating hydrocephalus in two sibs, one diagnosed prenatally by ultrasound. *Journal of Medical Genetics*, **24**, 204–6.

Witter, F. R. and Molteni, R. A. (1986). Intrauterine intestinal volvulus with hemoperitoneum presenting as fetal distress at 34 weeks' gestation. *American Journal of Obstetrics and Gynecology*, **155**, 1080–1.

Yagel, S., *et al.* (1986). Prenatal diagnosis of hypoplastic left ventricle. *American Journal of Perinatology*, **3**, 6–8.

Young, G., L'Heureux, P. R., Krueckeberg, S. T., Swanson, D. A. (1989). Mediastinal bronchogenic cyst: prenatal sonographic diagnosis. *American Journal of Roentgenology*, **152**, 125–7.

Young, I. D., McKeever, P. A., Brown, L. A., and Lang, G. D. (1989). Prenatal diagnosis of the megacystis–microcolon–intestinal hypoperistalsis syndrome. *Journal of Medical Genetics*, **26**, 403–6.

Zanke, S. (1986). Prenatal ultrasound diagnosis of acardius. *Ultraschall. Med.*, **7**, 172–5.

Zeitune, M., Fejgin, M. D., Abramowicz, J., Ben Aderet, N., and Goodman, R. M. (1988). Prenatal diagnosis of the pterygium syndrome. *Prenatal Diagnosis*, **8**, 145–9.

Zerres, K., *et al.* (1988). Autosomal recessive polycystic kidney disease. Problems of prenatal diagnosis. *Prenatal Diagnosis*, **8**, 215–29.

Zimmerman, H. B. (1978). Prenatal demonstration of gastric and duodenal obstruction by ultrasound. *Journal of the Canadian Association of Radiologists*, **29**, 138.

Acknowledgements

I wish to thank Mr Gordon Graham, Miss Marion Hoggan, and Professor Martin Whittle for their invaluable help in compiling the Glasgow database of prenatally diagnosable conditions. I also wish to acknowledge Blackwell Scientific Publications for permission to publish elements of the Table which had previously been included in Whittle and Connor (1989).

Index

LIBRARY
THE UNIVERSITY OF TEXAS
AT BROWNSVILLE
Brownsville, TX 78520-4991